the natural menopause SOLUTION

the natural menopause SOLUTION

Expert Advice for Melting Stubborn
Midlife Pounds, Reducing Hot Flashes, and
Getting Relief from Menopause Symptoms

The editors of Prevention® and Melinda Ring, MD

RODALE.

For women at midlife everywhere

Contents

Part IV:
Staying Healthy

Part V:
Putting It All Together

Acknowledgments

Many thanks to Sarí Harrar and Debra Gordon, our researchers/writers; to Melinda Ring, MD, our medical advisor; to Kimberly Fowler and Michele Stanten, our exercise experts; and to Susan McQuillan, our registered dietitian and recipe developer. Special thanks to the books team, including Andrea Au Levitt, Katie Wyszynski, Hope Clarke, Carol Angstadt, Chris Gaugler, Chris Krogermeier, and Sara Cox, and to our test panel coordinators, including Kelly Hartshorne, Tammy Strunk, Jessica Cassity, Molly Raisch, and Marielle Messing. Finally, our heartfelt appreciation goes to our dedicated test panelists, Eileen Fehr, Marie Fritz, Barbara Hunsicker, Carol Keene, Lori Klase, Mimi Kolb, Malissa Kuzma, Robin Laub, Cherylyn Rush, Alicia Schleder, Deborah Schrader, and Amy Wressell.

Part I

Why Go Beyond Hormones?

Chapter 1

Slimmer, Healthier, Happier . . . Naturally

*A*re you ready to melt stubborn midlife pounds, banish belly fat (at last!)—*and* get relief for perimenopausal and menopausal symptoms such as hot flashes, night sweats, insomnia, and low moods? *Don't* slash calories to a bare minimum. *Don't* spend hours in the gym. And *don't* reach for hormone replacement therapy (yet)—not until you've tried the research-proven and real-women-tested Natural Menopause Solution.

It's so simple, feels so good, and works on so many levels that you'll be amazed at the results. Here's what a few of the women who tried the plan told us.

- ◆ "I lost 5 pounds in the first 5 days," reports Robin Laub, 42, a busy first-grade teacher and a mother of two who went on to drop a total of

12 pounds in just 30 days—along with more than an inch each from her waist and hips. "I always said I could walk for 10 miles and not lose a single ounce. But the interval walks on the Natural Menopause Solution made a big difference. I feel good about myself again!"

- "I honestly didn't think anything would help my hot flashes," says Alicia Schleder, 55, who works for a utility company and has one daughter. "They've been cut in half on the plan." In addition, Alicia lost 11 pounds, saw her cholesterol fall 37 points, and moved her blood pressure into a healthier range. And she's feeling great: "It's like the old me is coming back, and I'm loving it."

- "I ate more, exercised less, and lost way more weight than on other programs I've tried. I'm totally thrilled," says Barbara Hunsicker, 58, a jewelry designer and a grandmother of three who lost 6 pounds in 4 weeks. "In the past, I barely lost weight on 1,200 calories a day. So when I heard we'd eat 1,500 calories in Phase 2 of the diet, I was a little worried. But there's something in the combination of the walking routine and the ingredients in this diet that made a big difference."

- "I'm sleeping soundly now and wake up feeling refreshed," says Carol Keene, 54, a human resources manager and a mother of two who fit the routine into a whirlwind schedule helping to plan her daughter's wedding. "I used to have several night sweats each night; now I'm down to just one little 'warm spell.' And my energy level is high—I never feel tired!" Carol lost 9 pounds and an inch each from her hips, waist, and thighs. "My daughter's wedding is soon—I'm going to look great in my mother-of-the-bride dress!"

DESIGNED FOR YOUR UNIQUE NEEDS

The Natural Menopause Solution begins with a specially formulated diet and exercise program—but it doesn't stop there, because as the editors of *Prevention* magazine, we know that a woman's health and wellness needs shift fundamentally in her thirties, forties, fifties, and beyond. Not only have we heard the stories from our millions of readers, but we've experienced it firsthand, too. Like you, we've had countless conversations about all the little changes we're noticing. We're talking about diet and exercise routines that suddenly don't work as well as they used to. Belly fat that won't budge no matter how many crunches we do. Strange mood swings, interrupted sleep, and cravings that pop up out of nowhere. Changes in our menstrual cycles. Shifts in key health indicators—blood pressure, cholesterol, blood sugar—that signal rising risk for serious trouble ahead like diabetes and heart disease. Oh, yes, and those hot flashes and night sweats.

We knew that by midlife, most women needed more than another conventional diet-and-exercise routine. So we went to work. Here at *Prevention* magazine, it's our mission to bring you only the most up-to-date, essential, well-researched, and practical information about health and wellness. So we read hundreds of medical studies each month. We're in constant contact with top experts in every area of women's health—from weight loss, fitness, and nutrition to complementary and alternative medicine to psychology to mainstream disease prevention and treatment. One expert, Melinda Ring, MD, medical director of Northwestern Integrative Medicine in Chicago, became the medical advisor for this book. We knew that thanks to an explosion of new research into midlife women's well-being, experts had a brand-new understanding of what was going on—and plenty of new tools and tricks for overcoming midlife weight, perimenopausal symptoms, low moods, and worrisome health changes, without necessarily reaching for that old standby, hormone replacement therapy (HRT).

Once upon a time, not so very long ago, doctors simply prescribed hormone replacement therapy (HRT) at menopause to counteract symptoms like hot flashes, sleepless nights, and more. Now we know so much more about safe and effective ways to stay slim, happy, healthy, and symptom free *naturally*—and that's exactly what you'll find in every aspect of the Natural Menopause Solution. While the landscape of midlife well-being has changed radically—and for the better—in the past decade, many women and their doctors simply weren't aware of all the exciting new developments in hormone-free solutions.

That's why our program also includes a comprehensive guide to easing menopausal and midlife symptoms—from night sweats and fatigue to hair loss and sexual discomfort. And you'll find a must-read section with the best thinking on ways to prevent the biggest health threats women face as they move through menopause, including diabetes, heart disease, brittle bones, strokes, and cancer. The bonus? On every level, this approach makes you feel great—boosting your mood, increasing your energy, reducing stress, and giving you the deep-down confidence that comes from knowing that you're in control of your health, your weight, your appearance, and your journey through perimenopause, menopause, and beyond.

MENOPAUSE AND MIDLIFE WELL-BEING

Menopause is a natural, years-long process—it's not a disease or a disaster. And it's not just about dwindling estrogen. A whole ballet company of hormones (powerful chemical "messengers" produced in your body's endocrine glands) gets in on this act, too.

When your cycles are running like clockwork, the dance begins each month with a rise in levels of gonadotropin-releasing hormone (GnRH)—which tells your pituitary gland to pump out follicle-stimulating hormone (FSH) and luteinizing hormone (LH). FSH prompts egg-containing follicles in your ovaries to mature. The follicles also contain cells that produce estrogen, which also begins to rise. Estrogen tells the lining of your uterus to thicken and triggers a burst of LH, which makes one follicle release an egg. Bingo! Ovulation! Now LH and estrogen levels sink as the old follicle begins pumping out progesterone. It readies the lining of the uterus for the arrival of a fertilized egg and also tells your body to stop making FSH and LH. If no fertilized egg arrives, progesterone levels also fall, and the lining is shed as your menstrual period. Then the whole cycle begins again.

But as early as your late thirties (or as late as your fifties), things change. You have fewer follicles and eggs, and the ones left aren't always top quality. It may take a bigger burst of FSH and LH to encourage one to mature—which is why those midcycle abdominal twinges called *mittelschmerz* (painful ovulation) can be downright excruciating. When follicles do mature, the amount of progesterone and estrogen they produce now fluctuates—leading to periods that may be lighter or heavier, longer or shorter, and to cycles that may be longer or shorter, too. Eventually, no follicles develop. Your ovaries stop making estrogen and progesterone. And your periods cease. Since you won't know right away that the last period you had was really The Last One, experts say that you can consider yourself postmenopausal when you've gone a full year without menstruating. (If you have spotting after a period-free year or more has gone by, contact your doctor to rule out health threats such as cancer.)

So far, it sounds like simply getting back those missing hormones would fix everything, doesn't it? Just 10 years ago, doctors still believed that the best remedy for a midlife woman's menopausal symptoms was HRT. In the 1990s, nearly 32 million HRT prescriptions were written annually; an estimated one in four menopausal women gave it a try. All that changed when the landmark Women's Health Initiative study found that combined estrogen/progestin HRT tripled heart disease risk, raised stroke risk from 9 to 31 percent, and boosted a woman's odds for breast cancer, too. Sales plummeted, and millions of women were left wondering how to cool their next hot flash (more about this in Chapter 2).

Fast-forward to today. The fall of HRT opened the door for new research into what's *really* happening at menopause—and how to cope safely and effectively. Now we're reaping the rewards. Newer forms of hormone therapy may be right if your symptoms are severe. But we're truly beyond hormones for two reasons. First, many—if not most—women can find relief via drug-free strategies. And second, we now know that hormone shifts aren't the only thing driving the big body-and-mind changes at midlife, opening the door to even more ways to spell relief.

A great example? Take extra pounds and belly fat. Many women complain about both in their forties and fifties, but the culprit's not just hormones. Your metabolism plays a bigger role than you might think. Truth is, women lose 5 to 7 pounds of lean, shapely, calorie-burning muscle *per decade* after age 25 or 30. Since muscle burns three times more calories

Beyond Plummeting Estrogen

New research shows that some hormones play a surprising role in many midlife symptoms and health risks. This news is changing conventional wisdom about relief and prevention. Three you should know about:

- **Cortisol:** New research shows that cortisol levels rise at menopause. Since cortisol fuels stress, anxiety, sleep problems, and weight gain, getting a grip with a soothing relaxation technique such as the yoga routine you'll follow with the Natural Menopause Solution can pay big dividends.

- **Inhibin:** Bone trouble starts early. Inhibin is another hormone released by your ovaries; it helps control FSH, a hormone that prompts eggs in your ovaries to develop during your menstrual cycle. But inhibin is also involved with developing and maintaining strong bones. Levels begin to drop before a woman reaches menopause—a great reason to be sure you're doing all you can to keep your bones healthy by getting enough calcium and vitamin D, as well as weight-bearing and strength-building exercise, all of which you'll find is part of our 30-Day Slim-Down, Cool-Down Diet.

- **Melatonin:** Is the sleep hormone also a menopausal hormone? In part, yes. Melatonin plays a part in keeping menstrual cycles regular. Levels drop with age, making this hormone a potential helper if you have sleep problems at midlife. (For details, see Chapter 8.)

than fat, that kind of loss sets you up for that midlife weight gain. And coupled with two hormonal shifts—falling estrogen and rising levels of the stress hormone cortisol—more of that fat than ever takes up residence just where you wish it wouldn't—at your midsection.

Belly fat is pervasive at midlife. Canadian researchers report, in a study of 174 women, that those approaching age 50 had *twice* as much visceral fat as women in their twenties. It's not just a fashion problem. More belly fat can mean longer, more severe, and more frequent hot flashes and night sweats. You're stuck in a vicious cycle: You're stressed out and low on energy because you're not sleeping; you're having those pesky hot flashes during the day; and you're tempted to grab a pack of cookies, a giant muffin, or a chocolate bar to bolster your energy or skip your next walk because you're just too tired. And, yes, that plays into low moods, too. Bad sleep, extra stress, and a lack of exercise can torpedo any woman's spirits.

The cycle also sets us up for serious, chronic health problems in the years ahead. As belly fat increases, it pumps chemicals into your bloodstream that make your body resistant to insulin, the hormone that tells your cells to absorb blood sugar. That's bad news, because a growing stack of research shows that insulin resistance makes weight loss much more difficult for midlife women. It also boosts your risk for heart disease, diabetes, and even some forms of cancer.

The good news? The Natural Menopause Solution breaks the cycle. Our 30-Day Slim-Down, Cool-Down Diet (in Part II) helps reverse insulin resistance, unlocking your body's ability to let go of excess pounds. Better sleep, fewer hot flashes, and more energy—learn how to get them all in our Natural Menopause Solutions section in Part III—make life feel good again. The disease-prevention strategies you'll find in Part IV strengthen bones and lasso rising blood pressure, blood sugar, and cholesterol levels—protecting your health now and for years to come. Finally, in Part V, you'll put it all together with the Natural Menopause Solution Journal and learn how to safely use HRT if you need it.

THE NATURAL MENOPAUSE SOLUTION ADVANTAGE

We've rolled all the research into an easy, feel-great eating plan that's chock-full of delicious and good-for-you foods. You'll feel full (no hunger on this diet!). Blast calories and fat without spending hours at the gym. Choose natural remedies proven to work (no more indecision in the health food store or confusion over conflicting claims on products). And have the peace of mind that comes from knowing that your health is improving at the same time.

Among the plan's unique, effective components are:

Our Slimming, Cooling Smoothie. Packed with a healthy dose of the Flash-Fighting Four ingredients—calcium, vitamin D, lean protein, and magnesium—this scrumptious daily smoothie helps you lose weight and feel your best. Research shows that women often skimp on these important nutrients. Getting your fill helps fight belly fat and insulin resistance, the metabolic glitch that makes weight loss difficult at midlife. Less belly fat means fewer hot flashes and night sweats because you've shed the heat-holding "blanket" that makes temperature regulation more difficult.

A "smart carb" meal plan to help you lose 21 percent more weight. Keeping blood sugar and insulin (the hormone that makes your body absorb blood sugar) lower and steadier has been proven to reverse insulin resistance—the shockingly common metabolic glitch affecting 30 to 60 percent of midlife women and the hidden culprit behind won't-budge pounds. A growing body of research shows that low-carb eating restores insulin sensitivity and boosts weight loss by as much as 21 percent when compared with higher-carb eating plans with the same number of calories.

Our superefficient and effective yoga-with-weights routine. Designed by a leading yoga instructor (who's at midlife herself), the Natural Menopause Solution yoga-with-weights routine takes just 20 minutes, but it delivers two things that midlife women really need: stronger muscles and stress-busting serenity. Going with yoga's soothing flow boosts your mood and reduces hot flashes—by 31 percent in one study at the University of California, San Francisco. (Reports of middle-of-the-night wake-ups and trouble returning to sleep fell 20 percent, too.) Meanwhile, strength training builds more shapely, toned muscle. And the more muscle you have (don't worry, you won't look like a bulky power lifter!), the more calories your body burns around the clock.

(continued on page 13)

Menopause FAQs

There's no Google Map, no global positioning system (GPS) app for your Smartphone (yet!) to tell you where you are in the years-long journey from regular menstrual periods to no periods at all. We'd sure love to see one! The hormone shifts that lead to menopause—your last-ever menstrual period—begin years earlier and can be quite subtle. Experts call the time leading up to your last period *perimenopause*. Once you've gone a year without a period, you're officially postmenopausal. Here's what you need to know about this important time of life.

What's the difference between perimenopause and menopause? Menopause is an event: your final menstrual period. Perimenopause includes the years of shifting hormones that precede menopause—usually about 4 to 7 years before your last period. That said, hormone changes, variations in your menstrual cycle, and symptoms like hot flashes and night sweats can start as early as your mid- to late thirties.

What's the average age for menopause? Female hormone shifts at midlife don't follow a strict timetable. The average age for a woman's final period is 51½, but menopause can happen naturally anytime between the ages of 42 and 58. Many factors—including smoking; having undergone chemotherapy, fertility treatment, a hysterectomy, or ovarian surgery; or even being of Latino or African American descent—can bring on an earlier menopause. In contrast, women of Chinese and Japanese descent may reach menopause a little later. Surprising factors that *won't* affect when you reach menopause: your age at your first period, whether or not you were ever pregnant or you breastfed, and whether or not you used oral contraceptives.

Can I predict when I'll hit menopause? You may be able to ballpark it by looking at when your mother and older sisters (if you have any) reached menopause, researchers from England's Institute of Cancer Research reported in 2011. A mom or a sister who had her last period at age 45 means that you're six times more likely to reach menopause early, too; the same goes for late menopause. If your mom reached The Change at age 54 or later, you're six times as likely to be headed for a later menopause yourself, and if your sister had a late menopause, your odds double.

How can I tell where I am in perimenopause? When women's health experts from the National Institutes of Health, the North American Menopause Society, and the American Society for Reproductive Medicine gathered a few years ago to sort out the stages of menopause, they agreed that "the end (menopause) is much easier to identify than the beginning." If you use your knowledge of your own menstrual cycle and notice hormone-related symptoms that may be starting, you can pinpoint your stage.

- **Late reproductive period (premenopausal).** Your cycles may be a few days shorter or longer than normal.

- **Early perimenopause.** Your cycles are at least 7 days shorter or longer than normal—so if your cycle used to be 31 days long, it might be 24 or 38 days now. You still have regular periods, however. You may start having hot flashes, night sweats, sleep problems, breast tenderness, and/or worse-than-usual or new premenstrual syndrome (bloating, mood changes, food cravings, and cramps).

- **Late perimenopause.** You've skipped two or more menstrual periods in a row and gone 60 or more days at a time without menstrual bleeding. Your periods may be lighter or heavier than usual. Hot flashes may start now if they haven't already. If you're already getting them, they may become longer, hotter, and/or more frequent.

- **Menopause.** Your last menstrual period. You'll have to wait a year to see if, indeed, your periods have stopped and you're officially postmenopausal, so you won't know at the time that this is your final period.

- **Early postmenopause.** The first 5 years after your last period. Hormone-related symptoms may continue. Meanwhile, bone loss accelerates at this time.

- **Late postmenopause.** More than 5 years after your last period. Your symptoms may have subsided, but about 10 percent of women continue to have hot flashes, sleep difficulties, and other menopausal symptoms into their seventies.

(continued)

Menopause FAQs (cont.)

Isn't there an easier way to tell if my symptoms are perimenopause? Yes. Canadian researchers who tracked the symptoms of women in the Perimenopausal Experiences Project say there's a good chance you're in perimenopause if you have at least three of these symptoms.

◆ New, heavy, and/or longer menstrual flow

◆ A menstrual cycle that's getting shorter

◆ Newly sore, swollen, or lumpy breasts

◆ New or worsening menstrual cramps

◆ Middle-of-the-night wake-ups for the first time

◆ Night sweats, especially during your period

◆ New or worsening PMS mood swings

◆ Weight gain that's not due to overeating or less exercise than usual

I've got other weird symptoms. Are they related to hormone changes? Maybe. Hot flashes and the other classic inconveniences are just the tip of the iceberg. Other symptoms that women report during perimenopause and beyond include headaches, sore and achy joints, dizziness, tiredness, itchy skin, breast tenderness, a change in sex drive, dry skin and hair, urinary problems such as incontinence, vaginal dryness, and painful intercourse. That said, it's worth mentioning anything unusual and troubling to your doctor; it could be a sign of another medical condition.

Can't a hormone test tell me what's going on? Tests of your levels of estrogen (it falls at some point during perimenopause) and follicle-stimulating hormone (FSH), which rises during perimenopause and menopause, may help your doctor find a cause if your periods become irregular or stop at an earlier-than-normal age. But home menopause tests and even a doctor's checkup are less useful for pinpointing where you are in perimenopause or predicting when you'll have your last period. A test is just a snapshot of your hormone levels at one point in time and can't factor in daily fluctuations that may make you seem closer to—or further from—The Change than you really are.

Interval walks that blast fat and calories—in just 30 minutes.
Test panelists who were longtime walkers said they got better results in
half the time with this special technique. By alternating short bursts of
fast walking with your regular pace, you burn more calories and body fat
than you would on a longer, steady-paced walk. Walking is also proven
to reduce hot flashes by as much as 49 percent and boost your mood, too.

Proven hot flash coolers. Soy? Flaxseed? Black cohosh? Yes, they
work for some women—we have the latest research on these classic remedies and much, much more. Like a mind trick that makes anything else
you try work better. Acupuncture. Muscle relaxation. And what you
should know about bioidentical hormone therapy and other medical
treatments if you're among the small percentage of women whose hot
flashes are stubborn and severe.

Sleep solutions for real life. We turned to research focused on
midlife women for strategies that really work and found plenty of promising options. From melatonin to massage, meditation to herbal tea, we
show you a range of slumber-improving strategies to try *before* you reach
for a sleeping pill. Small changes that won't mean rearranging your bedroom, your schedule, or your sleep habits can really work.

**Protection from diabetes, heart disease, brittle bones, and
more.** Your risk for these health threats rises at midlife—don't assume
that these are "men's diseases" or someone else's problem. You'll discover
how the healthy meals and feel-great moves of the 30-Day Slim-Down,
Cool-Down Diet are also proven lifestyle steps for lowering your chances
for developing one of these life-altering, and even life-threatening, conditions. Plus, you'll find additional prevention strategies if you're at risk.

These are the highlights of the many strategies and solutions that
you'll discover in the Natural Menopause Solution. It's your go-to source
for midlife health and happiness. In the pages to come, you'll find help
for everything from skin and hair changes to flagging energy and low
moods to lost libido and vaginal dryness. Add that to the benefits of our
30-Day Slim-Down, Cool-Down Diet—a trimmer waist; a healthier
weight; and a stronger, fitter, more serene you—and we can't imagine a
better place for you to be right now.

Happier and Healthier...
THE NATURAL MENOPAUSE SOLUTION WAY

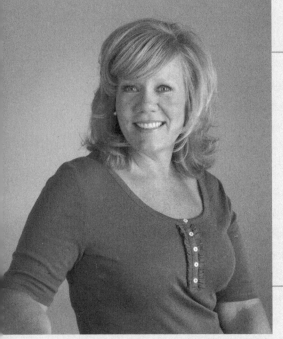

ROBIN LAUB

Age: 42

Pounds lost: 12

Inches lost: 4

Major changes: Better sleep, brighter moods, lowered blood pressure from a high 140/96 to a healthier 110/83, and improved total and LDL cholesterol levels.

"I Feel Good about Myself Again"

"Losing weight has become more difficult than it used to be," Robin told us when she started the program. A first-grade teacher and a mother of two, she reported: "I'm having some night sweats and more trouble sleeping. The stress of a full-time teaching job and raising a family only add to it."

But after just a few weeks on the program, Robin was sleeping through the night and waking up refreshed. "I did the yoga routine at night instead of having coffee, and it was so relaxing," she recalled. "I wasn't getting up several times a night to go to the bathroom anymore!" Her mood and energy levels improved, too. "The whole mood thing was big," she noted. "I had kind of been in a rut. Seeing the change in my weight helped me feel good about myself again. I felt I'd accomplished something when I lost several pounds in the first 5 days. And making time for myself every day for exercise—just getting out there and clearing my head—made a big difference."

Robin has always walked for exercise. But in the past she never found that it helped her lose weight. "I always said I could walk 10 miles a day and not lose an ounce, but the combination of the interval walks, the yoga-with-weights routine, and the eating plan changed all that," she says. "Dropping 12 pounds in a month is great! All of my clothes feel much better. I'm slipping into my summer pants and skorts more easily—and pulling out skinnier clothing from my wardrobe that I wouldn't have been able to wear a month ago."

Robin is out of the house by 6:30 in the morning. Her day doesn't end until 9:30 or 10:00 at night, when she finally has time to stop and relax. The short, effective Natural Menopause Solution exercise routines fit into small gaps in her busy days. Sometimes she took her interval walks on Sunday mornings before the family went to church, and she pulled her 3-year-old in a wagon behind her on weekend walks. "I'd borrow my older daughter's iPod, crank up some Top 40 songs—the Black Eyed Peas always put a kick in my step—and push myself. Sometimes I even jogged slowly on the fast-paced intervals to really step it up. I'd come home so sweaty, my girls would ask, 'Mommy, was it raining out?'"

Breakfast became one of Robin's favorite meals, thanks to scrumptious options like the Slimming, Cooling Smoothie ("It's absolutely delicious!") and the Open-Faced Omelet. "Some days there was so much food that I would pack some to take with me as a morning snack at work. My husband liked the dinners.

"The eating plan is easy," she continues. "Tonight the family ordered pizza, and I grilled some salmon and had it with broccoli and golden potatoes. It's my favorite meal now," Robin adds, referring to the plan's roasted salmon recipe, a crowd-pleaser with our test panelists. "This is something I can stick with. It fits into my life, and I'm not going to stop."

Chapter 2

Why Not Just Take a Pill?

There was a time when doctors handed out prescriptions for hormone therapy as if they were jelly beans. A time when nearly half of all women over the age of 50 were taking some form of hormone therapy—often for the rest of their lives. A time when the hormone therapy Prempro was the top-selling drug in the United States.

Not these days. Today, synthetic hormone therapy is no longer welcome in most women's medicine cabinets.

The story of how we got from there—when hormone therapy was compared to a pharmaceutical fountain of youth—to here—when hormone therapy is reviled in some circles—is, at its heart, a story of seeing what we wanted to see rather than looking beneath the surface to see what was really there.

SYNTHETIC FOUNTAIN OF YOUTH

Before the 20th century, there wasn't much call for menopausal treatments. Most women didn't live long enough to go through menopause. But once we cleaned up our act with safer water and milk and reduced the risk of death from childbirth and infection, and as medical care improved with vaccines and eventually antibiotics, more of us began living long enough to give rise to the era of Red Hot Mamas—and menopausal medicine.

The options for the hot flashes, the insomnia, and the mood disorders of the transition back then were, to say the least, limited. As early as 1899, women could swallow a product called Ovarin, made from dried and crushed cow ovaries, or inject a solution created from the testicles of dogs or guinea pigs to help with symptoms of the "climacteric."

Then science got involved. By the 1930s, the first official supplemental estrogens were introduced, some made from the urine of pregnant women, others from pregnant mares. This was in the days before the FDA required that drug manufacturers prove that their products not only worked but also were safe. (It wasn't until 1938 that the Food, Drug, and Cosmetic Act, which required that the FDA ascertain the safety of proposed drugs, was passed.)

In 1941, the FDA approved the first synthetic estrogen, one with the tongue-twisting name of diethylstilbestrol (DES) to treat menopausal symptoms. A year later, Premarin, a conjugated equine estrogen (i.e., made from horse urine), entered the market. Books were written touting its benefits and sales soared, doubling and tripling through the next 2 decades.

The first hint of a problem came in 1975, when investigators found that women taking supplemental estrogens like Prempro were developing uterine cancer at an alarmingly high rate. The reason? Estrogen causes the uterine lining to grow in preparation for pregnancy; without progesterone, which puts the brakes on such growth, cells lining the uterus continued to divide unopposed, eventually resulting in cancer.

In response, the FDA ordered estrogen manufacturers to add warnings to their products about the risk of uterine cancer, and sales plummeted. However, doctors soon realized that if women took supplemental progesterone with their estrogen, the risk evaporated. Add to that a National Institutes of Health (NIH) report in 1984 that estrogen therapy was the most effective means of preventing bone loss, and sales headed upward again.

THE RISE OF HORMONE THERAPY

By the early 1990s, more than 6 million postmenopausal women were using hormone therapy. Over the next decade, that number climbed to more than 15 million thanks to a single pill that combined estrogen and progestin (a synthetic version of progesterone).

There was just one problem: Not only did we not understand menopause itself and its role in women's health, but there was little, if any, evidence regarding the risks and benefits of the drug to the women taking it, particularly those who had taken the drug for years, even decades. There were also disturbing reports of blood clots and high blood pressure in younger women who took high doses of estrogen in the oral contraceptives available in the 1960s and '70s, and of blood clots and heart attacks in men who were given Premarin as part of a large cardiovascular trial designed to see if the estrogen could reduce their risk of heart disease.

All we had were observational studies—in which researchers look back at large groups of women who took the drug—that suggested hormone therapy not only cooled hot flashes, strengthened bone, and lubricated vaginal dryness but also improved heart health in women. For instance, a study published in the *Lancet* in 1981 looked at the medical records of women in a Los Angeles retirement community to see if there was any link between estrogen therapy and death from heart disease. The researchers found that the risk of dying from heart disease was 57 percent lower in the women taking estrogen compared with those who didn't use hormone therapy.

In 1992, the American College of Physicians recommended that *all* postmenopausal women be given hormone therapy to help prevent heart disease. Yet there had never been a prospective clinical trial—in which half of the participants receive the drug and half a placebo—to see if hormone therapy really *did* prevent heart disease. In essence, then, millions of women across the globe served as human guinea pigs.

The first large clinical trial designed to look at the potential effects of hormone therapy on cardiovascular disease wasn't published until 1998. The study was developed and paid for by Wyeth Pharmaceuticals, which sold the hormone therapies Premarin (estrogen only) and Prempro (estrogen and progestin). Called the Heart and Estrogen/Progestin Replacement Study (HERS), it involved 2,763 postmenopausal women with heart disease. Half of the women were assigned to take Prempro and half a placebo for an average of 4.1 years.

The trial found no difference in the number of heart attacks or deaths from heart disease between the two groups, suggesting that hormone therapy provided no benefit. In fact, in the first year of the study, more women taking the drug had heart attacks or other heart-related problems. However, the study also found that women receiving Prempro had lower levels of LDL cholesterol (the "bad" cholesterol) and higher levels of HDL cholesterol (the "good" cholesterol). Several smaller trials over the next few years had similar results. Researchers interpreted this to mean that if women already had heart disease, hormone therapy couldn't help. But what if they started taking it while their hearts were healthy? Could it keep them healthier longer?

THE WOMEN'S HEALTH INITIATIVE

To find out, the federal government agreed to fund one of the largest clinical trials ever conducted in women's health—the Women's Health Initiative (WHI). The trial involved 16,608 women who still had their uterus (and would get the combination hormone therapy Prempro) and 10,739 women ages 50 to 79 whose uterus had been removed (and would get the estrogen-only hormone therapy Premarin).

Three years after the study started, the arm involving the combination hormone therapy was stopped early when data showed that the women receiving the drug had a higher risk of heart disease, blood clots to the lungs, stroke, and breast cancer than the women taking a placebo. Later analysis found that those taking the combination drug who developed breast cancer were more likely to die of their disease than women who developed breast cancer but had never taken Prempro.

The risks of these conditions were small, however. Of 10,000 women taking the combination therapy, just 8 more than those not taking the therapy would develop invasive breast cancer, 7 more would have a heart attack or other coronary event, 8 more would have a stroke, and 8 more would have blood clots in the lung.

Eighteen months later, the estrogen-only part of the trial was also stopped early because of an increased risk of stroke in women receiving

When Hormones Help

This book is chock-full of natural remedies to address your menopausal symptoms. However, we still tell you when hormones might help. As Dr. Ring notes, for many women nothing quells hot flashes and improves vaginal dryness like estrogen. In fact, the WISDOM (Women's International Study of Long Duration Oestrogen After Menopause) trial, in which researchers followed about 5,600 health women ages 50 and older who received either estrogen–progestin or a placebo, found that hormone therapy significantly improved a woman's quality of life.

After 1 year, researchers reported in a 2008 article in the *British Medical Journal* that just 9 percent of women in the treatment group reported hot flashes compared with 25 percent in the placebo group. Women taking hormones also had nearly half as many night sweats, many fewer aches and pains, and far less insomnia. The major side effects reported by the women taking hormones were greater breast tenderness and vaginal discharge.

For more on hormones and how they can be used safely if you should need to take them, turn to Chapter 18.

the drug and no evidence of any health-related benefit. Of 10,000 women taking estrogen, 12 more would be expected to have a stroke compared with women not taking it, 6 more might develop a deep vein thrombosis, a blood clot in the legs that could break loose and travel to the lungs, where it might be fatal.

In the estrogen-only trial, however, women had no greater risk of developing breast cancer for at least 8 years after starting estrogen; in fact, there was some evidence that their risk of breast cancer was actually *lower* than the risk in women taking a placebo.

TIME TO MOVE BEYOND HORMONES

The news of the trials' outcomes hit the women's health world like a tsunami. Overnight, millions of women tossed out their hormones. Doctors' offices were deluged with calls from panicked patients who were terrified of the potential risks associated with the drug yet also concerned about the return of hot flashes and other menopausal symptoms that the drugs had kept at bay. Within 2 years, the number of prescriptions for oral hormone therapy plummeted by a third, from 87.3 million in 2000 to 59.6 million in 2003.

With their pills in the trash can, many women began to look for natural remedies that went beyond hormones to help them find relief and comfort. So did researchers. In *The Natural Menopause Solution,* we've pulled together the most up-to-date and credible studies on the most effective ways to cool down, slim down, and tame all your menopausal problems without reaching for HRT.

Chapter 3

The Natural Menopause Solution

*T*he Natural Menopause Solution is much more than a weight loss program. It's your road map for sailing through midlife happier, healthier, slimmer, *and* symptom free. We know— because we've been there!—that a woman's well-being is the sum of many parts. It's about having the energy and zest to live and love your life. Feeling good about your weight and your size. Enjoying the peace of mind that comes from knowing that you'll get a good night's sleep tonight and won't be sidetracked by major brain fog tomorrow. Knowing that you're in control of your health. And so much more.

You *can* have all of this. And you've come to the right place to find it. Using this book to reach your health, weight, and well-being goals couldn't be simpler. The plan has three parts—a diet-and-exercise program, symptom-relief remedies, and long-term strategies for sidestepping women's biggest health risks. These distinct, research-proven sections are designed to work together for total wellness.

THE 30-DAY SLIM-DOWN, COOL-DOWN DIET

How should you get started? We recommend beginning with the 30-Day Slim-Down, Cool-Down Diet, in Part II. It's the foundation that everything else is built upon, one that helps you not only lose weight but also maintain muscle, soothe menopausal symptoms, and protect your health. You'll discover an eating plan that will help you shed pounds, body fat, and inches—and that you can follow for years to come because it's filling, delicious, and meets your nutritional needs. The panel of women we recruited to test the program reported that their families also enjoyed the Natural Menopause Solution way of eating. No need to cook two meals!

You'll also be introduced to an incredibly effective exercise routine that gets the job done in mere minutes—burning calories, blasting fat, building muscle, and giving you an oasis of serenity that fits into your craziest, busiest days.

Test panelists reported that simply following this 30-day plan trimmed tummies, cooled hot flashes, and boosted energy and mood. It may be all you need to look and feel like your best self again. For a quick overview, turn to page 24.

NEED MORE SYMPTOM RELIEF? LOOK HERE

If you need more help with specific menopausal symptoms, turn to Part III. The broad range of proven remedies that you'll discover there will help you find relief at last. These solutions work on two levels: Some provide immediate relief, while others go to bat for the long-term prevention of symptoms. (What could be better?) And all of them go hand in hand with the 30-Day Slim-Down, Cool-Down Diet, so no worries about combining strategies.

(continued on page 26)

The 30-Day Slim-Down, Cool-Down Diet at a Glance

Phase 1: Days 1–5

Five days is all it takes to start losing weight and feeling great! In Phase 1, you will:

Sip a Slimming, Cooling Smoothie every morning. This flavorful blend of milk (regular, soy, or almond), pineapple, almond butter, flaxseed, and lime provides you with a healthy dose of our Flash-Fighting Four: calcium, lean protein, magnesium, and vitamin D. While the smoothie gives you a jump-start on these four important ingredients, it's not the last you'll see of them. Every day's menu includes foods featuring these nutrients, because we've discovered that they're essential for weight loss, symptom relief, and the prevention of health problems such as high blood pressure, brittle bones, and diabetes.

Eat three meals a day, for a total of 1,250 calories per day. Follow the quick, easy directions and you'll be sitting down to delicious, reduced-carbohydrate meals in minutes—at home and on the go. You'll love this introduction to flavorful Natural Menopause Solution eating!

Soothe stress with our 20-minute yoga routine. Take off your shoes and socks, settle onto your yoga mat, and experience the serenity of 10 flowing moves. This yoga plan is simple and safe, and it's perfect for beginners. Hidden bonus: It tones muscle while it relieves tension.

Walk for 20 to 30 minutes on 3 days. Tie up your walking shoes and hit the sidewalk, the trails at your favorite local park, or the treadmill. You'll burn calories, reduce stress, and get energized.

Phase 2: Days 6–30

Adding more choices to your eating plan and two powerful, time-efficient variations to the fitness routines you learned in Phase 1 will help ramp up your calorie burn. In Phase 2, you will:

Continue to enjoy foods featuring the Flash-Fighting Four. In addition to starting your day with the Slimming, Cooling Smoothie you've come to love, you'll incorporate foods rich in these vital nutrients in all your meals.

Add a daily 250-calorie snack or dessert. Choose from dishes such as Cheese and Olive Quesadillas, Baked Apples with Creamy Maple Sauce, and Chocolate Fondue.

Eat three meals a day of delicious Natural Menopause Solution foods. You're now eating a total of 1,500 calories a day. With menus balanced to reduce hunger and cravings and to optimize flavor, this plan will never feel like a diet.

Add intervals to your walks three to four times a week. Short bursts of speed blast up to three times more calories and fat than steady-state walks. You'll start with 20-minute interval walks and build to 30 minutes—and see big results with a small investment of time.

Add weights to your yoga routine. Pick up 2-pound dumbbells for most moves and you'll build more lean, shapely, calorie-burning muscle. After Day 15, you have the option to increase the weight if you'd like.

You'll find natural, drug-free remedies—including meditation, relaxation exercises, and supplements—that have been shown to help. But because this is a real-world guide intended to deliver real relief, we've also included a comprehensive discussion of medications and medical treatments for more severe symptoms. You'll discover the latest word on modern hormone replacement therapy, including progesterone cream and bioidentical hormones, with an up-to-date, well-informed discussion of the menopausal symptoms and health issues that these approaches best treat, as well as how to use the remedies safely and wisely. In addition, you'll discover hormone-free medication strategies for severe hot flashes, sleep problems, and other issues.

What's your biggest pet peeve at menopause? We have the solution. In Part III, symptoms are grouped by chapter into related clusters. But if you're not sure where you might find the cure to your worst midlife issues, see the opposite page for a list of symptoms and health concerns, arranged alphabetically, with page numbers for ready reference.

STAYING HEALTHY

Menopause is a health watershed for women. Shifting hormones conspire with other bodily changes (like more belly fat and less muscle) to raise your risk for major killers and disablers—like bone fractures, blood sugar problems, heart attacks, strokes, and cancer. New research shows that risks for all of these start to rise in the years before menopause. That tells us that prime time for prevention is, well, right now.

The sooner you take smart lifestyle steps to reduce your risk, the better your chances for sidestepping these illnesses—and the more powerful these simple, healthy, drug-free steps can be. Getting plenty of calcium and vitamin D plus bone-building exercise now (as you will on the 30-Day Slim-Down, Cool-Down Diet) can protect against osteoporosis, the brittle-bone disease that boosts your risk of having

The Natural Menopause Solution Symptom Solver

Acne. Zits? At your age? Unfortunately, yes. Turn to page 299 in Chapter 12 for advice to prevent or treat annoying acne.

Age spots. You don't have to live with those brown spots on your face or hands. Page 296 in Chapter 12 tells you how to get rid of them.

Anxiety. Those heart palpitations? The constant worrying? Don't let your anxiety ruin this time of life. See natural and medical remedies on page 248 in Chapter 9.

Belly fat. Our 30-Day Slim-Down, Cool-Down Diet starts on page 36, in Part II. It tackles belly fat with a mix of diet, exercise, and stress relief.

Depression. Your blue mood may be more than a temporary thing: Depression is far more common during the menopausal transition. See page 241 in Chapter 9 for advice on feeling better.

Fatigue. Do you feel like you're fighting through a haze of exhaustion all the time? Fatigue may be related to lack of sleep, depression, or another menopause-related condition. And once you've pinpointed the underlying cause of your fatigue and learned your options for treating it, turn to our 30-Day Slim-Down, Cool-Down Diet, starting on page 36, to help boost your energy.

Food cravings. Pregnancy and PMS-related food cravings were nothing compared with the irresistible urges you have now for all the worst kinds of foods. Happily, the combination of aerobic and

(continued)

The Natural Menopause
Solution Symptom Solver (cont.)

strength-training exercises on page 146, in Chapter 6, can help crave-proof your appetite.

Hair loss. Shifting hormones can reprogram your body's hair-growth patterns, but that doesn't mean you're destined to go bald. See page 305 in Chapter 12 for remedies.

Headaches. Like joint aches and pains, headaches in midlife are usually not directly caused by menopausal hormones but instead are often related to other issues such as stress-induced insomnia and sleep apnea. See pages 224 and 220 in Chapter 8 for ways to cope.

Heart palpitations. If you frequently feel like your heart is about to fly out of your chest, take a deep breath, and check out our easy natural strategies for calming the racing on page 253 in Chapter 9.

Hot flashes. It's the elephant in the menopause room. Slay it with the plethora of tips in Chapter 7, starting on page 188.

Incontinence. It's something women don't want to talk about—but it affects many of us at this time of life. Chapter 11, starting on page 282, tells you how to cope.

Insomnia. Can't sleep? Check out page 213 in Chapter 8 to find out why—and what you can do about it.

Joint aches and pains. From lower-back pain to arthritis to fibromyalgia, joint aches and pains in midlife can have many causes. Although not usually directly caused by the hormonal fluctuations of menopause, they can affect (and be affected by) other menopausal issues such as insomnia. See page 223 in Chapter 8 for more details.

a life-changing fracture. Knowing about the surprising diet shifts that improve your body's ability to process blood sugar can help you sidestep diabetes. (Hint: Eating more good fats and less "bad" saturated

Lost libido. How far down on your list is sex? If it's near the bottom, see page 261 in Chapter 10 for advice on reclaiming the sexual you.

Low energy. Wish you had more oomph? Test panelists told us they had more energy thanks to our 30-Day Slim-Down, Cool-Down Diet. Give it a try—it's in Part II of this book, starting on page 36.

Memory problems. If you can't remember where you put the keys, try the simple strategies on page 256 in Chapter 9 to sharpen your memory and snap out of hormone-related brain fog.

Nail problems. Peeling, weak nails? See page 303 in Chapter 12.

Night sweats. Just another name for hot flashes. See how to cool down the night on page 189 in Chapter 7.

Overweight. Got extra pounds that nothing will melt? Turn to Part II for our 30-Day Slim-Down, Cool-Down Diet. It's proven to tame stubborn midlife overweight with a diet featuring the Flash-Fighting Four ingredients, plus fat-blasting interval walks and a soothing, strength-building yoga-with-weights routine.

Painful sex. If sex hurts, something is wrong. See page 264 in Chapter 10 to identify potential problems and learn what to do about them.

Stress. Maybe it's the demands of midlife or the natural rise in stress hormones at this time of life. Stress may be common at perimenopause, but you can tame it. Try our yoga routine on page 170 in Chapter 6. These calming moves are proven to ease anxiety. Add our walking routine, on page 167, for more stress-busting power.

Urinary tract infections. Changing hormone levels can make these more common. See how to prevent them on page 286 in Chapter 11.

Wrinkles. We can't change the past, but we can hide it. See page 294 in Chapter 12 for advice on minimizing wrinkles.

fat, as you do on the Natural Menopause Solution, is as important as cutting out soda and cutting back on sugar-laden foods.) And tracking your blood pressure and cholesterol levels has never been more important. Research shows that despite an upswing in awareness of women's heart-health risks, many women—and their doctors—still shrug off early warning signs that, if heeded, could prevent heart attacks and strokes.

In Part IV, you'll discover smart ways to evaluate your risk today—and learn which health tests you really need. You'll find out why the 30-Day Slim-Down, Cool-Down Diet is also a great insurance policy for

Using Complementary and Alternative Medicine

Don't be thrown by studies on alternative options that seem to swing back and forth between positive and negative, advises Melinda Ring, MD, the medical expert for *The Natural Menopause Solution*. "I believe in evidence-based medicine, but I feel that the evidence required should be proportional to the potential for harm," she says. So, for instance, she doesn't need to see extensive studies on techniques like acupuncture, massage, and paced breathing to recommend them for her patients: "If there is decent data to support them, then I think they're worth trying."

She is more cautious with herbs and supplements, however, because they can have more "medicine-like effects," such as interacting with prescription and over-the-counter drugs or affecting your kidneys or liver. Unfortunately, there is little information about how safe herbs and most supplements are when used for months or even years.

That being said, don't read too much into negative studies on herbs or supplements. The studies might have used different formulations or doses or might have been conducted in women whose symptoms, age, and other parameters differ from yours. Another important thing to remember, Dr. Ring says, is that the quality of the supplement matters.

lifelong good health. And we'll show you additional measures to further reduce your risk.

Put it all together—from a flatter belly to a happier outlook, fewer menopausal symptoms, and a long and healthy future—and you get real peace of mind and a renewed zest for life. Get started today!

She's had female patients complain that the generic black cohosh they took had no effect on their hot flashes; once she switched them to a higher-quality product, they found relief.

That's why it's so crucial that you talk to your doctor about your desire to integrate alternative therapies into your menopausal regimen. If your doctor isn't knowledgeable about these treatments, you may want to seek out an integrative medicine specialist like Dr. Ring, who specializes in integrating the use of complementary and alternative medicine with conventional approaches. You can find a center for integrative medicine near you at www.imconsortium.org.

You might also look for a naturopath, a specially trained health professional who focuses on treating the entire person, not just the symptom or the disease. Naturopaths learn the same basic sciences as doctors do, but they also study holistic and nonmedical approaches to therapy. Make sure you find a well-qualified practitioner, however. That means one who studied at a naturopathic medical school for 4 years *after* college, followed by 4 years in training, and who passed a national licensing examination before being allowed to practice on his or her own. Not all states license naturopathic physicians, although the number is increasing. You can find an accredited naturopath near you through the American Association of Naturopathic Physicians at www.naturopathic.org.

Happier and Healthier...
THE NATURAL MENOPAUSE
SOLUTION WAY

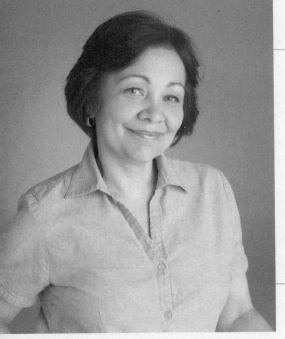

ALICIA SCHLEDER

Age: 55

Pounds lost: 11

Inches lost: 7¾

Major changes: Half as many hot flashes, lowered total cholesterol, LDL cholesterol, and blood pressure. Trimmed body fat percentage by nearly 4 percent.

"The Old Me Is Coming Back, and I'm Loving It"

Before she started the Natural Menopause Solution, "all I could do when I got home from work was feed the family and pets and hit the sofa for some TV time," Alicia admits. "But now I just keep moving. It's like the old me is coming back, and I'm loving it."

While many women see their hormone-related symptoms fade once they're past menopause, Alicia's have stayed with her ever since she reached menopause 5 or 6 years ago. "I get hot flashes in the summer, in the winter; and when I'm stressed, they're even worse—longer, hotter, more frequent. I didn't think anything would help. But after 30 days on this program, they're about cut in half. I had been having five to eight a day, and by the end of the program, it was two to four. And I'm not waking up in a sweat every night the way I used to, either."

Extra pounds crept up around menopause, too—and stayed until she lost 11 of them on the program. "I was never overweight until around menopause. I would try to lose weight by dieting and exercising, but it was hard to keep up. I'm short, just 5 feet 1 inch tall, so every pound really showed." Now her jeans are so loose, she has to wear a belt. "It's just so nice to put something on from the closet and it fits."

Alicia experienced a big personal loss just as she was starting the program. Her mom, who lived with Alicia and had been receiving hospice care at home, passed away. "It wasn't easy, but I decided to stick with the plan," she says. "I think the daily walks and yoga helped me with my grief—and kept me from eating all of the food that people brought to the house. It fit into my life even at a tough time. I'm proud of myself, and I know my mother would be proud of me, too."

Among Alicia's favorite foods on the plan was the Quick Tortilla Soup. "I would dry-roast a tortilla in a pan and crunch it up on top, mixed with cheese—the recipe called for a crunchy topping," she recalls. "The soup was a little spicy, and I love spicy food. The Veggie-Cheese Wrap and the Roasted Salmon with Green Beans and Potatoes were also major favorites. And my daughter loved the Indonesian salad, Gado Gado. We're both trying to eat healthier."

Alicia found the fast pace of the interval walks challenging at first. But that didn't stop her from changing her shoes and hitting the pavement at lunchtime for a brisk 20- to 30-minute stroll. "At first I would get out of breath pretty quickly, but I wanted to improve so much that I just kept trying. I listened to my body and didn't overdo it, but I kept pushing myself. And guess what? It got easier. And I got real results."

Part II

The 30-Day Slim-Down, Cool-Down Diet

Chapter 4

The Eating Plan

Roasted salmon with green beans and gold potatoes for dinner. Sausage, waffles, and muffins in the morning. A tart and sophisticated arugula salad with goat cheese or a slice of pizza at lunch. And a refreshing fruity smoothie once a day. (And did we mention wine and cheese, ice cream, and milk and cookies?)

Can eating these delicious foods really help you lose stubborn midlife weight, trim belly fat, *and* help banish menopausal symptoms? Our test panelists are proof that the answer is a resounding *yes!*

- Alicia Schleder lost 11 pounds—as well as 2 inches from her waist, more than 1 inch from her hips and ½ inch from each thigh. She's having half as many hot flashes, too. "My arms look more toned, and I'm much more flexible thanks to the yoga routine," she says.

- Amy Wressell's worst perimenopausal symptoms were stubborn pounds and trouble falling—and staying—asleep. Problems solved! Amy lost 7 pounds and trimmed her waist and hips by $2\frac{1}{2}$ inches each. "I've been sleeping very well," she reports. "I think it's the walking and yoga!"

- Lori Klase used to sweat through two to three hot flashes every day. After a few weeks on the Natural Menopause Solution, those pesky warm spells have diminished to two a week. Her weight loss success: She's $6\frac{1}{2}$ pounds lighter.

- Marie Fritz lost $4\frac{1}{2}$ pounds and 5 inches. Her "bad" LDL cholesterol fell 13 points—enough to lower her heart attack risk by 26 percent. And her blood pressure went from 110/80 to an even healthier 100/78. "My heartburn also went away," she says. "I know plenty of menopausal women who say heartburn is a big problem. I'm comfortable, finally!"

The eating plan portion of the 30-Day Slim-Down, Cool-Down Diet is built on recent scientific research that found that the healthiest of low-carbohydrate diets helps you conquer menopause-related excess pounds at last. It works its magic, in part, by reversing insulin resistance—a blood sugar–processing glitch that makes weight loss a vexing challenge for women in their forties, fifties, sixties, and beyond. It also targets abdominal fat—the deep and dangerous visceral fat that increases health risks and makes hot flashes more frequent and more severe. And this plan's focus on healthy, low-carb foods means you're also protecting yourself against heart disease, stroke, high blood pressure, diabetes, and thinning bones—five health risks that soar once a woman's hormones begin to shift at midlife.

In Part I of this book, you read all about emerging research that's uncovered the hidden causes of won't-budge weight and won't-leave belly fat—and their connections to menopausal symptoms and midlife health risks. In this chapter you'll discover how the delicious foods on the Natural Menopause Solution eating plan address these issues. The result? A slimmer, healthier, happier, and more energetic you.

SUCCESS SECRETS

How did we incorporate all of the exciting research into meals that taste good, are easy to put together, and—best of all—work on so many levels at once? The eating plan is unique and powerful because it delivers three secret weapons.

The right macronutrient balance. You get 15 to 20 percent of your daily calories from protein, 45 to 50 percent from carbohydrates, and 30 to 35 percent from fat. That's on par with the levels in a University of Nevada study and other studies that show a dramatic weight loss. This science-based balance helps your body burn more fat and process blood sugar more efficiently, and it even nurtures more calorie-burning around the clock. It overcomes the three major forces behind stubborn excess weight around menopause: insulin resistance, belly fat, and reduced muscle mass.

A superhealthy, supertasty mix of foods. Not every low-carb diet tastes this good—or is this good for you! Once we chose the optimal balance of nutrients for the 30-Day Slim-Down, Cool-Down Diet, registered dietitian Susan McQuillan translated the numbers on the page into delicious, health-enhancing meals for your plate and palate. She selected lean proteins, good fats, satisfying whole grains, low-fat and fat-free dairy products, and plenty of fruits and vegetables for menus and recipes. And she combined them in smart ways that ensure maximum flavor and satisfaction today, effective weight loss and fat loss over the next few weeks and months, and better health—strong bones, reduced risk for heart attacks and strokes, protection against cancer, and fewer bothersome menopausal symptoms—for years to come.

Slimming, cooling ingredients. Test panelists raved about the flavor of our specially formulated Slimming, Cooling Smoothie and how satisfied they felt afterward. Sipping one a day delivers a "booster shot" of four key nutrients—calcium, lean protein, magnesium, and vitamin D—that women's diets so often skimp on. These Flash-Fighting Four are the centerpiece of the eating plan because they help you lose weight with ease, trim more belly fat, maintain and build metabolism-revving muscle, reverse insulin resistance, protect your bones, bolster your cardiovascular system, and even play a role in putting hot flashes and night sweats on ice.

SLIMMING AND COOLING THE NATURAL MENOPAUSE SOLUTION WAY

There couldn't be an easier, yummier way to boost your intake of these four important nutrients than our thick-and-creamy signature smoothie. Create one in seconds flat by tossing milk (or fortified soy milk), fruit (fresh, frozen, or canned in juice), flaxseed, almond butter, and a splash of lime juice into your food processor or blender. Whip it up, pour a cupful into a glass, and enjoy. This beverage is a wonderful way to start the day, but you can drink it whenever you'd like (it makes a filling afternoon snack). Extra servings will keep in a covered pitcher in your refrigerator. That means fitting one in on your busiest mornings is no problem—just stir, pour into your travel mug, and you're good to go.

The smoothie is our way of highlighting the importance of our Flash-Fighting Four. But, of course, it's not the *only* place you'll find them. Every day the Natural Menopause Solution eating plan—meals, snack, and recommended supplements—fulfills your optimal daily requirement for calcium, lean protein, magnesium, and vitamin D. (For more information on recommended supplements, turn to page 63.) Here are the research-backed reasons why we think these fab four are so crucial for women at midlife and beyond.

Calcium: *Strong bones, protection from insulin resistance, healthier blood pressure, and easier weight loss*

Think you're getting enough of this essential, bone-building mineral? Chances are you're falling short. Women need 1,000 milligrams of calcium a day before age 50 and 1,200 milligrams a day thereafter. In one

Calcium without Dairy

If you don't do dairy at all—because you're a vegan who doesn't eat animal products or you just don't like moo juice and its offshoots—a healthy diet may be all that you need to maintain strong bones. In one study, the bone density of 105 postmenopausal vegan women and 105 nonvegan women of the same age found identical bone strength. The reason? The Vietnamese researchers who conducted the study, published online by the journal *Osteoporosis International,* suspect that it's the other sources of calcium in a vegan diet—after all, 4 ounces of tofu or a big serving of steamed collard greens has as much calcium as a glass of milk.

Looking for nondairy sources of calcium? Start with these:

FOOD	AMOUNT	CALCIUM (MG)
Blackstrap molasses	2 Tbsp	400
Collard greens, cooked	1 cup	357
Tofu, processed with calcium sulfate	4 oz	200–330
Calcium-fortified orange juice	8 oz	300
Soy or rice milk, commercial, calcium fortified, plain	8 oz	200–300
Commercial soy yogurt, plain	6 oz	80–250
Turnip greens, cooked	1 cup	249
Tofu, processed with nigari	4 oz	80–230
Tempeh	1 cup	215
Kale, cooked	1 cup	179
Soybeans, cooked	1 cup	175
Okra, cooked	1 cup	172
Bok choy, cooked	1 cup	158
Mustard greens, cooked	1 cup	152
Tahini	2 Tbsp	128
Broccoli, cooked	1 cup	94
Almonds	¼ cup	89
Almond butter	2 Tbsp	86
Soy milk, commercial, plain	8 oz	80

study of 10,000 midlife women, however, researchers at Boston's Brigham and Women's Hospital found that most got just 857 milligrams a day. That's a dangerous gap.

Why calcium matters at menopause. Low calcium intake boosts your risk for bone fractures—a special concern at midlife. After your mid-thirties, bone density begins to decline. As estrogen levels fall 2 to 3 years before your last period, you may lose 2 percent of precious bone density per year. And in the first 5 to 8 years after your periods stop and you enter menopause, you can lose 3 to 5 percent of bone mass every year—a silent weakening of your skeleton that puts you at risk for life-altering or even fatal bone fractures. Low calcium intake (along with low vitamin D) also raises your risk for insulin resistance by 36 percent, may hamper weight loss efforts, and seems to lock belly fat in place, too.

Weight loss edge. Can calcium really help you drop pounds? Yes—if you haven't been getting enough. In a study from Canada's Laval University, women who normally skipped calcium lost six times more weight and saw greater improvements in their cholesterol levels when they got 1,200 milligrams of calcium (plus vitamin D) daily, as compared with women who didn't get this dynamic duo. In one Virginia Tech study, women who consumed several servings of low-fat dairy products daily had less torso fat than those who got less. And women who drank fat-free milk after workouts lost more fat and gained more muscle than those who quenched their thirst with other beverages, according to a study at McMaster University in Hamilton, Ontario, that was published in the journal *Medicine & Sciences in Sports & Exercise*.

The reason? Calcium may help quell cravings. The combination of calcium, protein, and vitamin D in dairy can maintain and even help build muscle. This can help you lose weight and keep it off because muscle burns calories around the clock. More muscle = a higher metabolism. And there's growing evidence that calcium plus vitamin D prevents or helps reverse insulin resistance, too.

Menopause advantage. By helping your body burn off excess abdominal fat, calcium could help ease hot flashes. With less belly fat, your body temperature is easier to regulate without resorting to those hot flashes and night sweats to radiate heat fast.

Health bonus. Getting daily calcium (with vitamin D) may reduce your bone-fracture risk by an impressive 25 percent, according to a report in the journal *Lancet* about a study at Australia's University of Western Sydney.

Getting calcium (and vitamin D) from dairy could reduce risk for type 2 diabetes—which is caused by insulin resistance—by 15 percent, say Tufts University researchers, in a study published in the *Journal of Clinical Endocrinology & Metabolism*. The reason? Calcium, along with vitamin D, magnesium, and other nutrients in dairy, helps your cells maintain their insulin sensitivity.

Calcium-rich dairy products also put a lid on blood pressure. Minerals in milk pamper your arteries so they stay flexible. The most effective dietary strategy for blood pressure control is having two or more servings of low-fat or fat-free milk, yogurt, or even cheese— foods you'll enjoy on the Natural Menopause Solution, too. There's even evidence that calcium-rich dairy products protect against heart disease by improving the balance of heart-threatening LDL cholesterol and heart-protecting HDL cholesterol in your bloodstream.

Natural Menopause Solution's calcium-rich foods. Quick Tortilla Soup; Mushroom, Cheddar, and Walnut Pâté; Nutty Berry Fool. (And our Slimming, Cooling Smoothie, of course!)

Vitamin D: *Prevention of cancer, diabetes, and weak bones; metabolism support; possible ally against hot flashes*

Wonder what the odds are that you're not getting enough of this headline-grabbing vitamin? At least fifty-fifty. Half of all women (some experts say up to 75 percent) don't get enough.

Why vitamin D matters at menopause. Skimping on vitamin D raises the risk for diabetes, depression, heart disease, more serious infections, and several types of cancer. In one University of Toronto study of 512 women with newly diagnosed breast cancer, 76 percent had low levels of vitamin D. And researchers from the University of Rochester Medical Center reported in 2011 that women with breast cancer who had the lowest levels of vitamin D were 2½ times more likely to have more aggressive tumors.

Weight loss edge. Vitamin D tag-teams with calcium to help maintain strong muscle and bone when you're losing weight, as we described previously in the section on calcium.

Menopause advantage. It's unclear right now whether vitamin D has any direct effects on menopausal symptoms, but it may. Scientists at the Oregon Health and Science University note that studies suggest some women who get enough D may be less bothered by menopause-related muscle aches and pains. The researchers are even gearing up to see if vitamin D can help control hot flashes and night sweats. They note that a drop in levels of the brain chemical serotonin around menopause may be involved in the development of hot flashes (serotonin also affects temperature regulation). In lab studies, vitamin D helps maintain serotonin levels.

Health bonus. Topping off your tank is a brilliant move at any time of life but especially so around menopause. Vitamin D is the essential go-between that lets your body utilize calcium. This makes the vitamin an important player for healthy bones and healthy blood sugar processing (so you're not insulin resistant) and even guards against breast and colon cancer. D's got a unique ability to turn off a gene that promotes bodywide inflammation and turn on a segment of DNA that cools it down, which helps explain why this vitamin also helps guard against everything from colds to heart disease to cancer.

Trouble is, vitamin D is the "sunshine vitamin" produced by your skin in response to exposure to the sun's ultraviolet rays. Between indoor living (we spend 90 percent of our time in our homes, cars, and offices and in shopping malls these days) and a rise in the use of sunscreen, your skin probably doesn't have a chance to make enough D the way your ancestors' did. The 135 IU (international units) in your daily smoothie will help you reach your goal—as will the salmon, tuna, enriched dairy products, and soy milk in this eating plan. But be sure to take recommended supplements to hit your daily goal of 1,000 IU of D for most women.

The Natural Menopause Solution's vitamin D–rich foods. You'll enjoy 1½ to 2 servings of vitamin D–rich milk and yogurt daily, as well as salmon and tuna. Since getting optimal amounts of D from food is difficult, *The Natural Menopause Solution* medical advisor, Melinda Ring, MD, recommends that you also take a supplement containing 1,000 IU of D daily, though higher doses may be needed if you're deficient or don't get much sun exposure year-round.

Lean protein: *Satisfaction, more metabolism-boosting muscle, heart protection*

Are you getting enough protein? While many women do, that may not be the case as we move into and beyond menopause—or if we're trying to drop a few pounds. Skimping on protein may seem like a good way to cut calories, but in fact it can backfire (read on to find out why).

Eating the wrong kind of protein can be a problem, too. Loading your plate with fatty cuts of red meat and pork or with skin-on poultry floods your body with artery-clogging, diabetes-promoting saturated fat. It also deprives you of the health benefits of good fats found in protein choices like fish and nuts, not to mention the satisfying, cholesterol-controlling fiber found in beans.

Why your protein choices matter at menopause. In a Harvard School of Public Health study published in the journal *Circulation*, women who ate red meat once or twice a day not only took in more calories than those who stuck with healthier protein sources, but they were at higher risk for heart attacks and strokes, too. This is important news because heart disease and stroke risk rise steeply after menopause.

Weight loss edge. Protein contains an amino acid called leucine that's proven to help maintain muscle mass while you're on a weight loss diet. As you learned a few pages ago, maintaining muscle helps your body burn more calories at all times. In one study of 48 overweight women ages 40 to 56, those who ate more protein lost 20 percent more weight than those on an equal-calorie, higher-carb plan; and most of the weight loss was body fat, not muscle.

A meal plan with a little more protein and fewer carbs—like our 30-Day Slim-Down, Cool-Down Diet—also translates to a slower rise in blood sugar after meals in part because your body digests protein slowly. Staying off the blood sugar roller coaster can prevent cravings and between-meal hunger pangs.

Plant-based proteins also get starring roles in our plan. From white beans to lentils to navy beans, the Natural Menopause Solution includes plenty of recipes and meals featuring legumes. They're not only rich in satisfying protein, but they contain no saturated fat and deliver a big dose of soluble fiber, which fills you up so you eat less. They also help control blood sugar and cholesterol. Talk about brilliant multitasking!

Menopause advantage. Plant proteins—soy, beans, and peas—may have a special talent for cooling off hot flashes. Plenty of studies suggest that the plant estrogens in soy foods like tofu may help some women put the chill on hot flashes and night sweats. (For more about how it works and why soy doesn't help everyone, see Chapter 7.) What you may not know: Beans and peas also contain phytoestrogens. Though the amounts are smaller than those found in soy, they may help you stay cooler during the day and while you're sleeping.

Health bonus. Choosing lean cuts of meat instead of fatty stuff reduces your risk for metabolic syndrome and insulin resistance by 25 percent when compared with people who regularly consume red meat, fatty pork, and processed meats packed with preservatives and sodium, University of Minnesota researchers report in another study published in the journal *Circulation*. This, in turn, reduces your risk for diabetes and heart disease—plus it helps you lose weight. But lean protein does even more.

While chowing down on red meat may threaten bone density, lean sources of protein can help your body absorb calcium. Protein also keeps muscles strong, protecting against falls as you age and ensuring you'll be able to keep up bone-friendly exercise like walking and strength training.

The Natural Menopause Solution's protein-rich foods. You'll eat protein at every meal in dishes such as Homemade Turkey Sausage, Hearty Kale and White Bean Soup, Stir-Fried Ginger Shrimp and Veggies, and Roasted Turkey Breast and Vegetables.

Magnesium: *Better blood sugar and a healthier heart*

Half the magnesium in your body is stored in your bones; the rest helps support more than 300 important processes, from keeping your heartbeat steady to pampering muscles to regulating blood pressure and blood sugar. You need 320 milligrams of this important mineral daily, but chances are you're falling short. Most women get just 177 to 237 milligrams.

Why low levels of magnesium matter at menopause. You need magnesium on board now, more than ever, because even a small deficiency increases your odds for insulin resistance—which in turn raises your risk for diabetes, heart disease, and even some cancers. And as you've already learned, insulin resistance can foil your weight loss efforts, too.

Weight loss edge. One intriguing University of California, Davis, study found an association between low magnesium levels and higher body weight. A diet packed with processed foods is often low in this mineral, found in highest amounts in unprocessed edibles like almonds, peanuts, wheat bran, yogurt, bran flakes, brown rice, beans, lentils, peanut butter, and green leafy vegetables.

Menopause advantage. There's not much research-backed evidence that magnesium directly affects menopausal symptoms (though a few case studies suggest that it may cool hot flashes for some women). But menopausal women and their doctors note that magnesium can be calming and may help with anxiety and sleep problems during perimenopause. Stress depletes this vitamin, so making sure you have enough on board is especially important at this busy time of life.

Health bonus. If you take calcium supplements, adding magnesium will help you avoid bloating and constipation. It also plays an important role in blood sugar processing in your body—working with several enzymes to ensure that cells absorb their favorite source of fuel. Low levels make it harder for cells to respond to signals from insulin to absorb blood sugar (that's insulin resistance). In the Women's Health Study, women with the lowest magnesium levels had the highest insulin levels after meals and the highest risk for diabetes. High insulin levels also raise the risk for heart disease and stroke.

The Natural Menopause Solution's magnesium-rich foods. You'll enjoy Spiced Chicken with Lentils, Quinoa Salad with Apples and Walnuts, Mixed-Fruit Cup, Greek Spinach Scramble, and snacks like ice cream with cherries and almonds and a glass of wine with roasted almonds.

WEIGHT LOSS WITHOUT DEPRIVATION

If you love pasta, rice, bread, and potatoes, rejoice! Unlike *extreme* low-carb diets, which first gained popularity in the 1960s (and some of which are enjoying a comeback), this plan won't deprive you of comfort foods or sweet treats like fruit, cake, an afternoon cookie, or even a scoop of ice cream.

Carbs—found in everything from bread and noodles to apples, broccoli, and milk—are the foods that your body converts to blood sugar. Your brain, muscles, and body tissues rely on blood sugar for fuel. So you definitely need carbs. But not just any carbs. By steering clear of refined carbs (such as white bread and sugary drinks), emphasizing fiber-rich whole grains and fresh fruit and veggies, and combining these good complex carbs with protein and good fats, the Natural Menopause Solution eating plan will keep you energized. It won't trigger blood sugar spikes that lead to cravings and hunger pangs. And it won't "feed" insulin resistance, which can be made worse by a diet top-heavy with refined carbs.

But you won't need a magnifying glass to find the coconut rice, red quinoa, or Fig 'n' Flax Muffin on your plate because our carb portions are big enough to satisfy the most confirmed carb lover.

How is this nutrient balance different from other plans? A typical high-carb, low-fat diet gets about 65 percent of its calories from carbs (versus 45 to 50 percent on our plan), 20 percent from fat (versus 30 to 35 percent), and 15 percent from protein (versus 15 to 20 percent). The difference in the Natural Menopause Solution looks small on paper, but it's enough to move your blood sugar (and therefore your insulin levels) in a healthier and slimmer direction while providing *more* high-satisfaction foods so you can stay on track easily.

Rebalancing food groups so that you get slightly more fat and protein is emerging as the smartest strategy for weight loss. In one recent survey of 32,000 people on weight loss diets, lower-carb, higher-protein eating plans got better results than low-fat diets. You've just read why lean protein's so important. Well, there's evidence that fat is, too. Rates of overweight and obesity have increased drastically in the United States at the same time that the percentage of fat in our diets has dropped (from 45 percent 50 years ago to about 33 percent more recently, according to the USDA).

There's no need to fear fat, especially good fats like the omega-3 fatty acids in fish and walnuts and the monounsaturated fats in nuts, avocados, and olive oil. They boost satisfaction, reduce insulin resistance, and help discourage belly fat. Great reasons to savor! A daily dose of omega-3s has also been linked to another plus: better moods. In some studies, omega-3s have helped to ease mild depression.

THE DISTINCTIVE DIFFERENCE: WHAT'S NOT ON YOUR PLATE

Part of the magic's in what you *won't* be eating. We keep you away from obvious weight demons and health sappers like sugary soft drinks, empty-calorie cookies and bread, and crackers and pasta made with refined white flour. Avoiding refined sugar helps you control weight in two ways. Obviously, you subtract hundreds of empty calories a day from your diet if you've been indulging in sodas and sweets. You also get a handle on your blood sugar and insulin.

But you also won't see the gobs of saturated fat and sodium- and preservative-packed processed meats that some low-carb plans are built on. The reason? Even though any low-carb diet can help you lose weight in the short term, the red meats, bacon, lunch meats, and cheese that many plans feature *are uniquely dangerous for women's health at midlife and beyond*, new research shows. If your intuition always whispered that a giant steak topped with butter and blue cheese or a bacon cheeseburger (even without the bun) couldn't possibly be health food, you were right. Here's why.

Saturated fat boosts insulin resistance. And, studies suggest, so do salty, preservative-packed meats. Sodium raises your blood pressure. And experts are beginning to suspect that the chemical preservatives in cured meats interfere with the way our bodies process blood sugar. That's why the 30-Day Slim-Down, Cool-Down Diet features fish; lean poultry; "better" burgers made with skinless ground turkey; and tasty, healthy versions of sausage, bacon, and even ham.

That tweak really matters. For years, health experts have debated whether or not the famously meat- and cheese-packed versions of low-carb diets had negative effects on health. The answer came in 2010, when researchers from the Harvard School of Public Health released results of a study that tracked the meals and health of 85,000 women and 45,000 men for more than 20 years. Meat-rich, low-carb diets increased chances for an early death by 23 percent, while plant-rich cuisines reduced death risk by 20 percent. Women who ate the most vegetables were 23 percent less likely to die from heart disease, and those who ate the least meat were 31 percent less likely to die from colon cancer and 22 percent less likely to have fatal lung cancer, according to the study, published in the *Annals of Internal Medicine* in September 2010.

It's not the only study to point out the consequences of the best—and worst—low-carb diets. A National Cancer Institute study of a half million women and men found that women who ate the most red meat had a 36 percent higher risk for fatal cancers and a 50 percent higher risk for fatal heart disease than those who ate the least red meat. Processed meats packed with preservatives and sodium (which you won't find on this eating plan!) also increased risk, according to this study, which was also published in the *Annals of Internal Medicine*.

Don't misunderstand us. This plan has meat. Even the healthiest women in the Harvard study mentioned above ate meat several times a week. They just didn't overdo it. And neither will you. Keeping servings small, choosing lean types, and making smart substitutions—as you will on our diet—make all the difference. On the Natural Menopause Solution eating plan, you'll enjoy preservative-free, low-sodium versions of hearty fare like homemade turkey sausage (it's fast and easy to make, we promise!) and lean roast beef.

BITE BY BITE: BENEFITS OF THE REST OF THE NATURAL MENOPAUSE SOLUTION FOODS

We know that you're probably a world-class multitasker—juggling lots of balls (family, job, home, friends, faith, community, personal interests, and more) at the same time. You should expect nothing less from your diet, and the 30-Day Slim-Down, Cool-Down Diet delivers. In tandem with the exercise program (read all about it in Chapter 6), this eating plan helps ease menopausal symptoms and is your most powerful, first-line defense against serious women's health threats.

Each of the plan's five major food groups contributes something unique to these amazing benefits. Combined, the effect is even bigger. Pretty exciting! Two—lean protein and calcium-rich, low-fat dairy products—have already been discussed. Here's what you need to know about the rest.

Good fats: *Satisfaction, lower risk for heart disease and diabetes, an ally against belly fat*

Every day you'll eat plenty of satisfying and delicious good fats. These include omega-3 fatty acids found in fish, walnuts, flaxseed, and canola oil, as well as monounsaturated fats found in nuts, olive and canola oils, avocado, and, yes, even dark chocolate! Some luscious examples you'll soon be enjoying: Strawberry-Almond Smoothie, Crustless Quiche, Crab Salad, Vegetable and Quinoa Stew, and Cocoa-Nutty Brownie.

Weight loss edge. Good fats help you shed pounds in five important ways. They:

- **Target abdominal fat.** When Spanish researchers checked the body measurements of 59 women and men before and after they followed a low-carb eating plan featuring good fats or a high-carb, lower-fat plan for 4 weeks, they made an amazing discovery. On the low-carb plan, body fat shifted in a good way: Less was stored in volunteers' torsos by the end of the study. But the high-carb group saw more body fat become belly fat!

- **Reverse insulin resistance.** Good fats help your body regain its ability to "hear" insulin's commands. In one Swedish study of 162 people published in the journal *Diabetologia,* those following a diet high in monounsaturated fats saw insulin sensitivity improve by 9 percent. In contrast, those eating a diet high in saturated fat (the kind found in cheese, ice cream, butter, whole milk, and fatty meats) saw insulin sensitivity *decrease* by 12 percent. (Yes, you can enjoy ice cream on the Natural Menopause Solution eating plan!)

- **Help you get healthier blood sugar, fast.** In a study published in the *Journal of the American College of Nutrition,* researchers put 11 people with insulin resistance on one of three diets—a high-carb plan, a lower-carb plan packed with saturated fat, or one full of good fats. After a single breakfast, good-fat eaters had lower insulin and blood sugar levels than the high-carb group—perhaps because good fats slow the absorption of glucose into the bloodstream.

- **Increase satisfaction.** Is it the instant gratification from eating fat (like snacking on nuts or enjoying vegetables sautéed in olive oil)? Or might it be the long-term satisfaction because fat keeps you feeling full longer? Maybe it's both—and that explains why three times more people stuck with a good-fat diet than with a conventional high-carb, low-fat diet in one study from Brigham and Women's Hospital in

LEARN TO LOVE AVOCADOS

Savor a few slices of avocado in salads and sandwiches. Avocados are incredibly rich in heart-pampering monounsaturated fat and also contain respectable levels of an LDL-lowering compound called beta-sitosterol, the same stuff found in some cholesterol-lowering margarines.

Boston and the Harvard School of Public Health, published in the *International Journal of Obesity.*

◆ **Are easy to stick with for the long haul.** When 322 overweight women and men tried several weight loss plans—including a high-carb plan and a lower-carb plan with plenty of good fats—everyone lost pounds in the first 5 months. But 2 years later, the good-fat group had regained less than ½ pound on average, while others regained 2 to 3 pounds or more. What gave the good-fat eaters the edge? Every day they enjoyed several tablespoons of olive oil and a small handful of nuts—along with a diet packed with the rest of the healthy components you'll find in the Natural Menopause Solution eating plan.

Menopause advantage. These tasty fats are also menopause friendly. Here's how.

◆ **Omega-3s calm hot flashes and night sweats.** Found in fatty fish like salmon, as well as in walnuts and canola oil, omega-3s reduced daily hot flashes by about 40 percent—on par with hot-flash relief via hormone therapy and antidepressants, according to a study published in the journal *Menopause.*

◆ **Omega-3 fatty acids can help lift serious depression,** report University of Belfast researchers who reviewed 27 studies of the effects of these good fats on depression. Omega-3s—particularly a type called DHA (docosahexaenoic acid)—are associated with higher levels of the feel-good brain chemicals serotonin and dopamine and may also clamp down on depression-promoting inflammation. In addition, good fats may bolster other brain changes that brighten your mood, such as making cell walls healthier so that transmission of signals between cells is stronger.

Health bonus. Once considered luxuries, good fats are fast becoming essential elements of a healthy diet. Here's how they help.

- **Pamper your heart and arteries.** Omega-3 fatty acids lower your risk for irregular heart rhythms that cause strokes, trigger some heart attacks, and result in hundreds of thousands of deaths every year in the United States. These good fats can also help regulate blood pressure, keep arteries flexible, and even guard against a buildup of gunky plaque in artery walls by cooling off inflammation. Chronic inflammation, often caused by excess fat deep in the abdomen, pumps out chemicals that boost your risk for clogged arteries and heart attacks.

- **Guard against type 2 diabetes.** By reversing insulin resistance—the prime cause of type 2 diabetes—the good fats found in nuts, seeds, and olive and canola oil can also reduce your risk for this major blood sugar problem. After a year of following a healthy, low-carb diet with a few extra nuts or a little extra olive oil daily, 7 to 14 percent of people with insulin resistance saw the condition improve, according to a Spanish study published in the *Archives of Internal Medicine*.

Fruits and vegetables: *Low-calorie, high-nutrition satisfaction; powerful disease prevention*

Filling your plate with all sorts of veggies and fruits is an important strategy for losing weight and boosting health—and feeling full while you do it. Surveys of people who successfully lost pounds and kept them off consistently show that America's biggest losers make the supermarket produce department (as well as farmers' markets, the frozen fruit and

Should You Go Organic?

Eating any fruit and vegetables is better than avoiding produce. But choosing organic types when you can may be an even better idea. Some experts suspect that pesticides and other chemicals used in growing crops may be endocrine disruptors that mimic the way hormones like estrogen work in your body. For more on the best fruits and vegetables to buy in organic form, turn to page 363.

veggies aisle at the grocery store, and backyard vegetable patches) their go-to place when shopping for food. You'll do so on this diet—with dishes such as Stir-Fried Ginger Shrimp and Veggies, Baked Apples with Creamy Maple Sauce, and more!

Weight loss edge. Simply adding more vegetables and fruits to your diet can help you lose weight and keep it off. Here's how produce banishes extra pounds. It:

- **Fills you up, not out.** Low in calories but packed with fiber and water, fruits and vegetables are low-density, high-volume foods. They make you feel full with relatively few calories. Studies from Pennsylvania State University show that chunky vegetables in particular—in salads and soups, for example—have special talents for helping you eat less at meals, perhaps because they prompt your stomach to send signals to your brain that you couldn't possibly eat another bite!

- **Reverses insulin resistance by cooling off inflammation.** Excess abdominal fat sends out compounds that boost levels of bodywide inflammation and mutes cells' ability to obey insulin. Fruits and vegetables tone down inflammation. In one Harvard School of Public Health study of 486 women published in the *American Journal of*

Clinical Nutrition, those who consumed the most produce had the lowest levels of an inflammation marker called C-reactive protein. The result? Women who ate the most fruit were 34 percent less likely to be insulin resistant. Those who munched on the most veggies were 30 percent less likely.

◆ **Downshifts digestion for a slower, lower rise in blood sugar.** Fiber slows the release of sugar into your bloodstream. Enjoying produce at every meal doesn't just fill you up, it also keeps your post-meal blood sugar and insulin levels down.

Menopause advantage. In one study of 276 women, Korea University researchers found that those who ate the most green and yellow vegetables had slightly fewer hot flashes. The connection may be extra fiber; other studies have shown that women who eat more fiber have fewer hot flashes and night sweats.

Health bonus. It's almost impossible to overdo it when it comes to produce. And the more you eat, the greater the benefits.

◆ **Reduce cancer risk.** According to the American Institute for Cancer Research, filling your plate with fruits and veggies offers powerful protection against many cancers. Produce is packed with antioxidants that protect your DNA from damage that can lead to cancer. Cruciferous veggies like broccoli and cauliflower, green leafy vegetables like spinach and kale, all kinds of berries, beans, tomatoes, dark yellow and orange types like winter squash, and garlic may have special talents for guarding against cancer in this way. And by helping you reach and stay at a healthy weight, produce may also guard against a cancer risk that rises with higher levels of body fat—especially cancers of the colon, rectum, esophagus, endometrium, pancreas, kidneys, and breasts in postmenopausal women.

◆ **Slash heart and stroke risks.** Compared with women who ate just 1½ produce servings a day, those who feasted on 7 to 10 servings lowered their risk for heart and blood vessel problems by a whopping 55 percent and were 38 percent less likely to have a heart attack, according to a study at the Harvard School of Public Health published in the *American Journal of Clinical Nutrition*. Other studies show that having plenty of produce cuts odds for a stroke by 26 percent and can lower your blood pressure.

- **Clamp down on high blood pressure.** In a study of more than 40,000 women, Harvard School of Public Health researchers found that those who got the most fruits, vegetables, and whole grains were 24 percent less likely to have high blood pressure when compared with those who got the least. The reason? Eating lots of produce instead of processed foods lowers your intake of blood pressure–raising sodium and boosts levels of blood pressure–pampering minerals like potassium and magnesium.

Whole grains: *Better blood sugar; less inflammation; protection from strokes, high blood pressure, and more*

On the Natural Menopause Solution eating plan, "low carb" doesn't mean "no carb." You'll enjoy brown rice, whole grain muffins and wraps, and quick-cooking, flavorful grains like quinoa. How about Cranberry-Oat Breakfast Cookies, Pasta with Gorgonzola-Walnut Sauce, or a delicious Veggie-Cheese Wrap?

Weight loss edge. Like produce, whole grains contain several types of filling fiber, which can help control cravings by keeping your blood sugar lower and steadier.

- **Better insulin sensitivity.** Breads, crackers, and other foods made with refined white flour—processed to remove healthy fiber as well as the healthy nutrients and fats found naturally in whole grains—make blood sugar soar, then crash. Your body pumps out more insulin to force all that sugar into your cells, but refined carbs may interfere with how well your cells obey insulin's signals. In contrast, switching to whole grain bread improves insulin sensitivity, which has been shown to aid weight loss.

◆ **Steady blood sugar.** The fiber and bran in whole grains resist easy digestion, so it takes longer to convert a whole grain's starches into sugars. And some grains, such as oatmeal and barley, also contain resistant starches—a type of starch that acts like fiber, breaking down so slowly that it holds your blood sugar steady for hours on end. Barley, rye, oats, wheat germ, and other whole grains are also rich in lignans, a plant-based phytoestrogen that has beneficial effects for your blood glucose. One Danish study of more than 800 postmenopausal women, published in the *Journal of Nutrition*, found that women who ate the most whole grains had significantly higher blood levels of protective lignans. Other research has linked high blood levels of lignans to better insulin sensitivity and less abdominal fat, too!

Menopause advantage. Eating a high-fiber diet translates into fewer hot flashes, according to a University of California, Davis, study of 2,198 breast cancer survivors who experienced menopausal symptoms due to a natural drop in hormones or due to changes brought on by surgery or chemotherapy.

Health bonus. While it's important to cut back on refined grain products to avoid negative health consequences, it's just as important to fit whole grains into your meals daily to bolster good health. Here's why.

◆ **Cool inflammation.** Eating at least two whole grain servings a day reduced deaths from inflammation-related diseases by 30 percent over 17 years, reports the Iowa Women's Health Study.

◆ **Lower levels of heart-threatening LDL cholesterol.** Soluble fiber—the stuff found in oatmeal, barley, and rye—has special cholesterol-lowering skills. It forms a gel in your intestinal tract that

(continued on page 60)

Happier and Healthier...
THE NATURAL MENOPAUSE SOLUTION WAY

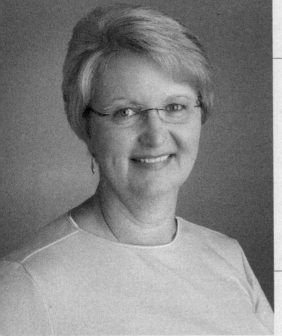

CAROL KEENE

Age: 54

Pounds lost: 9

Inches lost: 7½

Major changes: Half as many hot flashes, better sleep, lowered blood pressure from 134/96 to 126/82.

"I'm Finally Losing Fat"

Two years into menopause, Carol was frustrated with stubborn excess weight and inches that kept her two dress sizes higher than her goal. "Menopause changes everything with your weight and body shape," she says. "You think you have it all under control, you do all the things that helped you lose weight in the past, but nothing's happening! I found out that I had to do something new and different to get my body to respond."

That, Carol says, was her biggest *aha!* moment. "I discovered that when I make changes in what I'm eating *and* in the way I exercise, I can finally lose the fat. Before this, I was exercising for up to 1½ hours at a time several days a week, but my body wouldn't let go of the weight. It took the interval walking and the yoga with weights and the ingredients in the diet to change all that. I thought I needed even more activity, but what I really needed was to build muscle and boost the intensity with intervals," she says. "Then just keep on doing it. Being consistent counts, too."

Carol loves to cook—and eat—good food. So the creative and delicious Natural Menopause Solution recipes thrilled her. "So many diet plans take all of the taste out of the food, but not this one. I looked through the recipes and said to myself, 'There it is—there's the flavor I've been looking for.' It's in the olive oil, the spices, the red peppers, and so much more. It's not diet food. And it didn't leave me feeling hungry, either."

Take the recipe for Homemade Turkey Sausage. "It cooks up fast from scratch, and you get the flavor of sausage without all the fat, thanks to the sage and other spices," she says. "I made four and had three extra to store in the refrigerator or freezer and heat up in the microwave, which was so convenient."

Carol was also thrilled with the program's first lunch: a slice of pizza with chicken topping and a banana. "I was so happy! I walked out of work at lunchtime and told my assistant, 'I'm going out for pizza!' I ate my slice with a knife and fork, savoring each bite as if I were having a huge meal. Then I had my banana and thought, *'Yummmmm! This is wonderful!'*"

Carol started the program while she was busy helping to plan her daughter's wedding and was thrilled to find that she had more energy than ever. "We'll be on the go all day on most Saturdays, making wedding arrangements, and I'm not tired at all," she says. "One reason is that I'm sleeping soundly now. My night sweats have been reduced to just a warm spell that might wake me up once a night instead of several times each night."

Other menopause-related symptoms are better, too. "My hot flashes—I call them hot spells—are cut in half. I don't get a horrible, drenching sweat when I exercise. And I've noticed that on days when I didn't drink the Slimming, Cooling Smoothie, I would have a hot flash in the morning, but not on days when I had one," she notes. "I've looked a little swollen since hitting menopause, but now the puffiness in my arms and legs has gone down. I'm going to look great in my mother-of-the-bride dress at the wedding!"

traps cholesterol-rich digestive substances called bile acids. You then eliminate the bile acids instead of reabsorbing them. The result: To make more bile acids, your body must pull more LDL from your bloodstream, lowering levels there. Brilliant!

- **Slash your risk for heart disease and stroke.** Compared with people who had less than ½ serving of whole grains daily, those who had 2½ servings a day were 21 percent less likely to develop heart disease, said Wake Forest University Medical Center researchers who reviewed seven fiber studies involving 285,000 people. The study was published in the online edition of the journal *Nutrition, Metabolism & Cardiovascular Diseases*. Meanwhile, whole grains also lower your risk for stroke by up to 36 percent, your risk for heart failure by 29 percent, and your risk for high blood pressure by 11 percent.

- **Protect against diabetes.** When you have whole grains instead of breads, crackers, breakfast cereals, and grain side dishes made with refined grains, you get diabetes protection in two ways: Fiber slows the release of sugar into your bloodstream, while a rainbow of vitamins and minerals encourages better insulin sensitivity. No wonder just two servings a day cut the risk by 21 percent!

- **Guard against cancer.** Grains are a great source of plant estrogens, called phytoestrogens, which may help guard against the development of some types of cancer.

PUTTING IT ALL TOGETHER

Now that you've learned how all the components of the eating plan will help you slim down and cool down, it's time to eat! Remember, the 30-day program is divided into two phases.

In Phase 1 (Days 1 through 5), you'll eat 1,250 calories a day in three satisfying meals. The object of Phase 1? We want to introduce you to a whole new way of eating and give you a variety of foods to make and eat so that you can see for yourself how simple and satisfying it is. During this phase we recommend that you stick with the set meal plan as closely as possible.

In Phase 2 (Days 6 through 30), you'll add a daily 250-calorie snack, for a total of 1,500 calories a day. We want you to have plenty of fuel as you step up the intensity of your walking routine and add weights to your yoga sessions. We also want to ensure that your weight loss is steady and well paced to help preserve muscle and bone. Adding a snack also gives you more flexibility. You'll be able to stick with this plan even if a meal is delayed or you become extra hungry!

In both phases, the calorie counts for meals stay the same: Breakfast is about 350 calories; lunch and dinner are about 450 calories each. All meals feature the optimal mix of macronutrients: 15 to 20 percent lean protein (about 60 to 75 grams per day); 45 to 50 percent complex carbohydrates (about 150 to 170 grams per day); and 30 to 35 percent healthy fats (about 45 to 60 grams per day). (Snacks won't follow this rule.) Keep in mind, though, that all of these numbers are approximate. In fact, you may see that some of our recipes and/or daily menus exceed these guidelines occasionally or fall short of a specific nutrient every once in a while. That's okay as long as most meals most days fall more or less within these guidelines. The 30-Day Slim-Down, Cool-Down Diet is not about counting calories or grams of protein, carbs, or fat. It's about learning to feed your body the best mix of foods to help you lose weight, soothe menopausal symptoms, and prevent diseases common to women at midlife.

Finally, you'll enjoy a Slimming, Cooling Smoothie every day in both phases. Plus, you should have one other food per day that's a good source of each of the Flash-Fighting Four ingredients that together help you lose weight, control cravings, reduce belly fat, cool hot flashes, keep you energized, and prevent the major health threats that women face at, and after, midlife. (See box on page 64 for a list.)

THE NATURAL MENOPAUSE SOLUTION EATING PLAN "RULES"

We know flexibility's important to you, so it's built into this plan. Our "rules" are really guidelines to help you take the plan everywhere you go, easily, while still reaping the maximum benefits.

Rule #1. Feel free to substitute any food within the same food group. For instance, if you don't want an egg salad sandwich for lunch, have chicken salad, tuna salad, or salmon salad instead. If you don't want yogurt, substitute fat-free milk, low-fat cottage cheese, or a dairy-replacement food. If you don't eat meat, switch to a meat substitute such as tofu or tempeh.

Rule #2. You can also substitute one meal for another from within the same day's meal plan or from another day. In addition, lunches and dinners are interchangeable. For instance, you can enjoy Wednesday's breakfast on Monday, or swap Saturday's lunch with Saturday's dinner. But don't repeat the same meal too many times in the same week or you could miss out on important nutrients in your diet.

Rule #3. If you're eating out, order a meal that is similar to the one on your meal plan for that day or to one from any other day on the meal plan. Remember to keep your portion sizes small when you're not in charge of cooking and cannot control the ingredients.

Rule #4. If you prefer, break some of the meals into smaller parts, and save the rest to eat later. This may be helpful during Phase 1, especially if you're accustomed to having a snack. For example, if your breakfast includes ½ cup blueberries but your meal is satisfying enough without them, save them for an afternoon snack or for dessert after dinner. In Phase 2, you can choose either one full snack or dessert OR half portions of two different ones.

Rule #5. With the exception of milk or substitutes such as soy, rice, or almond milk that are included in your meal plans, all beverages should be calorie free: water, seltzer, coffee, tea. (You can add up to ¼ cup fat-free or low-fat milk to your coffee or tea and 1 or 2 teaspoons of sugar daily.) Decaffeinated and iced beverages are best if you are experiencing hot flashes. Although diet soda is calorie free, we don't recommend it; the research on artificial sweeteners is mixed.

Rule #6. In Phase 1, we're asking you to refrain from any alcoholic drinks. In Phase 2, you can choose to have a glass of wine or beer instead of a snack or dessert. But don't indulge in these "diet busters" more than once a week. (Alcohol can also trigger hot flashes, another reason to limit it.)

Rule #7. By cutting down on processed meats and other processed foods (which contribute the majority of sodium in our diets), the eating plan keeps sodium levels under 1,500 milligrams as often as possible and always under 2,300 milligrams, in accordance with the 2010 Dietary Guidelines, the USDA's "official" recommendations for healthy eating. Stick to low-sodium foods as much as you can.

Rule #8. Because even adding the Flash-Fighting Four to your diet may not give you enough of these important nutrients (and others you need for optimal health), you may want to take a multivitamin. Look for one labeled "for women over 50." Calcium is bulky, so it usually needs to be taken in a separate pill. Look for one with 500 to 600 milligrams of calcium citrate, 250 to 300 milligrams of magnesium, and 800 to 1,200 IU of vitamin D daily.

Where to Find the Flash-Fighting Four

As we noted, while the Slimming, Cooling Smoothie provides a booster shot of these four vital nutrients, in order to make sure that you get the optimal amount, you should have one other food per day that's a good source of each of the Flash-Fighting Four. If you follow the 30-day meal plan exactly, you'll see that we've already included these foods. But if you make any substitutions or decide to make your own menu, use these lists to help you get what you need.

Calcium

Dairy products, such as milk, yogurt, and cheese

Fortified dairy alternatives, such as soy milk and almond milk

Fortified breakfast cereals and fruit juices

Almonds and sesame seeds

Tofu processed with calcium

Broccoli and green leafy vegetables such as kale and collards

Vitamin D

Fortified milk and dairy products, such as yogurt and cheese, if made with fortified milk

Fortified soy milk and other dairy alternatives

Fortified breakfast cereals

Fish and shellfish, especially salmon and oysters

Lean Protein

Egg whites

Poultry, especially chicken and turkey breast

Fish and shellfish

Lean cuts of meat, such as beef sirloin, pork tenderloin, and leg of lamb

Legumes, including dried beans, lentils, and split peas

Fat-free and low-fat dairy products, such as milk, yogurt, and some cheeses

Soybeans and soy products, such as soy milk, soy yogurt, and tofu

Some grains, such as quinoa

Magnesium

Dairy milk

Soy milk

Bananas, pineapples, and oranges

Legumes, including black beans, chickpeas, soybeans, and lima beans

Green leafy vegetables, such as spinach

Nuts and nut butters, especially almonds, Brazil nuts, and cashews

Seeds, especially sunflower seeds and sesame seeds

Fortified breakfast cereals, including oatmeal

The
Slim-Down,
Cool-Down
Meal Plans

PHASE 1

In Phase 1, which lasts 5 days, you will be eating three meals per day. We recommend that you follow this meal plan as closely as you can in this phase. Of course, use the guidelines we've given to make substitutions for any foods you don't eat for any reason.

PHASE 2

In Phase 2, which lasts for the remainder of the 30-day program, you'll bump up your daily calorie intake by adding a snack from our list on page 79. In Phase 2, feel free to start experimenting with more substitutions for variety and convenience. Enjoy a breakfast, lunch, or dinner from any other day of the program, or use our advice when eating out. We've given you 10 days of menus for this phase to get you started.

Day 1

BREAKFAST

Homemade Turkey Sausage (page 91)

1½ cups cantaloupe cubes sprinkled with 1 tablespoon fat-free granola

Slimming, Cooling Smoothie (page 85)

362 calories, 20% protein, 49% carbohydrates, 32% fat

LUNCH

1 slice cheese pizza with chicken topping (⅛ of a 14" pie)

1 large banana

407 calories, 21% protein, 50% carbohydrates, 30% fat

DINNER

Roasted Salmon with Green Beans and Potatoes (page 122)

White Beans with Roasted Red Pepper (page 131)

1 small whole wheat roll

501 calories, 20% protein, 48% carbohydrates, 30% fat

Day 2

BREAKFAST

Mixed-Fruit Cup sprinkled with 1 tablespoon unsweetened coconut (page 87)

Slimming, Cooling Smoothie (page 85)

383 calories, 15% protein, 50% carbohydrates, 34% fat

LUNCH

Beef 'n' Broccoli Pasta Salad (page 101)

1 slice whole grain Italian bread spread with 2 teaspoons olive oil

526 calories, 20% protein, 46% carbohydrates, 33% fat

DINNER

½ serving Hearty Kale and White Bean Soup (page 117)

1 square piece Lavash bread

272 calories, 18% protein, 47% carbohydrates, 35% fat

Day 3

BREAKFAST

1 multigrain or high-fiber (frozen) waffle topped with ¼ cup sliced strawberries

1 hard-cooked egg white or 1 whole hard-cooked egg

Slimming, Cooling Smoothie (page 85)

291 calories, 16% protein, 50% carbohydrates, 33% fat

LUNCH

Quinoa Salad with Apples and Walnuts (page 97)

2 ounces sliced roasted chicken or turkey breast

½ cup steamed broccoli rabe

403 calories, 18% protein, 46% carbohydrates, 35% fat

DINNER

½ serving Spiced Chicken with Lentils (page 119)

1 toasted whole wheat pita (6½" round) brushed with 1½ teaspoons olive oil

¼ cup hummus

10 baby carrots

551 calories, 20% protein, 43% carbohydrates, 35% fat

Day 4

BREAKFAST

Fig 'n' Flax Muffin (page 92)

1 hard-cooked egg

Slimming, Cooling Smoothie (page 85)

424 calories, 15% protein, 50% carbohydrates, 35% fat

LUNCH

½ serving Arugula Salad Plate topped with hard-cooked egg white (page 96)

2 cups mixed berries

3 low-fat crackers

367 calories, 15% protein, 55% carbohydrates, 30% fat

DINNER

Stir-Fried Ginger Shrimp and Veggies (page 124)

½ cup cucumber slices + 8 baby carrots dressed with 1 teaspoon sesame oil + 1 tablespoon rice vinegar

491 calories, 22% protein, 46% carbohydrates, 31% fat

Day 5

BREAKFAST

Open-Faced Omelet (page 88)

Slimming, Cooling Smoothie (page 85)

315 calories, 17% protein, 51% carbohydrates, 32% fat

LUNCH

Veggie-Cheese Wrap (page 106)

1 cup apple slices

495 calories, 20% protein, 45% carbohydrates, 34% fat

DINNER

¾ serving Roasted Turkey Breast and Vegetables (page 114)

Sweet Potatoes with Orange and Walnuts (page 130)

430 calories, 20% protein, 50% carbohydrates, 30% fat

Day 6

BREAKFAST

1 cup cooked oatmeal with 2 tablespoons blueberries

2 hard-cooked egg whites or 1 whole hard-cooked egg

Slimming, Cooling Smoothie (page 85)

404 calories, 18% protein, 50% carbohydrates, 31% fat

LUNCH

Tuna salad sandwich on whole wheat bread

4 ounces low-fat plain yogurt

¼ cup sliced strawberries

457 calories, 20% protein, 46% carbohydrates, 34% fat

SNACK

5 shredded whole wheat crackers (such as Triscuits) with ⅓ cup hummus

241 calories, 10% protein, 52% carbohydrates, 37% fat

DINNER

French-Style Seafood Chowder (page 123)

414 calories, 18% protein, 44% carbohydrates, 30% fat

Day 7

BREAKFAST

Greek Spinach Scramble (page 89)

1/2 toasted whole wheat pita (61/2" round) brushed with 1 teaspoon olive oil

1/2 medium pear

Slimming, Cooling Smoothie (page 85)

354 calories, 15% protein, 49% carbohydrates, 36% fat

LUNCH

1 cup black bean or lentil soup (homemade or low-sodium canned)

1/2 avocado

1 ounce reduced-fat Swiss cheese

1 tomato, sliced

Small whole grain roll

441 calories, 18% protein, 47% carbohydrates, 35% fat

DINNER

Chicken Adobo (page 118)

1 cup brown basmati rice

1 cup zucchini and red pepper sautéed in olive oil

500 calories, 20% protein, 45% carbohydrates, 35% fat

DESSERT

1/2 cup light vanilla ice cream (regular, nonpremium ice cream such as Breyer's) topped with 1/2 cup pitted fresh cherries and 2 tablespoons chopped walnuts or almonds

217 calories, 10% protein, 59% carbohydrates, 31% fat

Day 8

BREAKFAST

Skillet-Baked Parmesan Eggs (page 90)

Slimming, Cooling Smoothie (page 85)

360 calories, 18% protein, 50% carbohydrates, 32% fat

LUNCH

Quick Tortilla Soup (page 103)

1 orange

444 calories, 18% protein, 50% carbohydrates, 32% fat

DINNER

½ serving Turkey Cutlets with Cranberry Wild Rice (page 115)

1 plain sweet potato drizzled with 1½ teaspoons olive oil

1 cup steamed green beans

411 calories, 20% protein, 44% carbohydrates, 35% fat

DESSERT

Nutty Berry Fool (page 141)

238 calories, 15% protein, 50% carbohydrates, 34% fat

Day 9

BREAKFAST

1 Cranberry-Oat Breakfast Cookie (page 93)

½ cup strawberries

2 egg whites

Slimming, Cooling Smoothie (page 85)

306 calories, 18% protein, 47% carbohydrates, 34% fat

LUNCH

Swiss cheese sandwich made with 2 ounces cheese, lettuce, and tomato, with 2 teaspoons mustard on 2 slices whole grain bread

1 apple

413 calories, 18% protein, 48% carbohydrates, 34% fat

HALF-SIZE SNACK

½ serving White Bean Spread on Toast (1 slice toast with 2 tablespoons bean spread) (page 138)

131 calories, 16% protein, 50% carbohydrates, 34% fat

DINNER

1 ounce boneless, skinless chicken breast

1 medium baked potato topped with 3 ounces plain low-fat yogurt, 2 tablespoons finely chopped green onion, and 1 tablespoon grated mozzarella cheese

Tomato-Avocado Salad (page 132)

433 calories, 20% protein, 49% carbohydrates, 30% fat

HALF-SIZE DESSERT

½ Cocoa-Nutty Brownie (page 140) with ½ cup low-fat (1%) milk or soy milk

124 calories, 18% protein, 45% carbohydrates, 37% fat

Day 10

BREAKFAST

1 oat bran muffin (2½" diameter), toasted

1 whole hard-cooked egg

Slimming, Cooling Smoothie (page 85)

412 calories, 15% protein, 50% carbohydrates, 35% fat

LUNCH

Crab Salad (page 99)

12 baked corn tortilla chips

1 cup cantaloupe cubes

495 calories, 20% protein, 46% carbohydrates, 34% fat

DINNER

$\frac{1}{2}$ serving Gingered Turkey Meat Loaf (page 116)

$\frac{3}{4}$ cup cooked brown rice

1 cup broccoli florets sautéed in 1 teaspoon olive oil with $\frac{1}{2}$ cup
sliced red bell pepper

375 calories, 20% protein, 50% carbohydrates, 30% fat

SNACK

Cheese and Olive Quesadilla (page 139)

1 glass (6 ounces) wine or 12-ounce light beer

250 calories, 16% protein, 19% carbohydrates, 21% fat, 44% alcohol

Day 11

BREAKFAST

1 slice whole grain toast topped with 1 ounce reduced-fat cream
cheese and 2 tablespoons sliced strawberries

2 hard-cooked egg whites

Slimming, Cooling Smoothie (page 85)

309 calories, 20% protein, 49% carbohydrates, 31% fat

LUNCH

Chicken Caesar salad made with 1 ounce grilled or roasted chicken
breast, 3 cups romaine lettuce, $\frac{1}{2}$ cup croutons, 2 tablespoons low-fat
Caesar salad dressing, and 1 tablespoon grated Parmesan cheese

1 cup Mixed-Fruit Cup (page 87) with 2 tablespoons unsweetened
coconut

460 calories, 20% protein, 45% carbohydrates, 35% fat

DINNER

Vegetable and Quinoa Stew (page 112)

1 ounce roasted chicken breast

477 calories, 18% protein, 50% carbohydrates, 33% fat

DESSERT

1 slice Pineapple-Carrot Loaf Cake (page 142)

¾ cup low-fat (1%) milk or soy milk

246 calories, 15% protein, 48% carbohydrates, 37% fat

Day 12

BREAKFAST

1 cup grapefruit sections with ¼ cup raspberries and 1 tablespoon dry-roasted sunflower seeds

2 hard-cooked egg whites or 1 whole hard-cooked egg

Slimming, Cooling Smoothie (page 85)

325 calories, 20% protein, 45% carbohydrates, 35% fat

LUNCH

Gado Gado (Hearty Indonesian Salad) (page 100)

452 calories, 18% protein, 44% carbohydrates, 38% fat

DINNER

Pasta with Gorgonzola-Walnut Sauce (page 113)

Green Bean and Tomato Salad (page 135)

402 calories, 17% protein, 48% carbohydrates, 35% fat

DESSERT

Baked Apples with Creamy Maple Sauce (page 144)

260 calories, 14% protein, 55% carbohydrates, 31% fat

Day 13

BREAKFAST

1 cup hot cooked wheat cereal topped with ¼ cup diced pear and 1 tablespoon finely chopped almonds

Slimming, Cooling Smoothie (page 85)

367 calories, 14% protein, 52% carbohydrates, 34% fat

LUNCH

1-ounce lean turkey burger with 1 ounce Cheddar cheese, 1 tablespoon low-sodium ketchup, and a small whole grain slider hamburger bun

Spinach and Orange Salad (page 98)

485 calories, 21% protein, 47% carbohydrates, 31% fat

SNACK

1 brown rice cake topped with 1 tablespoon almond butter and 2 sliced strawberries

1 cup low-fat (1%) milk or soy milk

246 calories, 18% protein, 38% carbohydrates, 44% fat

DINNER

Cod in Curry Broth with Rice (page 126)

½ serving Sweet Corn and Edamame Salad (page 134)

1 cup melon cubes

481 calories, 16% protein, 48% carbohydrates, 35% fat

Day 14

BREAKFAST

Lemon-Ricotta Pancake (page 94)

1 hard-cooked egg

Slimming, Cooling Smoothie (page 85)

426 calories, 18% protein, 47% carbohydrates, 35% fat

LUNCH

Pita Pizza (page 107)

1 cup sliced cucumber tossed with 2 tablespoons plain low-fat yogurt

406 calories, 18% protein, 47% carbohydrates, 35% fat

DINNER

2-ounce boneless pork chop or cutlet

½ cup unsweetened applesauce

1 cup succotash (corn and lima bean mix) tossed with 1 teaspoon olive oil

365 calories, 20% protein, 49% carbohydrates, 30% fat

DESSERT

4-ounce container dark chocolate pudding, topped with 1 tablespoon natural sliced or chopped almonds

1 glass (4 ounces) wine

269 calories, 7% protein, 62% carbohydrates, 30% fat, 41% alcohol

Day 15

BREAKFAST

Low-fat granola bar or energy bar

1 whole hard-cooked egg

Slimming, Cooling Smoothie (page 85)

334 calories, 15% protein, 51% carbohydrates, 33% fat

LUNCH

Grilled cheese sandwich with 2 slices whole grain bread, 2 ounces reduced-fat Cheddar cheese, and using 1 teaspoon light olive oil for skillet toasting

Tossed salad with 2 cups chopped romaine lettuce leaves, 1 finely chopped medium tomato, 8 thinly sliced green olives, and 1 tablespoon balsamic vinegar

½ large apple

466 calories, 20% protein, 44% carbohydrates, 36% fat

SNACK

1 container (6 ounces) lemon-flavored low-fat yogurt

4 graham cracker squares (2 full rectangles)

264 calories, 16% protein, 67% carbohydrates, 17% fat

DINNER

Roast Beef and Tomatoes with Basil Sauce (page 128)

½ cup corn kernels

White beans and artichokes made with ⅓ cup small white (navy) beans, and ½ cup drained artichoke hearts (frozen or packed in brine, not oil) served over 1 cup baby spinach leaves and sprinkled with balsamic or red wine vinegar

431 calories, 25% protein, 42% carbohydrates, 32% fat

Phase 2 Snack List

In Phase 2, you can have any one of the snacks or desserts below, each of which adds up to approximately 250 calories. Eat it whenever you'd like—to tide you over between breakfast and lunch, to satisfy midafternoon hunger pangs, to keep you full if you're having a late dinner, as dessert after lunch or dinner, or in the evening! You can even have half snacks at two different times of day.

- 1 glass (8 ounces) white or red wine (160–170 calories) with 1½ tablespoons dry-roasted unsalted almonds or 1 ounce reduced-fat cheese

- 1 beer (12 ounces) with 16 tiny twist pretzels

- 1 cup Pineapple Iced Tea with 1 ounce no-salt-added crispy soy chips. (To make Pineapple Iced Tea, combine ¾ cup pineapple juice with ½ cup brewed green, black, or jasmine tea and pour over ice in a tall glass. To vary the flavor, try mango or cranberry all-juice blends in place of pineapple juice.)

- 5 shredded whole wheat crackers (such as Triscuits) with 2 ounces reduced-fat cheese

- 7 shredded whole wheat crackers (such as Triscuits) with ⅓ cup hummus

- 1 cup low-fat (1%) milk with 2 small oatmeal-raisin cookies or 5 thin chocolate wafer cookies

- ½ cup vanilla ice cream (regular, nonpremium ice cream such as Breyers) topped with ½ cup pitted fresh cherries and 2 tablespoons chopped walnuts or almonds

- 1 small slice angel food cake (1/12 of cake) topped with 1 cup sliced strawberries and ¼ cup whipped cream or ⅓ cup vanilla pudding

Chapter 5

The Natural Menopause Solution Recipes

*A*re you ready for Beef 'n' Broccoli Pasta Salad? Stir-Fried Ginger Shrimp and Veggies? Cocoa-Nutty Brownies and Lemon-Ricotta Pancakes? You'll find these and dozens more of our delicious Slim-Down, Cool-Down recipes in this chapter. This food tastes so good, you'll have a hard time believing that it will also help you lose weight, ease menopausal symptoms, and protect your health.

Designed by registered dietitian Susan McQuillan, these recipes are packed not only with maximum flavor but also with maximum nutrition. They provide a healthy helping of our Flash-Fighting Four ingredients—calcium, lean protein, magnesium, and vitamin D. As you've already discovered, this fabulous foursome can help you shed stubborn pounds, bolster your metabolism, alleviate hot flashes and other midlife symptoms, and guard against bone loss, diabetes, heart disease, and other chronic health problems. The recipes also provide plenty of fruits and vegetables, a wide range of satisfying, delicious whole grains—including brown rice, quinoa, and whole grain pita—and good fats from avocado, nuts, salmon, and olive oil.

In addition to the recipes you'll need for our meal plan, this section offers bonus recipes that you can swap in or use anytime. These include delicious entrées such as Romaine-Fruit Salad with Creamy Orange Dressing, Pepper and Egg Sandwich, and Pasta with Garlicky White Clam Sauce. You'll also find yummy desserts (how about Pineapple-Carrot Loaf Cake with a cream cheese glaze?) and snack foods special enough to serve at your next party, such as Mushroom, Cheddar, and Walnut Pâté.

Our test panelists—and their families!—loved this food.

◆ "My favorite meal was the Roasted Salmon with Green Beans and Potatoes," said Carol Keene. "It was wonderful, quick, and easy—and full of flavor thanks to the rosemary and olive oil. And the meal cooked very quickly. It was done in less than 20 minutes. I set the table while the fish cooked, and it was done beautifully. My husband loved it, too."

◆ "I thought the Veggie-Cheese Wrap was fantastic," said Eileen Fehr. "I could have eaten it every single day for lunch. The combination of the crunchy cabbage, the creamy avocado, and the cheese and basil made it terrific. My husband loved the Gingered Turkey Meat Loaf. And the Homemade Turkey Sausage patties went together very quickly and tasted great, too."

◆ "The best thing was the Beef 'n' Broccoli Pasta Salad—wow!" said Cherylyn Rush. "The leftovers kept well in the refrigerator. In fact, my husband went looking for the leftovers the next day, but I'd taken them for lunch!"

◆ "I chose the meals I liked best and that were easiest for me to prepare," said Robin Laub. "I loved the salmon, so I had that a lot. I really enjoyed the chicken dishes, so I also had them frequently. The

Open-Faced Omelet with peppers and potatoes was delicious. In fact, the breakfasts were so big I would save part of them to eat as a mid-morning snack."

Preparing Slim-Down, Cool-Down Diet meals doesn't have to take a lot of time or be difficult. Actually, it can take *less* time than ordering a pizza and waiting for delivery or going out to a restaurant. To make meal prep as fast and easy as possible, deploy these strategies.

1. **Mix-and-match meals.** If you don't have time to put together a particular meal, choose one with a shorter prep time.

2. **Make a shopping list.** Page through the recipes, and then check your pantry and refrigerator. Write down all the ingredients you'll need before going to the store.

3. **Cook ahead.** On weekends, cook a double batch of a recipe, then refrigerate it for up to 3 days or freeze it. Pack up any leftovers and bring them for lunch the next day.

It's also easy to personalize the recipes to suit your tastes. If you or a member of your family is vegetarian, for instance, substitute a vegetarian protein for meat, poultry, or fish. If you don't eat dairy products, you'll find that most of the recipes work just as well with substitutes such as soy milk or soy cheese. If you have a gluten intolerance, go with gluten-free products and choose recipes featuring gluten-free grains such as quinoa. Once you get used to the mix of nutrients in the recipes, we encourage you to create some of your own favorites to stay slim, cool, and satisfied for life.

It Worked for Me!

**Amy Wressell, 52, lost 7 pounds and 8¼ inches—
and she's sleeping better.**

At 52, Amy suspects that she's in perimenopause—and all the signs point in that direction. Her cycles vary wildly, from 13 to 47 days. Lately she's found herself wide awake at 3 or 4 o'clock in the morning, too. "I don't like it," says this industry statistician and mother of two boys. "But in the last 3 weeks I've been sleeping very well—I think one reason is the Natural Menopause Solution exercise program. The yoga and the interval walks seem to be helping me."

The fitness routine also toned her waist and hips, subtracting a whopping 2½ inches from each. "I was wearing a size 12, but now I'm down to a size 10 or even a size 8," she says. "I have my skinny jeans on today, and I'll be shopping for new clothes soon. Losing nearly 7 pounds is great. Losing all of these inches is even better."

Amy says walking "felt kind of boring" in the past. But adding fast-paced intervals several times each week added a new dimension. "The time flew by," she says. "Keeping track of the intervals gave my mind something to do. And knowing the entire walk would be finished in 20 to 30 minutes motivated me to really go for it on the fast intervals."

Sensitive to gluten—a protein found in wheat and a few other grains— Amy easily modified the Natural Menopause Solution recipes to suit her dietary needs. "And I loved finding other grains right on the menu, like quinoa, so I didn't have to substitute all the time," she says. "Dishes without a grain component were even easier and so delicious. The kale and bean soup was great. The seafood chowder was really tasty and filling, too. I didn't feel hungry!"

High blood pressure runs in Amy's family. She and her doctor have been monitoring hers for a few years now, hoping that she wouldn't need medication. Then, eureka! Her numbers began to drop during her month on the plan. "It's great to see these healthy changes," she says.

Breakfasts

Slimming, Cooling Smoothie

Prep time: 5 minutes • *Total time:* 5 minutes
Makes 4 servings

Whether you use soy milk or regular low-fat (1%) milk, this eye-opener will get you off to a great nutritional start each day. Store the leftover smoothie mixture in the refrigerator, covered, and stir or reblend before pouring.

3 cups fortified plain soy milk or 1% milk

1 cup pineapple chunks (fresh or canned in juice)

2 tablespoons lime juice

2 tablespoons almond butter

2 teaspoons ground flaxseeds

1. Combine the milk, pineapple, lime juice, almond butter, and flaxseeds in a blender.

2. Whirl until smooth. For each serving, pour 1¼ cups of the smoothie into a large glass filled with ice.

   Per serving: 156 calories, 5 g protein, 21 g carbohydrates, 6 g fat, 0.5 g saturated fat, 3 g fiber, 103 mg sodium

Strawberry-Almond Smoothie

Prep time: 5 minutes • *Total time:* 5 minutes
Makes 2 servings

This smoothie is an entire breakfast in a glass. It won't be quite as smooth if you use whole almonds instead of almond butter, but it will still be delicious. The recipe makes a tall smoothie—if you like, have some for a quick breakfast and save the rest for a midmorning or afternoon snack. For a vegan smoothie, substitute soy milk and soy yogurt.

¾ cup (6 ounces) low-fat vanilla
    yogurt
½ cup 1% milk

1 cup fresh strawberries
2 tablespoons almond butter or
    dry roasted or raw almonds

1. Combine the yogurt, milk, strawberries, and almond butter or almonds in a blender.
2. Whirl until smooth, for about 1 minute.

Per serving: 202 calories, 8 g protein, 25 g carbohydrates, 9 g fat, 1 g saturated fat, 4 g fiber, 60 mg sodium

Mixed-Fruit Cup

Prep time: 10 minutes • *Total time:* 10 minutes
Makes 4 servings

You can use any combination of fresh fruit in season and substitute soy-based cheese for the cottage cheese if you like.

2 large bananas, sliced	1 tablespoon lemon juice
2 cups peach slices	1 cup 1% cottage cheese
1 cup strawberry slices	¼ cup chopped walnuts

1. Combine the bananas, peaches, strawberries, and lemon juice in a large bowl. Toss gently to mix.

2. Place ¼ cup cottage cheese in each of 4 serving bowls. Top with the mixed fruit and sprinkle with the walnuts.

Per serving: 193 calories, 10 g protein, 29 g carbohydrates, 6 g fat, 1 g saturated fat, 4 g fiber, 231 mg sodium

Open-Faced Omelet

Prep time: 10 minutes • *Total time:* 30 minutes
Makes 2 servings

To double the recipe, simply double the ingredients, but cook the eggs in 2 batches.

1 teaspoon olive oil, divided

1 small onion, finely chopped

1 green bell pepper, finely chopped

1 Yukon Gold potato, chopped

1/4 cup water

1/4 teaspoon salt, divided

1/8 teaspoon ground black pepper

1 roasted red pepper, finely chopped

1 egg

2 egg whites

1. Heat 1/2 teaspoon oil in a large nonstick skillet over medium heat. Add the onion and cook, stirring frequently, for 3 minutes. Add the green bell pepper and cook, stirring frequently, for 5 minutes. Stir in the potato and cook for 2 minutes, stirring occasionally. Add the water, 1/8 teaspoon salt, and the ground black pepper. Cover and cook for 5 minutes, or until the potato is tender. Stir in the roasted red pepper. Spoon the vegetables into a bowl and cover to keep warm.

2. Heat the remaining 1/2 teaspoon oil in a small skillet over medium-low heat. Lightly beat the egg, egg whites, and the remaining 1/8 teaspoon salt in a small bowl. Pour into the skillet. Cook for 1 minute, or until the egg is set around the edge. Run a thin spatula around the edge of the omelet, lifting to allow any uncooked egg to run under the cooked egg. Cover and cook for 2 minutes, or until there is no more runny egg.

3. Halve the omelet and transfer to individual serving plates. Top evenly with the reserved vegetables. Serve warm.

Per serving: 158 calories, 9 g protein, 20 g carbohydrates, 5 g fat, 1 g saturated fat, 3 g fiber, 522 mg sodium

Greek Spinach Scramble

Prep time: 10 minutes • *Total time:* 15 minutes
Makes 4 servings

Fresh spinach, a hint of feta cheese, and fresh dill turn ordinary scrambled eggs into healthier and more flavorful Mediterranean-style breakfast fare.

1 teaspoon olive oil	2 scallions, thinly sliced
1 egg	1 teaspoon chopped fresh dill or
4 egg whites	½ teaspoon dried
3 cups baby spinach leaves, chopped	1 ounce reduced-fat feta or goat cheese, crumbled

1. Heat the oil in a large nonstick skillet over medium heat. Stir together the egg and egg whites in a small bowl. Add to the skillet and cook, stirring gently, for 30 seconds.

2. Stir in the spinach, scallions, and dill. Cook, stirring occasionally, for 2 minutes, or until the mixture is heated and the eggs are just cooked through. Sprinkle with the cheese and serve.

Per serving: 68 calories, 7 g protein, 3 g carbohydrates, 3 g fat, 1 g saturated fat, 7 g fiber, 200 mg sodium

Make it a meal: Serve with half a medium pear and half a toasted 6½"-round whole wheat pita brushed with 1¼ teaspoons olive oil, along with a Slimming, Cooling Smoothie.

Meal per serving: 371 calories, 15 g protein, 56 g carbohydrates, 12 g fat, 2 g saturated fat, 9 g fiber, 475 mg sodium

Skillet-Baked Parmesan Eggs

Prep time: 10 minutes • *Total time:* 30 minutes
Makes 4 servings

If you have ramekins or au gratin dishes that can hold individual servings, divide the vegetables, eggs, and cheese among them and cook as directed.

$\frac{1}{4}$ cup fat-free reduced-sodium chicken broth

1 onion, finely chopped

1 green or red bell pepper, finely chopped

4 plum tomatoes, seeded and finely chopped

$\frac{1}{4}$ cup + 2 tablespoons chopped fresh basil

$\frac{1}{4}$ teaspoon salt

$\frac{1}{8}$ teaspoon ground black pepper

4 eggs

1 tablespoon grated Parmesan cheese

2 whole wheat pitas (6$\frac{1}{2}$" diameter), toasted and halved

1. Heat the broth to a simmer over medium-low heat in a medium nonstick skillet. Add the onion and cook in the broth, stirring occasionally, for 5 minutes or until tender. Add the bell pepper and cook, stirring frequently, for 5 minutes. Stir in the tomatoes, the $\frac{1}{4}$ cup basil, the salt, and the ground black pepper.

2. Use a spoon to make 4 large indentations in the vegetable mixture. Break an egg into each hollow. Sprinkle evenly with the cheese.

3. Cover and cook for 5 minutes, or until the eggs are set. Sprinkle with the remaining 2 tablespoons basil. Divide evenly among 4 small plates and serve with the pita halves.

Per serving: 204 calories, 12 g protein, 25 g carbohydrates, 7 g fat, 2 g saturated fat, 4 g fiber, 453 mg sodium

Homemade Turkey Sausage

Prep time: 10 minutes • *Total time:* 20 minutes
Makes 4 servings

If you have time, mix up this batch of seasoned sausage meat and refrigerate for up to 8 hours to let the flavors marry before cooking. This is a basic recipe; feel free to vary the seasoning to include other herbs, such as rosemary or parsley, or to increase the amount of herbs already used. To test the seasoning, pinch off and cook a small piece of the sausage mixture before shaping the patties.

½ pound 93% ground turkey

1 small onion, finely chopped

2 teaspoons olive oil, divided

½ teaspoon dried sage, crushed

½ teaspoon fennel seeds, crushed

¼ teaspoon salt

⅛ teaspoon ground black pepper

1. Combine the turkey, onion, 1 teaspoon oil, the sage, fennel seeds, salt, and pepper in a medium bowl.

2. Shape the sausage mixture into 4 equal patties.

3. Heat the remaining 1 teaspoon oil over medium heat in a medium nonstick skillet. Add the sausage patties and cook for 3 minutes. Turn the sausages, cover the skillet, and cook for 3 minutes longer, or until cooked through.

Per serving: 107 calories, 11 g protein, 2 g carbohydrates, 6 g fat, 1 g saturated fat, 1 g fiber, 187 mg sodium

Make it a meal: To each serving, add 1 cup cantaloupe cubes sprinkled with 2 tablespoons fat-free granola or other cereal, along with a Slimming, Cooling Smoothie.

Meal per serving: 352 calories, 18 g protein, 42 g carbohydrates, 14 g fat, 2 g saturated fat, 5 g fiber, 321 mg sodium

Fig 'n' Flax Muffins

Prep time: 20 minutes • *Total time:* 55 minutes
Makes 12 muffins

These are shortcut muffins made with a commercial cereal to keep the ingredient list short but still include a good mix of grains and flaxseed. You can use any type of flake, nugget, or puff-style flax cereal mixture, but the higher the protein content, the better. To freeze leftovers, double-wrap the muffins in plastic and foil, or single-wrap and store in a freezer-safe container.

1½ cups multigrain high-protein breakfast cereal with flax, crushed

1 cup fortified 1% milk or fortified plain soy milk

1½ cups whole wheat flour or spelt flour

1 tablespoon baking powder

½ teaspoon baking soda

½ teaspoon salt

½ cup packed light brown sugar

⅓ cup unsweetened applesauce

¼ cup light olive oil

4 egg whites

½ cup chopped dried figs

1. Preheat the oven to 400°F. Coat a 12-cup muffin pan with cooking spray.

2. Combine the cereal and milk in a large bowl. Let stand for 5 to 10 minutes. Meanwhile, whisk together the flour, baking powder, baking soda, and salt in a medium bowl.

3. Add the sugar, applesauce, oil, and egg whites to the cereal mixture and stir until well blended. Add the flour mixture and stir until just combined. Gently stir in the chopped figs. Spoon the batter evenly into the prepared muffin pan.

4. Bake for 18 to 20 minutes, or until a toothpick inserted in the center of a muffin comes out clean. Let cool on a wire rack for 15 minutes. Turn the muffins out onto a rack to cool completely.

Per muffin: 190 calories, 6 g protein, 32 g carbohydrates, 6 g fat, 1 g saturated fat, 4 g fiber, 325 mg sodium

Cranberry-Oat Breakfast Cookies

Prep time: 30 minutes • *Total time:* 1 hour

Makes 48 cookies

Make these crunchy, nutty cookies ahead of time, and freeze for those mornings when you are on the go and have to take your breakfast with you or you just don't feel like cooking. They also make a great snack.

2 cups old-fashioned oats

1/2 cup whole wheat pastry flour

1/4 cup ground flaxseeds

1 teaspoon baking soda

1 teaspoon ground cinnamon

1/2 teaspoon salt

1/4 teaspoon ground nutmeg

1 1/2 cups dried cranberries

1/2 cup sunflower seeds

3/4 cup unsalted almond butter or peanut butter

1/2 cup brown sugar

1/3 cup light olive oil

3 eggs

1 teaspoon vanilla

1. Preheat the oven to 375°F. Coat 2 baking sheets with cooking spray.

2. Mix together the oats, flour, flaxseeds, baking soda, cinnamon, salt, and nutmeg in a large bowl. Stir in the cranberries and sunflower seeds.

3. Stir together the nut butter, sugar, oil, eggs, and vanilla in a medium bowl until well blended. Add to the oat mixture, stirring until well blended.

4. Using your hands or 2 spoons, roll the dough into 1 1/2" rounds and place on the baking sheets. With a fork, press each round slightly to flatten.

5. Bake for 10 minutes or until lightly browned. Cool on a rack for 1 minute. Remove cookies to a rack to cool completely.

Per cookie: 92 calories, 2 g protein, 10 g carbohydrates, 5 g fat, 1 g saturated fat, 1 g fiber, 56 mg sodium

Lemon-Ricotta Pancakes

Prep time: 10 minutes • *Total time:* 40 minutes

Makes 6 pancakes

Instead of syrup, top your pancake with fresh fruit. In place of berries, you can use sliced bananas or chopped peaches or pineapple, or a mixture of all these fruits.

¾ cup all-purpose flour	1 egg
2 tablespoons toasted wheat germ	Grated peel of 1 lemon
2 tablespoons sugar	2 tablespoons lemon juice
2 teaspoons baking powder	1 teaspoon light olive oil
¼ teaspoon salt	2 cups sliced strawberries
¾ cup part-skim ricotta cheese	1 cup blueberries
¾ cup 1% milk	

1. Whisk together the flour, wheat germ, sugar, baking powder, and salt in a large bowl.

2. Stir together the ricotta, milk, egg, lemon peel, and lemon juice in a medium bowl. Stir into the flour mixture until just blended.

3. Heat the oil in a medium nonstick skillet over medium heat. For each pancake, add ¼ cup of the batter to the skillet. Cook for 2 minutes or until bubbles form on top of the pancake. Turn and cook for 1 to 2 minutes or until golden.

4. Toss together the strawberries and blueberries in a small bowl. Top each pancake with ½ cup of the berries.

Per pancake: 192 calories, 9 g protein, 30 g carbohydrates, 5 g fat, 2 g saturated fat, 3 g fiber, 325 mg sodium

Lunches

Arugula Salad Plate

Prep time: 30 minutes • *Total time:* 30 minutes
Makes 4 servings

If you can't find arugula, use watercress, baby spinach leaves, or a mix of salad greens. This is a lovely salad to serve if you're having company that appreciates good, healthy food.

2 tablespoons olive oil

1½ tablespoons balsamic vinegar

1 tablespoon honey

¼ teaspoon salt

⅛ teaspoon ground black pepper

1 can (15 ounces) no-salt-added chickpeas, rinsed and drained

1 can (15 ounces) red kidney beans, rinsed and drained

2 ribs celery, sliced

¼ cup finely chopped parsley

6 cups arugula leaves

4 ounces goat cheese, crumbled

2 scallions, thinly sliced

1 medium apple, chopped

4 dried apricot halves, finely chopped

¼ cup walnuts, toasted and chopped

1. Combine the olive oil, balsamic vinegar, honey, salt, and pepper in a small bowl.

2. Combine the chickpeas, kidney beans, celery, and parsley in a medium bowl. Add 2 tablespoons of the balsamic mixture and toss to coat well.

3. Divide the arugula, cheese, scallions, apple, apricots, and walnuts among 4 serving plates. Drizzle with the remaining dressing. Top with the bean mixture.

Per serving: 410 calories, 16 g protein, 42 g carbohydrates, 21 g fat, 8 g saturated fat, 9 g fiber, 510 mg sodium

Quinoa Salad with Apples and Walnuts

Prep time: 15 minutes • *Total time:* 40 minutes
Makes 4 servings

You can use regular white quinoa, but the red variety makes for a more attractive dish.

1 cup red quinoa, rinsed well

¼ cup orange juice

1 tablespoon lemon juice

1 tablespoon olive oil

2 tablespoons chopped fresh cilantro

2 tablespoons chopped fresh mint

½ teaspoon salt

⅛ teaspoon ground black pepper

2 apples, cored and finely chopped

½ cup chopped walnuts

¼ cup thinly sliced scallion or finely chopped red onion

4 cups mesclun or spring mix

1. Cook the quinoa according to package directions.

2. Combine the orange juice, lemon juice, oil, cilantro, mint, salt, and pepper in a large bowl.

3. Stir in the cooked quinoa, apples, walnuts, and scallion or onion. Toss well to combine. Divide the mesclun among 4 plates and top with the salad.

Per serving: 350 calories, 9 g protein, 48 g carbohydrates, 15 g fat, 2 g saturated fat, 8 g fiber, 336 mg sodium

Make it a meal: Add 2 ounces lean roast chicken, turkey, or other meat to each serving.

Meal per serving: 443 calories, 27 g protein, 48 g carbohydrates, 17 g fat, 2 g saturated fat, 8 g fiber, 378 mg sodium

Spinach and Orange Salad

Prep time: 15 minutes • *Total time:* 15 minutes
Makes 1 serving

To make more than 1 serving, simply multiply the ingredient amounts by the number of people you want to serve. In a pinch, you can use drained, canned, or bottled mandarin orange sections.

2 cups baby spinach leaves

1 orange, sectioned

¼ small red onion, thinly sliced

⅓ cup canned small white beans, such as navy, rinsed and drained

1 tablespoon balsamic vinegar

1 teaspoon olive oil

⅛ teaspoon ground black pepper

Toss the spinach leaves, orange sections, and onion in a salad bowl. Top with the beans and sprinkle with the vinegar and oil. Season with the pepper.

Per serving: 186 calories, 7 g protein, 35 g carbohydrates, 5 g fat, 0.5 g saturated fat, 9 g fiber, 273 mg sodium

Make it a meal: Serve with a 4-ounce turkey burger on a whole wheat bun.

Meal per serving: 451 calories, 33 g protein, 57 g carbohydrates, 14 g fat, 3 g saturated fat, 12 g fiber, 661 mg sodium

Crab Salad

Prep time: 20 minutes • *Total time:* 20 minutes

Makes 4 servings

You can substitute an equal amount of steamed or grilled scallops, shrimp, salmon, or another firm-fleshed fish for the crab in this recipe if you like.

2 tablespoons olive oil

1 tablespoon lemon juice or lime juice

½ teaspoon ground cumin

2 cups sliced jicama, cut into 2" x ¼" matchsticks

1 can (15.25 ounces) no-salt-added corn kernels

1 medium tomato, seeded and coarsely chopped

½ small red onion, finely chopped

¼ cup finely chopped cilantro

¾ pound cooked lump crabmeat

2 cups shredded romaine lettuce

1 avocado, peeled, pitted, and sliced

1. Whisk together the oil, lemon or lime juice, and cumin in a large bowl. Add the jicama, corn, tomato, onion, and cilantro. Toss to mix well.

2. Gently stir in the crabmeat.

3. Divide the lettuce, avocado, and crab salad among 4 plates.

   Per serving: 330 calories, 22 g protein, 30 g carbohydrates, 16 g fat, 2 g saturated fat, 8 g fiber, 334 mg sodium

Make it a meal: Serve with 12 baked tortilla chips.

   Meal per serving: 419 calories, 24 g protein, 44 g carbohydrates, 19 g fat, 3 g saturated fat, 10 g fiber, 527 mg sodium

Gado Gado (Hearty Indonesian Salad)

Prep time: 30 minutes • *Total time:* 30 minutes
Makes 4 servings

This colorful arranged salad combines a mixture of steamed and raw vegetables topped with a sweet-and-spicy dressing that can be made with any type of nut butter. The protein comes from the tofu or hard-cooked eggs, but you can also substitute shredded or finely chopped leftover chicken or meat. Just about any type of food tastes great with this dressing.

DRESSING

⅓ cup almond butter, peanut butter, or any other nut butter

2 tablespoons low-sodium soy sauce

2 tablespoons honey

1 teaspoon finely chopped fresh ginger

⅛ teaspoon salt

Pinch of red-pepper flakes (optional)

½–¾ cup boiling water

SALAD

1¼ pounds small gold or red-skinned potatoes, quartered

1 pound green beans, cut into 2" pieces

8 ounces firm tofu, cut into bite-size pieces

2 hard-cooked eggs, halved lengthwise

2 cups shredded red cabbage

1 cup shredded carrot

1. *To make the dressing:* Combine the nut butter, soy sauce, honey, ginger, salt, and red-pepper flakes, if using, in a blender or a food processor. With the machine running, add the boiling water through the lid. Process until very smooth. Set aside.

2. *To make the salad:* Simmer the potatoes in a large saucepan covered with water for 10 minutes or until just tender. Add the green beans to the pan for the last 3 minutes of cooking time. Drain well.

3. Arrange the potatoes, green beans, tofu, eggs, cabbage, and carrot on a large platter. Stir the dressing and drizzle over the salad. Serve at once. If making ahead, store the salad and the dressing separately in the refrigerator.

Per serving: 452 calories, 20 g protein, 52 g carbohydrates, 21 g fat, 3 g saturated fat, 8 g fiber, 540 mg sodium

Beef 'n' Broccoli Pasta Salad

Prep time: 10 minutes • *Total time:* 40 minutes
Makes 4 servings

A creamy basil dressing binds the ingredients in this hearty one-dish meal. Another time, substitute asparagus, green beans, or sugar snap peas for the broccoli. If you're traveling with your salad, pack the salad and the dressing separately and store in the refrigerator until ready to go. Add the dressing just before eating.

8 ounces bow-tie, rotelle, or other small pasta

3 cups broccoli florets

6 ounces top round or sirloin steak

½ teaspoon salt, divided

1 cup low-fat plain yogurt

¼ cup light mayonnaise

1 cup fresh basil leaves

1 tablespoon balsamic vinegar

1 roasted red pepper, thinly sliced

1 small red onion, halved and thinly sliced

¼ cup finely chopped sun-dried tomatoes packed in olive oil

1. Prepare the pasta according to package directions. Add the broccoli florets for the last 3 minutes of cooking time.

2. Meanwhile, preheat the broiler. Place the steak on a broiler pan and sprinkle with ¼ teaspoon salt. Broil 4" from the heat source for 8 minutes, or until a thermometer inserted in the center registers 145°F for medium-rare. Transfer to a cutting board and let stand for 5 minutes before thinly slicing across the grain.

3. Combine the yogurt, mayonnaise, basil, vinegar, and the remaining ¼ teaspoon salt in a blender or a food processor. Process until smooth.

4. Combine the pasta, broccoli, steak, roasted pepper, onion, and tomatoes in a large bowl. Toss with the yogurt mixture until coated.

Per serving: 414 calories, 26 g protein, 55 g carbohydrates, 10 g fat, 3 g saturated fat, 4 g fiber, 544 mg sodium

Romaine-Fruit Salad with Creamy Orange Dressing

Prep time: 15 minutes • *Total time:* 15 minutes
Makes 4 servings

If you're traveling with your lunch, prepare and pack the salad ingredients separately from the dressing, and combine everything when you are ready to eat. We chose kiwi, pineapple, and apple, but you can use any combination of fruit you like.

1 cup 0% plain Greek yogurt

⅓ cup orange juice

2 teaspoons light olive oil

2 teaspoons poppy seeds (optional)

Pinch of salt

4 kiwifruit, peeled, halved, and thinly sliced

2 cups pineapple chunks

1 apple, cored and finely chopped

8 cups torn romaine lettuce

½ cup walnuts, pecans, or almonds

1. Whisk together the yogurt, orange juice, oil, poppy seeds, if using, and salt in a medium bowl. Add the kiwi, pineapple, and apple. Toss gently to coat.

2. Divide the lettuce, fruit salad, and nuts among 4 plates.

   Per serving: 264 calories, 10 g protein, 37 g carbohydrates, 11 g fat, 1 g saturated fat, 7 g fiber, 107 mg sodium

Make it a meal: Serve with 1 cheese stick and 20 small pretzel twists.

   Meal per serving: 443 calories, 18 g protein, 65 g carbohydrates, 15 g fat, 3 g saturated fat, 8 g fiber, 969 mg sodium

Quick Tortilla Soup

Prep time: 10 minutes • *Total time:* 40 minutes
Makes 4 servings

You can make this vegetarian soup with any type of beans, even lima beans or chickpeas. For a more traditional tortilla soup, substitute 2 cups of shredded cooked chicken or turkey breast for the beans. You can also try a mix of beans and poultry.

2 teaspoons olive oil

4 scallions, chopped

2 cloves garlic, minced

1 green bell pepper, chopped

1 medium zucchini, chopped

1 teaspoon ground cumin

1/2 teaspoon chili powder

1 tablespoon no-salt-added tomato paste

4 cups low-sodium vegetable broth

2 tablespoons lime juice

1/4 teaspoon salt

2 cans (15 ounces each) no-salt-added small red beans or pinto beans, drained

1/4 cup finely chopped cilantro

1/2 avocado, finely chopped

4 ounces baked tortilla chips, crushed

1 1/3 cups reduced-fat shredded Monterey Jack cheese

1. Heat the oil in a large saucepan over medium heat. Add the scallions and cook, stirring frequently, for 5 minutes, or until tender. Add the garlic and cook for 1 minute. Add the green pepper, zucchini, cumin, and chili powder. Cook for 5 minutes or until the pepper is tender.

2. Stir in the tomato paste, broth, lime juice, and salt. Simmer for 10 minutes. Stir in the beans and simmer for 5 minutes longer.

3. Ladle the soup into 4 bowls and sprinkle with the cilantro. Divide the avocado, crushed tortilla chips, and cheese among the bowls.

Per serving: 375 calories, 18 g protein, 40 g carbohydrates, 16 g fat, 6 g saturated fat, 10 g fiber, 772 mg sodium

Make it a meal: Serve with 1 orange.

Meal per serving: 444 calories, 20 g protein, 57 g carbohydrates, 16 g fat, 6 g saturated fat, 13 g fiber, 773 mg sodium

Chicken Salad Pita

Prep time: 10 minutes • *Total time:* 10 minutes
Makes 4 servings

If you're packing your lunch, be sure to pack the pita and the chicken salad separately. Fill the pita pockets when you're ready to eat.

¼ cup low-fat plain yogurt

2 tablespoons mayonnaise

1 tablespoon fresh dill or
    1 teaspoon dried

⅛ teaspoon salt

1½ cups chopped cooked chicken
    breast

½ avocado, chopped

1 rib celery, finely chopped

¼ cup chopped black olives

2 whole wheat pitas
    (6½" diameter)

1. Combine the yogurt, mayonnaise, dill, and salt in a medium bowl. Add the chicken, avocado, celery, and olives. Stir to mix.

2. Cut the pitas crosswise to make 4 open pockets. Divide the chicken salad evenly among the pockets.

Per serving: 267 calories, 21 g protein, 17 g carbohydrates, 13 g fat, 2 g saturated fat, 4 g fiber, 472 mg sodium

Make it a meal: To each serving add 8 cherry tomatoes and a medium banana.

Meal per serving: 393 calories, 23 g protein, 48 g carbohydrates, 13 g fat, 2 g saturated fat, 8 g fiber, 505 mg sodium

Pepper and Egg Sandwich

Prep time: 10 minutes • *Total time:* 20 minutes
Makes 1 sandwich

If you're bringing your lunch to work, pack the pepper and egg mixture separately from the pita. Combine the two and gently heat in a microwave oven when you're ready to eat. This sandwich also makes a great portable breakfast.

1 teaspoon olive oil
$\frac{1}{2}$ small green bell pepper, sliced
$\frac{1}{2}$ small onion, thinly sliced
2 eggs, lightly beaten

$\frac{1}{8}$ teaspoon salt
Pinch of ground black pepper
1 whole wheat pita (6$\frac{1}{2}$" diameter)

1. Heat the oil over medium heat in a small nonstick skillet. Add the bell pepper and onion. Cook, stirring, for 5 minutes, or until the vegetables are just tender.

2. Add the eggs, salt, and black pepper. Cook, stirring, for 1 minute, or until the eggs are scrambled and cooked through.

3. Cut a $\frac{1}{2}$" slice from the top of the pita to open it. Fill with the pepper and egg mixture.

Per sandwich: 327 calories, 18 g protein, 33 g carbohydrates, 15 g fat, 3.5 g saturated fat, 5 g fiber, 727 mg sodium

Veggie-Cheese Wrap

Prep time: 10 minutes • *Total time:* 10 minutes
Makes 1 wrap

If you have any leftover vegetables in your refrigerator, feel free to add them to this hearty wrap.

1 large (10") low-carb, high-fiber wrap

1 cup spinach leaves

$\frac{1}{4}$ cup torn basil leaves

$\frac{1}{4}$ cup coleslaw

$\frac{1}{8}$ avocado, thinly sliced

2 ounces low-sodium mozzarella cheese or reduced-fat Swiss cheese, thinly sliced

1 roasted red pepper, thinly sliced

1 plum tomato, seeded and thinly sliced

1. Lay the wrap on a work surface. Cover with the spinach leaves and basil to within 1" of the edges. Top with the coleslaw, avocado, cheese, bell pepper, and tomato.

2. Fold a side of the wrap partway over the filling. Fold it down, about 2" from the top and 2" from the bottom. Roll the wrap tightly from the folded side.

3. To pack your sandwich to go, wrap it in aluminum foil or plastic wrap. Cut the wrap in half just before eating, if desired.

Per wrap: 442 calories, 26 g protein, 43 g carbohydrates, 19 g fat, 9 g saturated fat, 24 g fiber, 822 mg sodium

Pita Pizzas

Prep time: 10 minutes • *Total time:* 30 minutes
Makes 4 pizzas

You can use any type of ground poultry or ground meat to top these pizzas.

1 teaspoon olive oil

6 ounces ground turkey or chicken

½ teaspoon dried oregano

½ teaspoon ground allspice

¼ teaspoon salt

⅛ teaspoon ground black pepper

4 whole wheat pitas (6½" diameter)

1 cup garlic hummus

2 ounces goat cheese or feta cheese, crumbled

1 red bell pepper, finely chopped

¼ cup finely chopped fresh mint leaves (optional)

1. Preheat the oven to 400°F. Position the oven rack in the lower third of the oven. Coat a large baking sheet with cooking spray.

2. Heat the oil in a medium nonstick skillet over medium heat. Add the turkey or chicken, oregano, allspice, salt, and black pepper. Cook, stirring often, for 7 minutes, or until the meat is no longer pink.

3. Place the pitas on the baking sheet. Spread ¼ cup of the hummus over each pita. Top with the turkey mixture. Sprinkle with the cheese and the bell pepper.

4. Bake for 10 to 12 minutes, or until the cheese melts and the pita is toasted. Sprinkle with mint, if using.

Per serving: 406 calories, 19 g protein, 50 g carbohydrates, 17 g fat, 4 g saturated fat, 8 g fiber, 920 mg sodium

Make it a meal: Serve with 1 cup cucumber slices tossed with 2 tablespoons low-fat plain yogurt.

Meal per serving: 438 calories, 21 g protein, 56 g carbohydrates, 17 g fat, 5 g saturated fat, 8 g fiber, 938 mg sodium

Crustless Quiche

Prep time: 10 minutes • *Total time:* 55 minutes
Makes 4 servings

Since quiche can be served either warm or at room temperature, you can make it ahead and carry it to work for lunch. Warm up a slice in a microwave oven or simply take it out of the refrigerator and let it stand at room temperature for 30 minutes before eating.

5 ounces ($\frac{1}{2}$ of 10-ounce box) frozen kale, thawed and well drained	1 cup part-skim ricotta cheese
1 cup corn kernels	$\frac{1}{4}$ teaspoon salt
4 eggs	$\frac{1}{8}$ teaspoon ground black pepper
	$\frac{1}{8}$ teaspoon ground nutmeg

1. Preheat the oven to 350°F. Lightly oil a 9" pie plate.

2. Combine the kale and corn in a medium bowl. Stir in the eggs, cheese, salt, pepper, and nutmeg until well mixed. Place in the pie plate.

3. Bake for 30 to 35 minutes, or until a wooden pick inserted in the center comes out clean. Let stand for 10 minutes before serving.

   Per serving: 199 calories, 15 g protein, 12 g carbohydrates, 11 g fat, 5 g saturated fat, 2 g fiber, 304 mg sodium

Make it a meal: Serve with 1 sliced tomato sprinkled with basil and 1 toasted whole wheat pita round (6½" diameter) brushed with 1 teaspoon olive oil.

   Meal per serving: 432 calories, 23 g protein, 52 g carbohydrates, 17 g fat, 6 g saturated fat, 8 g fiber, 650 mg sodium

Nacho Lunch

Prep time: 15 minutes • *Total time:* 25 minutes
Makes 4 servings

If you're traveling with your lunch, pack the chips and toppings separately. Warm the bean topping in a microwave oven, if you have one, and assemble the nachos when it's time to eat.

1 teaspoon olive oil

1 small onion, chopped

2 cloves garlic, chopped

1 can (19 ounces) pinto beans, drained and rinsed

1 tomato, chopped

1 tablespoon finely chopped cilantro

$\frac{1}{8}$ teaspoon salt

4 ounces baked corn tortilla chips

1 cup shredded sharp Cheddar or Monterey Jack cheese

1 avocado, chopped

$\frac{1}{2}$ cup 0% plain Greek yogurt

10 pimiento-stuffed olives, thinly sliced

1. Heat the oil over medium-low heat in a large nonstick skillet. Add the onion. Cook, stirring occasionally, for 5 minutes or until tender. Add the garlic and cook for 1 minute. Stir in the beans. Cook, stirring, for 5 minutes, until the beans are heated through. With a potato masher or a fork, crush half of the beans. Remove from the heat and stir in the tomato, cilantro, and salt.

2. Divide the chips among 4 serving plates. Divide the hot bean mixture, cheese, and avocado evenly among the chips. Spoon 2 tablespoons of the yogurt over each plate of nachos and sprinkle with 1 tablespoon of the olives.

Per serving: 407 calories, 18 g protein, 38 g carbohydrates, 21 g fat, 6 g saturated fat, 10 g fiber, 666 mg sodium

Make it a meal: Serve with seltzer water with fresh lime and a small apple.

Meal per serving: 460 calories, 18 g protein, 52 g carbohydrates, 21 g fat, 6 g saturated fat, 13 g fiber, 667 mg sodium

Dinners

Vegetable and Quinoa Stew

Prep time: 15 minutes • *Total time:* 45 minutes
Makes 4 servings

Turmeric and cumin add a hint of authentic Indian flavor to this hearty, quickly prepared vegetarian main dish. If you like your food spicier, double the amount of red-pepper flakes.

1 pound butternut squash, peeled and cut into 1" cubes (about 3 cups)

1 medium tomato, seeded and finely chopped

½ teaspoon ground turmeric

½ teaspoon ground cumin

4 cups water

½ cup uncooked red or white quinoa

2 cans (15 ounces each) no-salt-added chickpeas

½ cup coconut milk

2 tablespoons light olive oil

1 teaspoon mustard seeds

2 cloves garlic, finely chopped

¾ teaspoon salt

¼ teaspoon red-pepper flakes

2 tablespoons lime juice

1 tablespoon honey

½ cup finely chopped cilantro

1. Combine the squash, tomato, turmeric, cumin, and water in a large pot or Dutch oven. Heat to boiling over medium-high heat. Reduce the heat to low, cover, and simmer for 15 minutes.

2. Meanwhile, cook the quinoa in a small saucepan according to package directions.

3. Uncover the pot, stir in the cooked quinoa, chickpeas, and milk, and simmer for 10 minutes, or until the squash is very tender.

4. Meanwhile, in a small saucepan, heat the oil over medium-low heat until very warm. Add the mustard seeds. When the seeds start to pop, remove the pan from the heat and add the garlic, salt, and red-pepper flakes. Stir and add this mixture to the stew. Stir in the lime juice, honey, and cilantro. Serve warm.

Per serving: 431 calories, 13 g protein, 62 g carbohydrates, 17 g fat, 8 g saturated fat, 13 g fiber, 493 mg sodium

Pasta with Gorgonzola-Walnut Sauce

Prep time: 15 minutes • *Total time:* 25 minutes
Makes 4 servings

If you love veined cheeses, you'll love this hearty pasta dish. If you don't love veined cheeses, substitute goat cheese or sharp Cheddar for the Gorgonzola or blue cheese.

2 cups whole grain corkscrew pasta, such as fusilli or rotelle

2 teaspoons olive oil

½ cup chopped walnuts

2 cloves garlic, minced

½ cup dry white wine or fat-free reduced-sodium chicken broth

3 ounces Gorgonzola or blue cheese, crumbled

¼ cup finely chopped parsley

1. Prepare the pasta according to package directions.

2. Meanwhile, heat the oil in a small skillet over medium heat. Add the walnuts and cook, stirring occasionally, for 5 minutes, or until lightly toasted. Stir in the garlic and cook for 1 minute. Transfer to a large serving bowl.

3. Heat the wine or broth over medium-low heat in the same skillet. Add the cheese and cook, stirring, for 4 minutes or until melted.

4. Add the pasta, cheese mixture, and parsley to the bowl; toss to coat well.

Per serving: 354 calories, 12 g protein, 36 g carbohydrates, 19 g fat, 5 g saturated fat, 5 g fiber, 445 mg sodium

Roasted Turkey Breast and Vegetables

Prep time: 20 minutes • *Total time:* 1 hour
Makes 8 servings

If you use a turkey breast with the skin on, brush the herb and oil mixture under the skin and be sure to remove the skin before eating. If you use a rolled or tied breast, it may take slightly longer to cook. Don't have all the herbs? No problem! Just use a selection of any of the three you have.

1 boneless, skinless turkey breast half (about 1½ pounds)

2 pounds zucchini, halved lengthwise and cut into 1" pieces

1 pound baby carrots

6 plum tomatoes, quartered

2 onions, cut into wedges

¼ cup olive oil

4 cloves garlic, minced

1 tablespoon lemon juice

1 tablespoon dried rosemary, crumbled

½ teaspoon dried thyme, crumbled

½ teaspoon salt

1. Preheat the oven to 400°F. Coat a 13" x 9" roasting pan with cooking spray.

2. Place the turkey breast in the center of the pan. Surround it with the vegetables.

3. Combine the oil, garlic, lemon juice, rosemary, thyme, and salt in a small bowl. Brush all over the turkey and pour the remainder over the vegetables. Stir the vegetables to coat.

4. Roast for 20 minutes. Brush the turkey with oil from the pan and gently stir the vegetables. Roast for 15 minutes more, or until a thermometer inserted in a breast registers 165°F. Transfer the turkey to a platter and let stand for 10 minutes before slicing. Surround the turkey with the vegetables to serve.

Per serving: 240 calories, 26 g protein, 17 g carbohydrates, 8 g fat, 2 g saturated fat, 5 g fiber, 227 mg sodium

Turkey Cutlets with Cranberry Wild Rice

Prep time: 10 minutes • *Total time:* 1 hour
Makes 4 servings

Enjoy this streamlined Thanksgiving dinner any time of the year! For a change of pace, you can substitute chicken, veal, or pork cutlets for the turkey without changing any other ingredients.

RICE

1 cup wild rice

2 tablespoons olive oil

2 tablespoons orange juice

1/3 cup dried cranberries, chopped

1/3 cup dry-roasted unsalted sunflower seeds

1/4 teaspoon salt

1/8 teaspoon ground black pepper

TURKEY

1 tablespoon olive oil

1 tablespoon orange juice

1/2 teaspoon dried sage

1/2 teaspoon salt

1/8 teaspoon ground black pepper

4 thin turkey cutlets (4 ounces each)

1. *To make the rice:* Prepare the rice according to package directions. Stir in the oil, orange juice, cranberries, sunflower seeds, salt, and pepper.

2. *To make the turkey:* Meanwhile, combine the oil, orange juice, sage, salt, and pepper in a shallow bowl. Add the turkey and turn to coat. Marinate for 15 minutes.

3. Preheat the broiler. Coat a broiler pan with cooking spray. Arrange the turkey cutlets on the pan. Drizzle with any remaining marinade.

4. Broil 4" from the heat source for 6 minutes, turning once, or until just cooked through. Serve the cutlets on top of the rice.

Per serving: 357 calories, 32 g protein, 22 g carbohydrates, 17 g fat, 2 g saturated fat, 3 g fiber, 542 mg sodium

Make it a meal: Serve turkey and rice with 1 cup steamed green beans.

Meal per serving: 401 calories, 35 g protein, 32 g carbohydrates, 17 g fat, 2 g saturated fat, 7 g fiber, 543 mg sodium

Gingered Turkey Meat Loaf

Prep time: 12 minutes • *Total time:* 1 hour 22 minutes
Makes 6 servings

Seasoning vegetables—such as onions, garlic, carrots, and fresh ginger—helps maximize the flavor of this meat loaf while minimizing the use of salt. For lunch, make a sandwich using a slice of leftover meat loaf on high-fiber bread with a little ketchup, and serve with a tossed vegetable salad on the side.

1¼ pounds lean ground turkey breast

1 cup old-fashioned or quick oats

½ cup reduced-sodium chicken broth

1 egg

1 cup finely shredded carrots

1 onion, finely chopped

2 cloves garlic, minced

1 teaspoon finely chopped fresh ginger

½ teaspoon salt

⅛ teaspoon ground black pepper

¾ cup (12 ounces) unsalted tomato sauce, heated

1. Preheat the oven to 350°F. Line an 11" x 7" baking pan with aluminum foil overlapping the sides.

2. Stir together the turkey, oats, broth, egg, carrots, onion, garlic, ginger, salt, and pepper in a large bowl just until combined. Shape into an 8" x 3" loaf and place in the pan. Fold the extra foil up over the top of the loaf to loosely cover.

3. Bake for 50 minutes or until a thermometer inserted in the center registers 165°F and the meat is no longer pink. Remove from the oven and let stand for 15 minutes before slicing. Serve with the tomato sauce.

Per serving: 197 calories, 28 g protein, 16 g carbohydrates, 3 g fat, 0.5 g saturated fat, 3 g fiber, 330 mg sodium

Make it a meal: Serve the meat loaf with Sweet Pepper Rice and 1 cup broccoli sautéed in 1 teaspoon olive oil.

Meal per serving: 470 calories, 34 g protein, 58 g carbohydrates, 13 g fat, 2 g saturated fat, 8 g fiber, 353 mg sodium

Hearty Kale and White Bean Soup

Prep time: 15 minutes • *Total time:* 1 hour
Makes 4 servings

If you want to make your own sausage for this robust one-dish meal, use the recipe for Homemade Turkey Sausage patties. Halve the recipe, mix in a pinch of red-pepper flakes, if you like, and shape the sausage mixture into tiny meatballs rather than patties. Then just follow the directions below.

2 tablespoons olive oil, divided

4 ounces fresh, hot or mild, Italian-style turkey or chicken sausage, sliced

1 onion, finely chopped

3 large cloves garlic, finely chopped

2 teaspoons chopped fresh sage or 1 teaspoon dried

1 cup cooked or canned cannellini beans, rinsed and drained

2 cans (14$\frac{1}{2}$ ounces each) or 4 cups low-sodium chicken broth

2 cups water

8 cups shredded kale or 5 ounces ($\frac{1}{2}$ of 10-ounce box) frozen chopped kale

$\frac{1}{2}$ cup grated Parmesan cheese

2 whole wheat pitas, toasted and halved

1. Heat 1$\frac{1}{2}$ tablespoons oil in a large saucepan over medium heat. Add the sausage and cook for 5 minutes, stirring often, until browned. Transfer to a plate.

2. Add the onion to the saucepan and cook, stirring, for 5 minutes. Add the garlic and sage and cook, stirring, for 30 seconds. Add the beans, broth, water, and kale. Simmer for 15 minutes.

3. Use a potato masher to mash some of the beans and thicken the broth. Stir in the reserved sausage. Simmer for 10 minutes.

4. Ladle the soup into individual bowls and sprinkle evenly with the cheese. Brush the toasted pitas with the remaining $\frac{1}{2}$ tablespoon oil. Serve half a pita with each portion of the soup.

Per serving: 399 calories, 20 g protein, 38 g carbohydrates, 20 g fat, 7 g saturated fat, 8 g fiber, 548 mg sodium

Chicken Adobo

Prep time: 10 minutes • *Total time:* 35 minutes
Makes 4 servings

An unusual, and unusually delicious, combination of vinegar, soy sauce, and garlic makes up the broth that flavors the chicken. This traditional Filipino dish can also be made with cubes of lean pork tenderloin or a mixture of pork and chicken.

1 tablespoon olive oil	¾ cup distilled white vinegar
¾ pound boneless, skinless chicken breast, cut into 1" pieces	¼ cup low-sodium soy sauce
	4 large cloves garlic, finely chopped
2 cups water	1 bay leaf

1. Heat the oil in a large saucepan over medium heat. Add the chicken and cook, stirring constantly, for about 3 minutes or until lightly browned. With a slotted spoon, transfer the chicken to a bowl.

2. Add the water, vinegar, soy sauce, garlic, and bay leaf to the saucepan. Heat to a boil over medium-high heat. Reduce heat to medium-low and simmer for 15 minutes. Return the chicken to the pan and simmer for 5 minutes longer or until the chicken is no longer pink. Remove the bay leaf.

Per serving: 146 calories, 19 g protein, 2 g carbohydrates, 6 g fat, 1 g saturated fat, 0 g fiber, 637 mg sodium

Make it a meal: Serve with ¾ cup cooked brown basmati rice and 1 cup zucchini and red bell pepper cooked, stirring frequently, in 1 tablespoon olive oil.

Meal per serving: 440 calories, 24 g protein, 40 g carbohydrates, 22 g fat, 3 g saturated fat, 4 g fiber, 645 mg sodium

Spiced Chicken with Lentils

Prep time: 15 minutes • *Total time:* 1 hour 15 minutes
Makes 4 servings

You can also make this dish with turkey drumsticks instead of chicken parts.

2 tablespoons olive oil

4 small bone-in chicken breasts, skin removed

1/2 teaspoon salt

1/4 teaspoon ground black pepper

2 medium onions, chopped

4 carrots, chopped

2 ribs celery, chopped

4 cloves garlic, sliced

3/4 cup dried lentils

1 can (14.5 ounces) reduced-sodium chicken broth

1 can (14.5 ounces) diced tomatoes

2 tablespoons finely chopped fresh sage or 1 tablespoon dried

2 teaspoons ground cumin

1 tablespoon red wine vinegar

1. Heat the oil in a nonstick Dutch oven or a large pot over medium heat. Add the chicken, salt, and pepper. Cook for 5 minutes, turning once, or until browned. Remove the chicken to a plate and set aside.

2. Add the onions, carrots, celery, and garlic. Cook over medium heat for 5 minutes, or until softened. Stir in the lentils and broth. Heat to a boil, reduce the heat to low, and cover and simmer for 20 minutes. Stir in the tomatoes, sage, cumin, and vinegar.

3. Return the chicken to the pot and bring to a simmer. Cover and simmer over low heat for 30 minutes, or until the lentils are tender and saucy and the chicken is cooked through. Add a little more broth or water, if needed.

Per serving: 430 calories, 33 g protein, 41 g carbohydrates, 14 g fat, 3 g saturated fat, 16 g fiber, 885 mg sodium

Chicken Stew with Almond Couscous

Prep time: 15 minutes • *Total time:* 45 minutes

Makes 4 servings

This simple recipe shows how you can cut back on animal protein and include more beans as a source of plant protein in your diet. To make this a vegetarian dish, eliminate the chicken and add at least twice the amount of chickpeas. Substitute vegetable broth for the chicken broth in both the stew and the couscous.

STEW

1 tablespoon olive oil

1 onion, finely chopped

2 cloves garlic, finely chopped

2 teaspoons ground cumin

1 teaspoon paprika

1 teaspoon finely chopped fresh ginger or $\frac{1}{4}$ teaspoon dried

$\frac{1}{2}$ teaspoon ground cinnamon

$\frac{1}{2}$ teaspoon salt

$\frac{1}{8}$ teaspoon ground black pepper

$\frac{1}{2}$ pound boneless, skinless chicken breast, cut into 1" pieces

1 cup no-salt-added chickpeas, drained

1 cup baby carrots, halved

1 medium zucchini, halved lengthwise and cut into $\frac{1}{2}$"-thick slices

$2\frac{1}{2}$ cups low-fat unsalted chicken broth

$\frac{1}{3}$ cup raisins

12 medium green olives (any type), sliced

2 tablespoons no-salt-added tomato paste

$\frac{1}{4}$ cup finely chopped cilantro

COUSCOUS

$\frac{3}{4}$ cup low-fat unsalted chicken broth

1 tablespoon olive oil

$\frac{1}{4}$ teaspoon salt

$\frac{3}{4}$ cup uncooked instant couscous

1 teaspoon grated lemon peel

$\frac{1}{4}$ cup natural almonds, finely chopped

1. *To make the stew:* In a large pot, heat the oil over medium heat. Add the onion and cook, stirring frequently, for 5 minutes or until tender. Stir in the garlic, cumin, paprika, ginger, cinnamon, salt, and pepper. Cook for 1 minute, stirring occasionally. Add the chicken and cook, stirring, for 1 minute longer.

2. Stir in the chickpeas, carrots, zucchini, broth, raisins, olives, and tomato paste. Heat to a boil over medium-high heat. Reduce the heat to low, cover, and simmer for 20 minutes, or until the vegetables are tender. Stir in the cilantro and serve over the couscous.

3. *To make the couscous:* Bring the broth, oil, and salt to a boil in a small saucepan. Stir in the couscous; cover and remove from the heat. Let stand for 5 minutes; fluff with a fork. Stir in the lemon peel and almonds.

Per serving: 474 calories, 28 g protein, 60 g carbohydrates, 15 g fat, 2 g saturated fat, 8 g fiber, 747 mg sodium

Make it a meal: Serve the stew with ½ cup sliced cucumbers sprinkled with balsamic vinegar.

Meal per serving: 487 calories , 28 g protein, 62 g carbohydrates, 15 g fat, 2 g saturated fat, 8 g fiber, 749 mg sodium

Roasted Salmon with Green Beans and Potatoes

Prep time: 20 minutes • *Total time:* 45 minutes
Makes 4 servings

If you like, you can substitute asparagus for the green beans and new potatoes for the Yukon Gold.

1½ pounds Yukon Gold potatoes, cut into 1½" chunks

¾ pound green beans

2 tablespoons olive oil, divided

2 tablespoons chopped fresh rosemary or 2 teaspoons dried, divided

2 cloves garlic, finely chopped

½ teaspoon salt, divided

4 small salmon fillets (3 ounces each), preferably center cut

1. Preheat the oven to 450°F. Toss the potatoes, beans, 1½ tablespoons oil, 1 tablespoon rosemary, the garlic, and ¼ teaspoon salt in a 17" x 11" baking dish. Roast for 10 minutes, stirring once.

2. Push the vegetables to the sides of the pan. Place the salmon fillets, skin side down, in the center. Brush the fillets evenly with the remaining ½ tablespoon oil and sprinkle with the remaining 1 tablespoon rosemary and ¼ teaspoon salt.

3. Roast for 10 minutes, or until the vegetables are tender and the salmon is just cooked through. Divide the salmon and vegetables among 4 plates.

Per serving: 346 calories, 22 g protein, 38 g carbohydrates, 13 g fat, 2 g saturated fat, 7 g fiber, 344 mg sodium

French-Style Seafood Chowder

Prep time: 20 minutes • *Total time:* 55 minutes
Makes 4 servings

Cod, pollack, salmon, catfish, and shellfish top the American Heart Association's list of fresh seafood that contribute healthful omega-3 fatty acids to a diet and are also low in mercury and other environmental contaminants. This tasty chowder is a one-dish meal.

¼ cup extra-virgin olive oil

1 onion, chopped

2 ribs celery, chopped

2 cloves garlic, minced

1½ pounds Yukon Gold potatoes, peeled and cut into ½" cubes

1 can (14.5 ounces) no-salt-added diced tomatoes

2 cups water

1 bottle (6 ounces) clam juice

¾ cup dry white wine or vermouth or reduced-sodium chicken broth

½ teaspoon fennel seeds

¼ pound cod, pollack, or catfish fillet, cut into bite-size pieces

¼ pound scallops, halved if large

¼ pound shelled, deveined shrimp

1. Heat the oil over medium heat in a large pot. Add the onion, celery, and garlic and cook for 5 minutes or until tender. Stir in the potatoes. Cover and cook for 5 minutes.

2. Add the tomatoes, water, clam juice, wine or broth, and fennel seeds. Cover and simmer over low heat for 20 minutes. Add the cod, scallops, and shrimp. Simmer for 2 minutes or until the seafood is opaque.

Per serving: 414 calories, 20 g protein, 49 g carbohydrates, 15 g fat, 2 g saturated fat, 6 g fiber, 517 mg sodium

Stir-Fried Ginger Shrimp and Veggies

Prep time: 25 minutes • *Total time:* 55 minutes
Makes 4 servings

You can substitute broccoli florets or trimmed and chopped asparagus or zucchini for the snow peas and use any color bell pepper. Don't confuse canned coconut milk, which is used in this recipe, with the coconut milk sold in cardboard containers in the dairy department alongside regular milk.

1½ cups water

½ cup canned light coconut milk

1 cup brown basmati rice

2 teaspoons cornstarch

2 tablespoons dry sherry

2 tablespoons reduced-sodium soy sauce

⅔ cup low-sodium chicken broth

2 tablespoons light olive oil, divided

1 pound peeled, deveined shrimp

3 cloves garlic, minced

1 tablespoon finely chopped fresh ginger

1 can (8 ounces) water chestnuts, drained and sliced

2 cups snow peas, trimmed

1 large red, orange, or yellow bell pepper, thinly sliced

1. Bring the water and coconut milk to a boil in a medium saucepan over medium-high heat. Stir in the rice. Reduce the heat to low, cover, and simmer for 20 minutes or until the liquid is absorbed.

2. Meanwhile, stir together the cornstarch, sherry, and soy sauce in a small bowl. Stir in the broth until smooth. Set aside.

3. Heat 1 tablespoon oil in a large skillet or a wok over medium-high heat. Add the shrimp and cook for 4 minutes, stirring constantly, until they are pink and opaque. Use a slotted spoon to transfer the shrimp to a bowl.

4. Add the remaining 1 tablespoon oil to the skillet. Add the garlic and ginger and cook for 1 minute. Add the water chestnuts, snow peas, and pepper. Cook, stirring constantly, for 2 minutes.

5. Return the shrimp to the skillet. Stir the reserved soy sauce mixture and add it to the skillet. Cook, stirring constantly, until the sauce thickens and coats the shrimp and vegetables. Divide the rice among 4 plates. Top with the shrimp mixture.

Per serving: 415 calories, 27 g protein, 50 g carbohydrates, 12 g fat, 3 g saturated fat, 7 g fiber, 448 mg sodium

Cod in Curry Broth with Rice

Prep time: 10 minutes • *Total time:* 45 minutes
Makes 4 servings

Seasoning is especially important when you are cutting back on salt and still expect rich flavor from your foods, so don't skimp on herbs and spices and other sodium-free flavors like citrus. A sprinkling of fresh basil and cilantro, combined with a squeeze of lime juice, gives this dish an authentic Southeast Asian taste. You could just as easily make this dish with chunks of boneless chicken breast or pork tenderloin, shrimp, or another firm-fleshed fish such as salmon in place of the cod.

1 cup brown basmati rice

2 tablespoons light olive oil

1 small onion, thinly sliced

2 cloves garlic, finely chopped

2 teaspoons curry powder

1 can (14.5 ounces) low-sodium chicken broth

4 cups chopped Swiss chard or baby spinach leaves

$\frac{1}{4}$ cup chopped fresh basil

$\frac{1}{4}$ cup chopped fresh cilantro

1 tablespoon lime juice

8 ounces skinless cod fillet, cut into bite-size pieces

1. Prepare the rice according to package directions.

2. Meanwhile, heat the oil over medium heat in a medium saucepan. Add the onion and cook for 5 minutes or until tender. Stir in the garlic and curry powder and cook for 1 minute. Add the broth. Heat to a boil, reduce the heat to low, and cover and simmer for 20 minutes.

3. Add the Swiss chard or spinach, basil, cilantro, and lime juice. Simmer over low heat, uncovered, for 2 minutes. Add the cod pieces. Cover and simmer for 3 minutes, or until the fish is opaque.

4. Divide the rice and cod mixture among 4 bowls.

Per serving: 360 calories, 17 g protein, 39 g carbohydrates, 15 g fat, 3 g saturated fat, 1 g fiber, 142 mg sodium

Pasta with Garlicky White Clam Sauce

Prep time: 10 minutes • *Total time:* 25 minutes
Makes 4 servings

This is a classic pasta recipe with the added twist of using chopped spinach in place of parsley. To experiment with other green leafy vegetables, substitute kale or collard greens for the spinach. If you like, you can toss in some chopped fresh parsley as well.

8 ounces dry fusilli, rotelle, rotini, or other spiral-shaped pasta

3 tablespoons olive oil, divided

2 tablespoons finely chopped garlic, divided

8 cups spinach leaves, finely chopped

¾ cup fat-free reduced-sodium chicken broth or white wine

2 cans (6.5 ounces each) chopped clams, with liquid reserved

2 tablespoons lemon juice

½ teaspoon dried oregano, crumbled

½ cup grated Parmesan cheese

1. Prepare the pasta according to package directions, boiling until tender.

2. Meanwhile, heat 1 tablespoon oil in a large saucepan over medium heat. Add 1 tablespoon garlic and cook, stirring, for 1 minute. Add the spinach a little at a time as it cooks down, stirring often. Cook for 3 minutes or until the spinach is wilted. Transfer to a large bowl.

3. Add the remaining 2 tablespoons oil and 1 tablespoon garlic to the pan. Cook over medium heat for 1 minute, stirring occasionally. Add the broth or wine, the liquid from 1 can of clams (discard the remaining liquid or save for another use), lemon juice, and oregano. Heat to a boil over medium-high heat. Reduce heat and simmer for 5 minutes.

4. Add the clams and pasta to the saucepan. Cook for 1 minute, tossing. Transfer to the bowl with the spinach. Top with the Parmesan cheese.

Per serving: 404 calories, 20 g protein, 51 g carbohydrates, 15 g fat, 4 g saturated fat, 5 g fiber, 858 mg sodium

Roast Beef and Tomatoes with Basil Sauce

Prep time: 15 minutes • *Total time:* 1 hour
Makes 6 servings

Eye round, top round, bottom round, top sirloin, round tip, and filet (mignon), or tenderloin, are the leanest cuts of beef that are sold as roasts. Some cuts are larger than others, so you will have to cut them down further or adjust your cooking time to accommodate the larger size.

BEEF

2 tablespoons olive oil

1½ pounds eye round roast

6 plum tomatoes, halved
    lengthwise

2 teaspoons Italian seasoning

½ teaspoon salt

¼ teaspoon ground black pepper

BASIL SAUCE

2 cups fresh basil leaves

1 large clove garlic

¼ teaspoon salt

1 tablespoon olive oil

½ cup fat-free reduced-sodium
    chicken broth

1. *To make the beef:* Preheat the oven to 375°F.

2. Heat the oil in a medium roasting pan over medium-high heat. Add the beef and cook for 5 minutes, turning often, until browned on all sides. Remove from the heat.

3. Add the tomatoes to the pan, cut side up. Sprinkle the roast and tomatoes with the Italian seasoning, salt, and pepper.

4. Roast for 40 to 45 minutes, or until a thermometer inserted in the center registers 145°F for medium-rare. Let stand for 10 minutes before slicing.

5. *To make the sauce:* While the beef is roasting, process the basil, garlic, and salt in a blender or a food processor until smooth. With the machine running, gradually add the oil and broth. Serve the sauce with the beef and tomatoes.

Per serving: 224 calories, 27 g protein, 3 g carbohydrates, 11 g fat, 2 g saturated fat, 1 g fiber, 426 mg sodium

Make it a meal: Serve with ½ cup corn kernels and white beans and artichokes made by heating ⅓ cup small white (navy) beans with ½ cup drained artichoke hearts (frozen or packed in brine, not oil), served over 1 cup baby spinach leaves and sprinkled with balsamic or red wine vinegar.

Meal per serving: 431 calories, 38 g protein, 46 g carbohydrates, 13 g fat, 3 g saturated fat, 17 g fiber, 528 mg sodium

Sweet Potatoes with Orange and Walnuts

Prep time: 10 minutes • *Total time:* 55 minutes
Makes 4 servings

You can double this recipe, if need be.

4 small sweet potatoes, scrubbed

1 cup peeled and finely chopped orange sections (from 1 to 2 oranges)

¼ cup finely chopped walnuts

¼ cup orange juice

2 tablespoons honey

1 tablespoon olive oil

1. Preheat the oven to 400°F. Pierce the potatoes all over with a fork and place on a baking sheet.

2. Bake for 45 minutes or until tender.

3. Meanwhile, combine the orange sections, walnuts, orange juice, honey, and oil in a small bowl.

4. Split the potatoes open lengthwise and mash the flesh within the skin with a fork. Divide the orange mixture among the potatoes.

Per serving: 250 calories, 4 g protein, 43 g carbohydrates, 8 g fat, 1 g saturated fat, 6 g fiber, 72 mg sodium

White Beans with Roasted Red Pepper

Prep time: 10 minutes • *Total time:* 15 minutes

Makes 4 servings

If you have fresh basil, dill, or any other fresh herb on hand, feel free to add it to the mix.

1 can (15 ounces) no-salt-added cannellini beans or navy beans, drained

1 roasted red pepper, finely chopped

2 tablespoons lemon juice

2 teaspoons olive oil

$\frac{1}{4}$ cup chopped parsley

1. Heat the beans in a small saucepan over medium-low heat until just warmed through, about 5 minutes. Stir in the red pepper.

2. Meanwhile, in a small bowl, stir together the lemon juice, oil, and parsley. Add the beans and red pepper and toss gently to mix. Serve warm.

Per serving: 81 calories, 3 g protein, 11 g carbohydrates, 3 g fat, 0.5 g saturated fat, 3 g fiber, 90 mg sodium

Tomato-Avocado Salad

Prep time: 10 minutes • *Total time:* 10 minutes
Makes 1 serving

This simple salad recipe serves 1, but all you have to do is double, triple, or quadruple the ingredients to make multiple servings. If you like, you can toast the pine nuts in a small dry skillet over medium heat for several minutes or until golden brown.

1 medium tomato, sliced

$\frac{1}{4}$ cup finely chopped avocado

2 teaspoons lemon juice

$\frac{1}{8}$ teaspoon salt

$\frac{1}{8}$ teaspoon ground black pepper

2 tablespoons chopped fresh basil

1 tablespoon pine nuts

Arrange the tomato slices on a salad plate. Top with the avocado. Sprinkle with the lemon juice, salt, pepper, basil, and pine nuts. Serve at once.

Per serving: 142 calories, 3 g protein, 10 g carbohydrates, 11 g fat, 1 g saturated fat, 4 g fiber, 300 mg sodium

Make it a meal: Serve with roasted or grilled chicken and a baked potato topped with yogurt, scallions, and Parmesan cheese.

Meal per serving: 470 calories, 33 g protein, 55 g carbohydrates, 15 g fat, 3 g saturated fat, 9 g fiber, 520 mg sodium

Sweet Pepper Rice

Prep time: 5 minutes • *Total time:* 15 minutes

Makes 6 servings

1 tablespoon olive oil

1 small onion, finely chopped

1 red or yellow bell pepper, chopped

3 cups cooked brown rice

Heat the oil in a medium skillet over medium heat. Add the onion and cook, stirring, for 5 minutes or until tender. Stir in the pepper and rice and cook, stirring, for 5 minutes or until heated through.

Per serving: 213 calories, 4 g protein, 39 g carbohydrates, 5 g fat, 1 g saturated fat, 4 g fiber, 4 mg sodium

Sweet Corn and Edamame Salad

Prep time: 10 minutes • *Total time:* 15 minutes
Makes 4 servings

This crisp and quick-to-throw-together side salad is a nutritious accompaniment to any light, Asian-inspired meal.

½ cup shelled, frozen green soybeans (edamame)

1 tablespoon light olive oil

1 tablespoon rice wine vinegar or lemon juice

1 tablespoon low-sodium soy sauce

1 can (15 ounces) no-salt-added corn kernels, drained

½ cup finely chopped red bell pepper

¼ cup thinly sliced scallions

¼ cup finely chopped cilantro

1. Cook the soybeans in a small saucepan of boiling water to cover for 5 minutes, or according to package directions. Drain well and allow to cool.

2. In a medium bowl, stir together the oil, vinegar or lemon juice, and soy sauce until blended. Add the soybeans, corn, pepper, scallions, and cilantro. Toss well. Refrigerate until ready to serve.

Per serving: 160 calories, 6 g protein, 26 g carbohydrates, 6 g fat, 1 g saturated fat, 4 g fiber, 139 mg sodium

Green Bean and Tomato Salad

Prep time: 10 minutes • *Total time:* 20 minutes
Makes 4 servings

This simple salad is so versatile—serve it warm or at room temperature, or make it ahead of time and serve cold.

4 cups green beans, trimmed and cut into 1½" lengths

1 tablespoon lemon juice

1 tablespoon balsamic vinegar

1 teaspoon dried oregano

¼ teaspoon salt

⅛ teaspoon ground black pepper

2 medium tomatoes, cored and finely chopped

1. Steam the beans until tender-crisp, about 4 minutes.

2. Meanwhile, in a medium bowl, stir together the lemon juice, vinegar, oregano, salt, and pepper. Add the tomatoes and toss gently to coat.

3. Drain the beans and add to the bowl with the tomato mixture. Toss gently. Serve at once or refrigerate until ready to serve.

Per serving: 48 calories, 2 g protein, 11 g carbohydrates, 0 g fat, 0 g saturated fat, 4 g fiber, 156 mg sodium

Snacks and Desserts

Mushroom, Cheddar, and Walnut Pâté

Prep time: 10 minutes • *Total time:* 20 minutes
Makes 6 servings

If you're a blue cheese lover, substitute Gorgonzola, blue cheese, or any other veined variety for the Cheddar.

1 tablespoon olive oil

8 ounces mushrooms, stemmed and finely chopped

1 clove garlic, minced

1 teaspoon dried thyme

$\frac{1}{8}$ teaspoon salt

$\frac{1}{4}$ cup chopped walnuts

2 ounces Neufchâtel cream cheese

2 ounces shredded reduced-fat Cheddar cheese

3 cups mixed cut-up raw vegetables, such as celery sticks, zucchini slices, radish slices, fennel slices, and red bell pepper chunks

1. Heat the oil over medium heat in a small skillet. Add the mushrooms, garlic, thyme, and salt. Cook for 5 minutes, stirring, until the mushrooms begin to release their liquid. Cook for 10 more minutes, or until most of the liquid evaporates.

2. In a blender or a food processor, combine the walnuts, cream cheese, and Cheddar cheese. Add the mushroom mixture. Pulse with an on-off motion, scraping down the sides of the container, if necessary, until the mixture is well blended. Scrape into a small bowl.

3. Spread 3 tablespoons pâté on $\frac{1}{2}$ cup assorted raw vegetables per serving. Refrigerate leftover pâté for up to 5 days.

Per serving: 123 calories, 6 g protein, 5 g carbohydrates, 10 g fat, 3 g saturated fat, 2 g fiber, 178 mg sodium

Make it a meal: Serve with a grape spritzer made with 6 ounces of grape juice topped off with seltzer or 1 glass (6 ounces) of wine.

Meal per serving: 220 calories, 6 g protein, 30 g carbohydrates, 10 g fat, 3 g saturated fat, 2 g fiber, 193 mg sodium

White Bean Spread on Toast

Prep time: 5 minutes • *Total time:* 15 minutes
Makes 6 servings

Serve this dip when company comes, or keep it in the refrigerator for a quick after-noon snack. When you feel hungry, take out a serving and warm it up in a micro-wave oven before spreading it on toast.

2 tablespoons olive oil

2 large cloves garlic, minced

1 can (15 ounces) no-salt-added cannellini beans, rinsed and drained

1 tablespoon fresh or dried rosemary

$\frac{1}{4}$ teaspoon salt

$\frac{1}{8}$ teaspoon ground black pepper

5 ounces soft goat cheese

6 slices whole grain Italian bread, toasted and halved

1. Heat the oil over medium heat in a small saucepan. Add the garlic and cook for 1 minute. Stir in the beans, rosemary, salt, and pepper. Cook for 5 minutes, stirring occasionally, until warmed through.

2. Transfer the bean mixture to a blender or a food processor and add the cheese. Process until smooth, scraping down the sides of the container, if necessary. Transfer to a bowl and serve warm with the bread.

Per serving: 262 calories, 11 g protein, 32 g carbohydrates, 10 g fat, 4 g saturated fat, 4 g fiber, 478 mg sodium

Cheese and Olive Quesadillas

Prep time: 10 minutes • *Total time:* 15 minutes
Makes 2 servings

Quesadillas are simple and filling, and they go great with wine, light beer, or a juice spritzer. You can use reduced-fat Swiss, Monterey Jack, or any other type of reduced-fat cheese you like.

1 large (10") whole wheat wrap

2 ounces grated reduced-fat
   Cheddar cheese

6 pimiento-stuffed olives, thinly
   sliced

1. Place a large skillet over medium heat. Lay the wrap in the skillet. Sprinkle evenly with the cheese and olives.

2. Fold the wrap in half and press gently with a spatula. Cook for 4 minutes, turning once, or until lightly browned and crisp underneath. Transfer to a cutting board and let stand for 5 minutes.

3. Cut the quesadilla in half. Cut each half in half again for a total of 4 triangles.

Per serving: 199 calories, 11 g protein, 20 g carbohydrates, 9 g fat, 3 g saturated fat, 2 g fiber, 692 mg sodium

Make it a meal: Serve 2 triangles with a spritzer made with 6 ounces pomegranate cranberry juice topped with seltzer over ice, 1 glass (6 ounces) red or white wine, or 1 bottle (12 ounces) light beer.

Meal per serving: 276 calories, 11 g protein, 38 g carbohydrates, 9 g fat, 3 g saturated fat, 2 g fiber, 709 mg sodium

Cocoa-Nutty Brownies

Prep time: 15 minutes • *Total time:* 45 minutes
Makes 20 brownies

No one would ever guess that these rich, sweet, chocolatey bites are made with olive oil. If you are allergic to nuts, you can either leave them out or substitute dry-roasted unsalted sunflower seeds.

¾ cup all-purpose flour	½ cup granulated sugar
⅓ cup unsweetened cocoa powder	½ cup packed light brown sugar
2 tablespoons toasted wheat germ	½ cup light olive oil
½ teaspoon baking powder	1 teaspoon vanilla
½ teaspoon salt	½ cup chopped walnuts
2 eggs	

1. Preheat the oven to 325°F. Lightly oil and flour an 8" x 8" x 2" baking pan.

2. In a small bowl, whisk together the flour, cocoa powder, wheat germ, baking powder, and salt.

3. In a medium bowl, with an electric mixer on medium-high speed, beat the eggs, granulated sugar, and brown sugar for 1 minute. On medium speed, beat in the oil and vanilla until blended. On medium-low speed, gradually beat in the flour mixture until blended. Stir in the walnuts. Spread the batter evenly in the prepared pan.

4. Bake for 30 minutes or until a pick inserted in the center comes out clean. Transfer the pan to a wire rack to cool completely. When cool, use a knife to make 4 lengthwise cuts and 5 crosswise cuts for a total of 20 brownies.

Per serving: 138 calories, 2 g protein, 16 g carbohydrates, 8 g fat, 1 g saturated fat, 1 g fiber, 79 mg sodium

Make it a meal: Serve with 1 cup 1% milk or soy milk.

Meal per serving: 241 calories, 10 g protein, 28 g carbohydrates, 11 g fat, 3 g saturated fat, 1 g fiber, 187 mg sodium

Nutty Berry Fool

Prep time: 10 minutes • *Total time:* 10 minutes
Makes 4 servings

You can substitute thinly sliced ripe peaches, nectarines, or plums or other berries for the raspberries and blueberries in this old-fashioned, make-ahead, creamy fruit dessert. You can also substitute dry-roasted unsalted sunflower seeds for the nuts if you prefer.

¼ cup heavy cream

12 ounces 0% plain Greek yogurt

3 tablespoons honey

2 cups blueberries

1 cup raspberries

3 tablespoons finely chopped walnuts

Fresh mint for garnish (optional)

1. Whisk the cream in a small bowl until stiff.

2. Stir together the yogurt and honey in a medium bowl until well blended. Gently fold in the whipped cream until just blended.

3. Fold the berries into the yogurt mixture or layer the berries and the yogurt mixture in 4 clear dessert dishes or parfait-style glasses. Refrigerate until ready to serve. Just before serving, sprinkle with the nuts and garnish with the mint, if using.

Per serving: 238 calories, 10 g protein, 32 g carbohydrates, 10 g fat, 4 g saturated fat, 4 g fiber, 39 mg sodium

Pineapple-Carrot Loaf Cake

Prep time: 20 minutes • *Total time:* 1 hour 10 minutes
Makes 16 slices

Some desserts are naturally more healthful than others, and carrot cake is one of them. As carrot cake is traditionally prepared, not only the vitamin A from the carrots makes it nutritious but also the oil that's used instead of butter, and the magnesium-rich nuts and canned pineapple.

CAKE

1 cup all-purpose flour

2 tablespoons toasted wheat germ

1 teaspoon baking powder

1 teaspoon baking soda

$\frac{1}{4}$ teaspoon salt

1 teaspoon ground cinnamon

$\frac{1}{2}$ teaspoon ground allspice

$\frac{1}{4}$ teaspoon ground nutmeg

$\frac{1}{2}$ cup granulated sugar

$\frac{1}{2}$ cup packed light brown sugar

$\frac{1}{2}$ cup well-drained crushed pineapple canned in water or juice, or finely chopped fresh pineapple

2 eggs

$\frac{1}{2}$ cup light olive oil

1 teaspoon vanilla extract

2 carrots, grated (1 cup)

$\frac{1}{4}$ cup finely chopped walnuts (optional)

GLAZE

2 ounces low-fat cream cheese, at room temperature

1 tablespoon granulated sugar

$\frac{1}{4}$ teaspoon vanilla extract

1 tablespoon low-fat milk

1. *To make the cake:* Preheat the oven to 350°F. Lightly oil an 8½" x 4½" loaf pan.

2. In a small bowl, whisk together the flour, wheat germ, baking powder, baking soda, salt, cinnamon, allspice, and nutmeg until well blended. Set aside.

3. In a large bowl, with an electric mixer on medium speed, beat together the granulated sugar, brown sugar, pineapple, eggs, oil, and vanilla until well mixed. Reduce the speed to low and gradually beat in the flour mixture. Stir in the carrots and walnuts. Turn the batter into the oiled loaf pan.

4. Bake for 40 to 45 minutes, or until a wooden pick inserted in the center of the cake comes out clean. Transfer the pan to a rack to cool completely. When completely cool, spread the glaze over the cake, allowing some to drip down the sides. Refrigerate the cake until ready to serve.

5. *To make the glaze:* While the cake is baking, prepare the glaze. In a small bowl or a cup, mix together the cream cheese, sugar, and vanilla until well blended. Stir in the milk until smooth. Spread the glaze evenly over the top of the cake.

6. To serve, use a serrated knife to cut the cake into 16 very thin (½") slices.

    Per slice: 169 calories, 2 g protein, 22 g carbohydrates, 8 g fat, 2 g saturated fat, 1 g fiber, 179 mg sodium

Make it a meal: Serve 1 slice cake with ¾ cup 1% milk or soy milk.

Meal per serving: 246 calories, 8 g protein, 31 g carbohydrates, 10 g fat, 3 g saturated fat, 1 g fiber, 259 mg sodium

Baked Apples
with Creamy Maple Sauce

Prep time: 10 minutes • *Total time:* 25 minutes in microwave oven;
   1 hour 10 minutes in conventional oven

Makes 4 servings

Some apples are good for baking, while others are better for eating out of hand or in salads. Good baking varieties include Granny Smith, Gala, Cortland, Rome, Gravenstein, Braeburn, Pippin, and Winesap.

4 medium to large baking apples

½ cup chopped walnuts or pecans (optional)

¼ cup uncooked instant or old-fashioned oats or muesli cereal

2 tablespoons apple juice

¼ teaspoon ground cinnamon

⅛ teaspoon ground nutmeg

1 cup 0% plain Greek yogurt

3 tablespoons pure maple syrup

1. With a paring knife or a vegetable peeler, pare away the skin halfway down from the top of each apple. Cut out the core of each, leaving about ½" intact at the bottom.

2. Combine the nuts (if using), oats, apple juice, cinnamon, and nutmeg in a small bowl. Divide among the apples, pressing into the core and allowing the mixture to overflow slightly, if necessary.

3. *To make in a microwave oven:* Place the apples in a microwave-safe baking dish just large enough to hold them upright. Pour ¼ cup water into the dish. Microwave at full power for 10 to 12 minutes or until the apples are tender.

4. *To make in a conventional oven:* Preheat the oven to 425°F. Place the apples in a lightly oiled baking dish. Pour ¼ cup water into the dish. Cover loosely with aluminum foil. Bake for 40 to 60 minutes or until the apples are tender.

5. Stir together the yogurt and maple syrup in a small bowl. Divide among the warm apples.

Per serving: 260 calories, 9 g protein, 39 g carbohydrates, 10 g fat, 1 g saturated fat, 4 g fiber, 23 mg sodium

Chocolate Fondue

Prep time: 15 minutes • *Total time:* 25 minutes
Makes 4 servings

You can use any fruit you like, but bananas and strawberries are always a hit with fondue. If you are doing some of the preparation in advance, wait to cut up the banana until just before serving so it doesn't have time to turn brown. Use a small fork or toothpicks for dipping the fruit and the cake into the Chocolate Fondue.

1 small banana

2 cups strawberries, halved

1 slice angel food cake ($\frac{1}{12}$ of a tube cake), cut into 1" pieces

3 ounces semisweet chocolate chips

$\frac{1}{3}$ cup fortified evaporated skim milk

$\frac{1}{4}$ teaspoon vanilla, mint, or almond extract

1. Cut the banana into $\frac{1}{4}$"-thick slices. Arrange the fruit and cake on 4 individual serving plates.

2. Combine the chocolate chips and milk in a small saucepan. Cook over medium heat, stirring often, for 3 minutes or until bubbly. Continue cooking, stirring often, for 5 minutes, or until the mixture is very smooth and slightly thickened. Stir in the extract. Divide among 4 small bowls and serve with the fruit and cake for dipping.

   Per serving: 200 calories, 4 g protein, 35 g carbohydrates, 7 g fat, 4 g saturated fat, 3 g fiber, 120 mg sodium

Make it a meal: Serve with iced coffee made with 6 ounces 1% milk and $\frac{1}{4}$ cup brewed regular or decaf coffee over ice.

Meal per serving: 272 calories, 10 g protein, 44 g carbohydrates, 8 g fat, 5 g saturated fat, 3 g fiber, 196 mg sodium

Chapter 6

The Exercise Plan

When 12,000 American women were asked in an online poll what they'd do if they had an extra hour a day, more than 20 percent said "exercise." We know what they're talking about. Between a job, a family, the responsibilities of a home and possibly a pet (or two), community commitments, friends, and—lest we forget—your spouse or significant other, finding moments for movement can seem daunting. A 25-hour day would come in very handy, indeed!

But we're here to tell you that you can get the physical activity you want and need in the time you have. It's a busy woman's dream come true: a walking routine that delivers *more* calorie-burning, fitness-boosting, energy-raising results in *less* time. Plus a yoga routine that incorporates strength training so that you can tone your upper body, lower body, and core—and feel that deep-down sense of serenity and relaxation that only yoga brings, in just 20 minutes.

When the 12 midlife women on our test panel tried the exercise component of the 30-Day Slim-Down, Cool-Down Diet, the results amazed them. Our walking routine—a mix of steady-paced walks and interval walks that alternate short, fast bursts of speed with slower-paced walking—helped Robin Laub, a busy mother of two and first-grade teacher, get past her "walking plateau." Before the program, she says, no matter how long she walked, the weight wouldn't budge. On the program, she lost 12 pounds in just 1 month!

Alicia Schleder credits the plan's yoga-with-weights program for her increased flexibility, newly toned arms, and an 11-pound weight loss. "My arms are definitely less flabby, and I feel stronger all over," says Alicia. "The yoga plan looks easy, but it's very challenging in a good way." Not only did Alicia see amazing physical changes on the program, she also found that she had more energy and less stress.

On the Natural Menopause Solution exercise plan, you'll take advantage of America's favorite exercise—walking—with a time-saving, fat-blasting twist. Thanks to the new science of interval walking, you'll burn more calories and torch more body fat in 20 minutes than you could on a brisk but steady 40-minute stroll! We asked walking expert Michele Stanten, an American Council on Exercise–certified fitness instructor, a former fitness director of *Prevention* magazine, and author of *Walk Off Weight,* to develop this walking plan specifically for time-strapped midlife women—and it really delivers.

We weren't finished. We wanted a plan that would also help you recharge your metabolism by rebuilding sleek, toned muscle. And our wish list included time for yoga so you'd experience the deep calm that fights food cravings and eases vexing menopausal symptoms from hot flashes and night sweats to insomnia, forgetfulness, and low moods. For that we turned to Kimberly Fowler, a yoga instructor, owner of YAS Fitness Centers in Southern California, author of *The No OM Zone* (and a midlife woman herself), to develop a time-saving yoga-with-weights routine exclusively for the Natural Menopause Solution.

In as few as 40 minutes a day, you'll get an effective walking routine, a muscle-building strength-training workout, *and* a calming dose of yoga. Do one segment before work, another on your lunch break or after dinner. This plan is short enough to work into the busiest schedule—and effective enough to help you lose weight, sail through menopause, and conquer the big health threats that women face at midlife and beyond.

THE WONDERS OF WALKING

No form of exercise is easier than walking—but don't underestimate its power to help you slim down, feel great, and stay healthy. Whether you're a longtime fan of foot-powered fitness or new to walking, you may be surprised to learn that tweaking the world's oldest workout with 20-minute interval walks pumps up the rewards.

Taking an interval walk is exhilarating and fun, as you alternate brief bursts of fast walking with your normal brisk pace. Pushing beyond your comfort zone for a few seconds at a time is worthwhile because it calls on your body's anaerobic energy-producing system—something most of us don't use very often unless we're climbing a set of steps or a steep hill quickly. How is it different? Walking at a steady pace, which is what most walkers do most of the time, uses your body's aerobic system. It uses oxygen to burn carbohydrates and fat for energy. In contrast, the anaerobic system powers your muscles solely by burning carbohydrates already stored in your muscle cells. Experts call this HIIT—high-intensity interval training. It hits the spot when it comes to losing pounds and inches!

By pushing yourself harder for very brief periods of time, you use up these stored carbs, called glycogen, so your muscle cells have to sip more blood sugar to replenish their supply. Simple enough, but the benefits of calling on your anaerobic system are far-reaching and seem custom-tailored to help midlife women lose more weight, reduce insulin resistance, increase physical energy, and encourage the development of more calorie-burning muscle.

That's because intervals prompt your body to build more of the microscopic "power plants," or mitochondria, which produce energy inside muscle cells. You have hundreds of mitochondria inside every active cell in your body. But their numbers and efficiency dwindle with age (one reason it's tougher keeping up with your kids, lifting heavy grocery bags, or walking all day on vacation!). Intervals can increase the number of mitochondria you have on board by a whopping 40 to 50 percent in as few as 6 weeks, report researchers from Canada's York University in a study published in the *Journal of Applied Physiology*. But that's not all. Intervals also pump up the activity of an enzyme involved with fat-burning inside mitochondria, say experts at the Pennington Biomedical Research Center in Louisiana. So these little power plants work better, too.

The result? Your body gets better at burning stored carbs and fat—so you have more muscle power, more energy, *and* lose more weight. And as we've already mentioned, interval training works its magic in just 20 minutes—getting results you won't achieve with a much longer, steady-paced walk.

So why isn't every walk on your workout schedule an interval walk? Truth is, this kind of workout is so effective that your muscles need time to recover and replenish. You'll do three interval walks a week. In between you'll do steady-paced walks or have a rest day. Steady-paced walks burn calories and offer a multitude of health benefits—from reduced risk for heart disease to hot flash relief to a powerful mood boost.

Looking for more motivation to lace up your walking shoes? Consider the following:

Weight loss edge. Walking not only helps you maintain muscle and burn more body fat, but it specifically targets belly fat. In one Canadian study, women who walked for an hour daily trimmed belly fat by 20 percent in $3\frac{1}{2}$ months. Less tummy pooch plus more toned muscle means your clothes will be fitting better even before you see changes in the number on the bathroom scale.

Adding intervals also increases insulin sensitivity, say researchers at Australia's University of New South Wales. That may help explain why, in their 2008 study published in the *International Journal of Obesity*, women lost overall body fat and abdominal fat after doing 20-minute

CELL PHONES CAN BE HAZARDOUS TO YOUR HEALTH

Skip cell phone chats while you're walking. In one University of Illinois study, walkers who talked while they "walked" through virtual streets were 15 percent more likely to be in an accident than those who listened to music. They also crossed intersections 25 percent slower—even with a hands-free phone. Carry one for safety, but chat only with your walking buddies!

interval workouts three times a week for 15 weeks. In contrast, women who exercised twice as long but at a steady pace didn't lose body fat at all!

Menopause advantage. Walking just three times a week can ease the heightened stress and sleep problems that so often crop up as a woman's hormones begin shifting around menopause. In one recent Canadian study published in the journal *Menopause,* women who walked for 45 minutes 3 days a week for 16 weeks reported brighter moods during the day and better snoozing at night.

Regular, moderately intense activity, meanwhile, can even cool off bothersome hot flashes and night sweats. In one Australian study that tracked 438 women for 8 years, regular exercisers were 49 percent less likely to report hot flashes than those whose physical activity levels were low. A Swedish study reached the same conclusion about the power of movement to aid the body's temperature-regulation system. Exercise may help by reducing stress—so that moments of tension don't set off a cascade of stress hormones that can trigger a hot flash. It may also help by increasing levels of feel-good endorphins, which also help your body regulate its core temperature (without making you wonder out loud: "Is it hot in here, or is it just me?").

Regular strolls can also guard against memory glitches and fuzzy thinking, boost your energy, and relieve stress and depression—all issues for many midlife women. In 2010, researchers at Southern Methodist University released a review finding that exercise works as well as, and sometimes better than, antidepressants for some people. Other research suggests that physical activity helps your brain react more mildly to stress by increasing levels of a protective compound called galanin. Less brain strain when faced with everyday ups and downs could keep a low mood from spiraling into depression.

Health bonus. Walking is a potent health protector. When researchers at the Harvard School of Public Health followed 200,000 nurses for more than 30 years, they discovered just how amazing putting one foot in front of the other can be—women who walked for ½ hour most days of the week reduced their risk for heart disease, stroke, and type 2 diabetes by up to 40 percent and slashed their breast cancer risk by 20 to 30 percent. Walking for 4 hours a week can reduce the risk for hip fractures by an impressive 41 percent, according to Harvard Medical School researchers. This is important because your risk for thinning bones and skeletal fractures rises sharply at menopause. (Read more about the essential, health-protecting benefits of exercise in Part III.)

YOGA FOR A CALM, COOL, AND COLLECTED YOU

There's nothing like a gracefully flowing yoga routine to bring you home to yourself. As each moment unfolds, the harmony of breath and posture in the 11 easy poses in the Natural Menopause Solution yoga routine lets you settle into a deep pool of calm. Feels great. In recent years, research is catching up with something midlife women have been noticing for a long time: This kind of serenity also eases troubling menopause symptoms like insomnia, hot flashes, night sweats, achy muscles and joints, and even problems with finding your mental focus. By easing stress (you'll feel like you've just had a great massage or spent a couple of days on vacation at the beach!), yoga can also help you conquer emotional eating so that weight loss is faster and easier, too.

Weight loss edge. Yoga poses don't just keep muscles strong and supple and help your joints stay flexible. A regular routine can help you lose weight for deeper reasons. In one study that tracked the weight and health habits of 15,500 midlife women and men, researchers at the Fred Hutchinson Cancer Center in Seattle found that those who were overweight and practiced yoga regularly were more likely to lose weight over 10 years than those who hadn't.

Yoga also helped the study participants maintain their weight—a feat that can be much more difficult over the years than losing pounds in the first place! Those with a regular yoga practice were 85 percent more likely to maintain their weight over 10 years than those who didn't practice it regularly.

The connection? Yoga tunes you in to body sensations and, as a result, promotes more mindful eating, so you're more likely to eat when you're physically hungry (instead of in response to emotions) and to stop when you're full (instead of munching without thinking about it).

Menopause advantage. The word *yoga* means "union" or "yoke" in Sanskrit, the ancient language of India. Uniting your breath with some of yoga's most relaxing poses creates relaxation so deep that it can switch off or turn down the volume on a variety of menopausal symptoms that are triggered by tension.

When midlife women with plenty of hot-flash experiences—they were coping with 4 severe hot flashes per day, and up to 30 moderate to severe hot flashes per week!—practiced yoga several times a week in a University of California study, they got big improvements. The number of hot flashes fell by 30 percent—and by up to 68 percent for some women—and the severity of their hot flashes eased by an average of 34 percent (for one woman, hot flashes became 78 percent less intense). Reports of middle-of-the-night wake-ups and trouble returning to sleep fell by 20 percent, too. Most had never tried yoga before volunteering for the experiment, but nearly 70 percent kept it up after the study ended.

Studies at Pennsylvania State University and the University of Washington in Seattle have yielded similar results, using some of the same poses you'll find in the Natural Menopause Solution yoga routine such as Cobbler Pose, Seated Wide-Angle Pose, Bridge Pose, and—the most relaxing of all—Corpse Pose. Yoga may cool off hot flashes by calming down the body's sympathetic nervous system—the part of the nervous system responsible for the high-stress "fight or flight" response to everything from a missed deadline to a near-miss on the highway at rush hour—and activating the body's calming parasympathetic nervous system.

That's important, because stress can trigger the exaggerated body changes that happen during a hot flash, as blood vessels dilate in your skin to release heat. And by turning on the body's "relaxation response" as it dials back stress, yoga's been shown in other research to also help ease insomnia. In one Harvard Medical School study, people who practiced yoga and breathing exercises before bed slept longer, spent less time wide-eyed and awake during the night, and woke up feeling refreshed.

And if you've been having trouble remembering where you left your car keys lately, here's more good news: Yoga may even sharpen your memory and thinking skills. It did just that in a study of 108 perimenopausal women conducted in India—the birthplace of yoga. The researchers suspect that by easing your brain into a state of "alert rest," yoga improves the way your little gray cells process information even when declining estrogen levels interfere with razor-sharp recall and quick thinking. In other words, practicing yoga can put you back on top of your mental game.

Health bonus. Yoga delivers some serious benefits for your mind and your body. Recent research shows that this ancient art can help with everything from chronic pain and stiff knees to low moods and poor sleep. In fact, yoga may work even better than taking a walk (though we think doing both is best!) for easing low moods. Boston University researchers have found that yoga has a unique ability to boost a depression- and anxiety-banishing brain chemical called gamma-aminobutyric acid (GABA), according to a 2010 study published in the *Journal of Alternative and Complementary Medicine.* All of these benefits help explain why yoga's at the forefront of mind-body techniques that are gaining a place in mainstream medicine.

STRENGTH TRAINING FOR SEXIER, STRONGER, CALORIE-TORCHING MUSCLES

Don't underestimate the power of those 2-pound hand weights that you'll begin using in Phase 2 of the exercise plan. Combining strength-building moves with yoga poses works your muscles in far more challenging ways than a conventional routine does. (You'll feel it the next day—we did!) And starting light protects you from injury; as weight training gains popularity, injuries are rising in midlife women and men who pick up too much weight too soon.

Maintaining muscle mass and building more of this sleek, strong, metabolically active stuff are the prime reasons to include strength training in your exercise routine. Muscle isn't just more toned and compact than fat (so you look slimmer and trimmer). It also burns three times more calories around the clock. It doesn't take much strength training to build your supply. In a University of Alabama at Birmingham study, women and men who followed a 3-day-a-week strength-training program for 6 months lost 6 pounds of fat, gained 4½ pounds of muscle, and saw their metabolism rise by 12 percent.

Here's how grabbing your weights helps with weight loss and more.

Weight loss edge. Strength training is the only way to reverse the age-related loss of muscle mass and drop in metabolism that happen naturally beginning in our thirties and forties. Do nothing and you could lose 5 to 7 percent of your muscle mass per decade and see your metabolism fall by 3 to 5 percent—which means eating the same amount of food would cause weight gain. Building new muscle, in contrast, could help you burn up to 100 extra calories every time you work out, Boston University researchers estimate.

More muscle can also help you move faster during steady-pace and interval walks. Strengthening your quadriceps muscles—the long, powerful muscles in the front of your thighs—can increase your walking speed 15 percent. That's enough to take you from a 17-minute-mile to a 15-minute-mile speed. It also means going faster and farther during your interval walks so you can burn more calories without devoting more time to exercise.

We hope you make strength training a part of your exercise routine for life. For starters, it can help you maintain a lower, healthier weight. In an Arizona Cancer Center study that followed 122 midlife women for 6 years, those who strength-trained regularly were 22 percent less likely to gain weight and fat compared with those who did not.

Menopause advantage. While little or no research has looked into the specific benefits of strength training for menopausal symptoms, one benefit is obvious: help with hot flashes. Strength training has a unique ability to help you lose more belly fat. And with less of this "blanket" holding in heat, your body won't have to resort to hot flashes and night sweats to keep cool.

Health bonus. By building more muscle and using it, you can reduce insulin resistance and increase insulin sensitivity significantly—by 30 percent in one Tufts University study of midlife women. Having more active muscle on board means your body can absorb blood sugar more easily and burn stored sugar and fat with ease, too. That's great for weight loss, and it also reduces your risk for type 2 diabetes. Strength training seems to *encourage* healthy blood sugar processing.

And building strength builds a strong heart. It can help you lower your blood pressure by 3 to 5 points and rebalance your cholesterol, too. In a University of Athens study of more than 1,500 women, those who got the most resistance training and aerobic activity every week had the highest HDL and the lowest LDL and triglyceride levels. That's especially important for women; before menopause, our heart-protecting HDL is naturally higher than men's, but it tends to plummet as our hormones shift. Keeping your HDL high is as crucial for a healthy ticker as is keeping your LDL and triglyceride levels low. (For more on this essential topic, turn to Chapter 13.)

Working your muscles also tugs on your bones, creating stress that encourages healthy bone density that in turn reduces your risk for fractures. Bone loss accelerates in the first few years after your menstrual period stops permanently, so it's good to know that strength training can slow down, stop, or even reverse it. In an Italian study published in the *Journal of Aging and Health*, postmenopausal women who strength-trained three times a week for 6 months lost significantly less bone than women who didn't work out. A University of Arizona study of 140 post-menopausal women even found gains in bone density with strength training especially in women's hips, where the bones support more weight than anywhere else in your body.

WALKING + YOGA + WEIGHTS = BIGGER BENEFITS

Each element of our exercise plan is a winner. Adding them all together *multiplies* the results. For example, you'll build more muscle by strength training, then you'll use that extra muscle while you walk (and all day long as you move around). So you'll use more calories and be able to go faster during interval walks. Yoga and walking can help you sleep better *and* cool hot flashes and night sweats. That reduces stress. Less emotional stress means you're less likely to be gripped by irresistible cravings for high-fat, high-calorie foods. Lower stress levels also discourage your body from storing excess calories deep in your midsection. And reducing belly fat reduces insulin resistance, which makes weight loss easier for many women at midlife.

But don't take our word for it. Research shows that combining strategies à la Natural Menopause Solution lets you achieve the following:

Trim more belly fat. In one small but well-designed Korean study published in 2010 in the *International Journal of Sport Nutrition and Exercise Metabolism*, women who walked and performed a simple strength-training routine 3 days a week slimmed their midsections 25 percent more than those who just walked. In a study of 112 postmeno-pausal women at Wake Forest University in North Carolina, those who followed a weight loss diet and exercised lost 27 percent of their abdominal fat—more than those who just dieted.

Reverse insulin resistance further. Perhaps because they lost more deep abdominal fat, women in the Wake Forest study got the biggest decreases in their insulin levels—a sign that their bodies had become more insulin-sensitive. As you discovered in Chapter 2, improving insulin sensitivity goes hand in hand with improvements in fat-burning in your muscle cells and can translate into better weight loss results.

Improve cholesterol and blood pressure numbers the most. Compared with walkers, the women in the Korean study mentioned above who performed a combined walking and strength routine also saw bigger increases in heart-protecting HDL cholesterol, bigger decreases in heart-threatening triglycerides (a blood fat), and bigger reductions in blood pressure, too.

Build more muscle. Reining in the calories you eat is the best way to lose weight. After all, opting for a grilled-chicken salad instead of a bacon cheeseburger could save you hundreds of calories, while burning off 500 calories would require more than an hour of extra walking. But adding exercise to the equation ensures that you'll lose more of that weight as body fat and at the same time build your supply of toned, metabolism-boosting muscle. That's important, because muscle burns about three times as many calories as fat all day long. In one University of Rhode Island study, women who followed a strength-training routine and a healthy weight loss diet increased their muscle mass slightly and lost more fat, while the diet-only group lost precious muscle mass. And in a study at the University of Pittsburgh, women who dieted without exercising lost three times more lean body mass (which includes muscle) than those who added a walking routine.

Crave-proof your appetite every day. Vigorous aerobic exercise *plus* strength training reduce levels of the body's "I'm hungry, let's eat" hormone, ghrelin, report researchers from Loughborough University in the United Kingdom in the *American Journal of Physiology— Regulatory, Integrative and Comparative Physiology.* Either one alone helps, but researchers at the University of Nebraska have found that getting both on a regular basis (as you will in the 30-Day Slim-Down, Cool-Down Diet) helps control cravings and over-the-top hunger far better. Exercise also controls hunger and cravings by raising levels of the appetite-suppressing hormone peptide YY. If you've had trouble with not feeling full after meals, exercise has another special talent that can help you: In the online journal *PLoS Biology*, Brazilian researchers reported recently that aerobic exercise can also make brain cells involved with appetite regulation more sensitive to your body's "I'm full" hormone, leptin. Since you'll alternate between vigorous interval walks and our strength-building yoga-with-weights routine, you'll get a daily dose of protection against cravings.

THE PLAN THAT FITS YOUR LIFE

If you're anything like us, you know from experience that starting an exercise plan is easy. But after a few weeks, the demands of everyday life start to get in the way. Thanks to our time-saving interval walks and to our multitasking yoga/strength-training routine, you'll get great results in as little as 40 minutes a day. But time-saving moves are just one reason that this is *the* plan you can stick with. You'll also love it for these reasons.

- **Offers anytime, anyplace ease.** You can walk on vacation, on your lunch hour, and even before diving into a shopping expedition at the mall. With an inexpensive mat and a set of light hand weights, our yoga-with-weights routine goes anywhere, too. All you need is a patch of floor in a quiet room. This flexibility breeds success: Stanford University researchers found in one study of midlife women (and men), published in the journal *Circulation*, that new exercisers who did their workouts at home were 45 percent more likely to stick with it for a year than were those who had to travel to a gym.

- **Is gentle on your joints and muscles.** Staying injury free means more time for exercise, less lost to recovery. That makes walking, yoga, and light-weight strength training a brilliant choice. Walking exerts one-half to two-thirds *less* force on impact with every step than running does. Injury rates are eight times lower, too. And you can do our easy yoga moves at any age and at any weight, even if you're not particularly flexible.

- **Fits your budget.** You can outfit yourself for the complete Natural Menopause Solution exercise program even on a tight budget—good news if you're trying to save money. Wondering whether spending more gets you more? Not necessarily. Budget-priced shoes were rated as good as or sometimes superior to expensive models for support and comfort in one study published in the *British Journal of Sports Medicine.*

- **Makes you feel great.** While almost any form of exercise gives you a postworkout emotional lift, walking makes you feel good while you're doing it—and the benefits begin within minutes, report University of Illinois researchers in a study published in the *Journal of Behavioral Medicine.* Meanwhile, as we've already learned, yoga increases levels of GABA in the brain, helping to lift depression and anxiety. When exercise feels this good, you can't wait to do it again!

GET READY: THE GEAR GUIDE

A little preparation will help you get the most from your walking and yoga routines and will let you feel terrific doing them. You only need a few pieces of gear, some of which you may already have.

Walking shoes. If you make one investment in your health for this program, make it affordable shoes that are designed specifically for the type of walking you'll be doing most often. A good pair of walking shoes can cost from $60 to $120, but don't make the expensive mistake of thinking that a higher price means a better shoe. In one study from the University of Dundee in Scotland, testers rated a midpriced shoe as good as or better than an expensive model for support, cushioning, and comfort.

But don't just pull your latest pair of sneakers out from under the bed. Real walking shoes can help you prevent injury, avoid pain, and stay comfy because they're built to support the heel-toe motion of walking. The rounded or beveled heel and the extra heel cushioning in a walking shoe help you roll smoothly through your step, propelling you forward. (In contrast, running shoes have more cushioning at the midfoot because runners' feet strike the ground in a more flat-footed way. If you already have running shoes, though, or plan to run as well as walk, it's fine to use a running shoe for walking.) We don't, however, recommend using toning walking shoes for your workout.

It's smart to buy walking shoes in person rather than online so that you can try them on. Come with your socks (read on for recommendations from our walking expert Michele Stanten), visit a specialty store to have access to a wider variety of walking shoes (and a better chance to snap up some good deals during sales or end-of-season clearance events), and shop in the evening when your feet are biggest. You're sure to get the most comfortable fit that way. Ask to have your feet measured—more birthdays, more pounds, and childbearing can all lead to a larger foot size, so don't assume that the size 8 you wore when you were 25 is still your size. And because athletic shoes are sometimes sized a little differently from everyday shoes, be ready to try on a bigger or smaller size if a style you like doesn't fit right.

You're almost done—but not quite. Once you've narrowed your choices to just a few, give 'em a whirl. Many walking and running shoe stores have an in-house treadmill you can use to test-drive your selections. If they don't, ask if you can walk outside for a test walk. At the very least, walk around the store. The right shoe should feel good right

Quick Tip
WALKING IN A WINTER WONDERLAND

Find a way to walk in winter—at home, at a shopping mall, on a treadmill at the gym. Or you can choose a day when the skies and sidewalks are clear. Just be sure to bundle up and slip on a pair of ice grippers (such as Yaktrax) in case you hit an icy patch outdoors. In one Vanderbilt University study, women were the least active in December, January, and February—burning a whopping 10 percent fewer calories per day than they did in the summer.

out of the box and without a break-in period. If a shoe pinches, rubs, or slips at the heel, it's not the walking shoe for you.

Walking socks. Forget about those old cotton ankle socks in the back of your drawer. Socks made from a synthetic wicking material keep your feet dry, comfortable, and blister free and are worth getting at $3 to $12 per pair. Fabrics recommended by Michele include CoolMax, Dri-Fit, and a lightweight wool developed for active use such as Icebreaker and SmartWool. Newer socks may combine more than one of these materials for even better performance.

Be sure to check the sock size—socks that are too tight can cause blister problems, while socks that are too big can bunch up. And you may want to look into special features available in some "performance" socks, such as extra padding in the heel and at the ball of the foot for walkers; extra-thin socks that keep your feet cool; odor control; blister protection via special gels embedded in the material; and rumple-free, anatomically correct socks designed to fit your left and right feet.

Comfortable, weather-appropriate clothing. A T-shirt and a pair of stretchy shorts, sweatpants, or yoga pants are all the gear you'll need for walks and our yoga routine. Add sunglasses and a hat with a brim to keep the sun off your face and out of your eyes. For outdoor walks in cool weather, add a jacket. In rain, make it a breathable waterproof jacket with a brim on the hood, or wear a waterproof hat with a brim to keep rain out of your eyes. You may want to invest in two pairs of walking shoes if you plan to walk outdoors in all weather so that one can dry out completely. This helps prevent blisters, smelly feet, and fungal infections.

What about a sports bra? It's optional, but you may want one for walks and for your yoga routine. Up to 60 percent of women experience breast pain during exercise, something that the correct support can alleviate. Look for a sports bra made from a wicking material so you stay cool and comfortable. In one British study, sports bras with separate, molded cups were best at reducing pain. And this type of sports bra stops motion in all directions, not just up and down. Straps that adjust in the front make adjustments easier. And be sure it's not too tight—if it restricts your breathing, it's not the bra for you. *(continued on page 164)*

Happier and Healthier...
THE NATURAL MENOPAUSE SOLUTION WAY

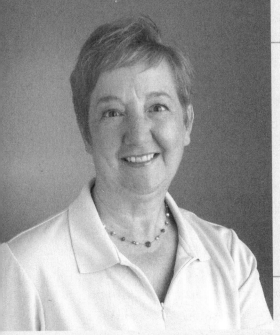

BARBARA HUNSICKER

Age: 58

Pounds lost: 6½

Inches lost: 5¼

Major changes: Ate more and exercised less but still lost 2¼ inches from her waist. Lowered total cholesterol and body-fat percentage.

"Interval Walking Got Me Pumped and Moving"

Barbara's clothes are "a tad looser." She feels "thinner and more upright." And even her massage therapist noticed the difference. "I am totally thrilled with the results," she says. "On this program I exercised for less time than usual. I ate more food than I would on other diets. And I still lost over 6 pounds in a month—great for a body that doesn't like to give up weight easily!"

She credits the Flash-Fighting Four in the eating plan and the energizing interval walks for her unprecedented success. "Normally I'll stick with

1,200 calories, but this time I was eating 1,500 calories in Phase 2 and losing more weight than in the past. Something was better this time. The interval walks really got me pumped and moving."

Barbara enjoyed a Slimming, Cooling Smoothie every day and even brought her smoothies on a trip to visit her son in Washington, DC. "I made up a batch and stored the container in a thermal bag with ice. It kept beautifully," she recalls. In fact, she loved the smoothies so much that she decided to keep them in her daily menus after the program ended. "I've already had one this morning," Barbara notes a week after the test panel ended. "The dairy and the almond butter in the recipe are so satisfying. It also makes a very filling afternoon snack."

Another portable favorite was the Pita Pizza. "It travels well. Just make the turkey topping ahead of time and add when you're ready to eat." She also discovered that she could translate the principles of the diet—plenty of produce, lean protein, good fats, and low-fat or fat-free dairy—into meals away from home. "If I was out golfing, I could order a salad with salmon for lunch."

Already a dedicated walker, Barbara found the 20-minute interval walks challenging at the beginning. "I carried a little timer with me to time the intervals," she says. "At first I did a 20-minute interval walk. The first few minutes were a brisk warmup, then every 30 seconds there was a rapid burst. I walked really fast, then would calm down to my regular but still brisk pace for the next 30 seconds, then I'd do another fast burst. It was difficult at first, but by the last week I was doing the full 30 minutes at an even brisker pace."

The intensity of the intervals led to a weight loss breakthrough. "I've been a walker for a long time—it's what I turn to first for fitness," Barbara says. "I really liked the intensity of the interval walking. I think it's a big reason I lost weight. In the past I would walk briskly for 45 to 60 minutes and lose 1 to 2 pounds in a month—nothing like the 6 pounds I lost on this plan. I'll definitely keep this up!"

A timer. You'll need a watch with a second hand, a sports watch with a timer, or another timing device to keep you on track during your interval walks. Carrying one means you'll always know when it's time to start a fast-paced interval and when it's time to slow down. A wristwatch with a second hand may be all you need, or you may prefer a sports watch that allows you to preprogram your interval length. When you hit Start, some models will beep to let you know when to start and stop.

A yoga mat. Whether you spend $15 or $150, a good yoga mat cushions you from a hard floor (and prevents rug burns!), giving you more support than a carpet. And rubbery, nonslip mats make your yoga routine easier, safer, and more comfortable. Mats come in many colors, designs, and materials, so pick one you'll enjoy.

Two-pound weights. Dumbbells or hand weights are great for building strength. You'll need a pair of 2-pound weights on Day 6 of the yoga-with-weights routine. After Day 15, you have the option of moving up to slightly heavier weights (such as 3-, 4-, or 5-pound weights) if you can easily perform the routine with 2-pound weights. You can find dumbbells in many discount stores: Some have a grippy rubber coating; others are bare metal. Choose a set that you like and that fits your budget. Hold off on buying the heavier weights until you see how challenging the routine is with the 2-pound dumbbells.

You may also want to keep a blanket or two and/or a bolster or a cushion (or two) on hand during the yoga routine, in case you need to add support so that every pose feels comfortable.

PUTTING IT ALL TOGETHER

Okay, we've convinced you that each element of the exercise plan will help you lose weight, ease menopause symptoms, and stay healthy. You've collected all the gear you need, and now you're ready to get moving! Like the eating plan, the 30-day program is divided into two phases. You'll gradually increase time and intensity with each phase and see the benefits increase, too. Here's what you'll be doing.

Phase 1: Days 1–5

◆ **Follow the 20-minute yoga routine every day.** In Phase 1, you'll do the routine without weights so that you can experience the stress-soothing benefits and become familiar with the 11 flowing moves.

◆ **Walk for 20 to 30 minutes at a brisk pace on 3 days.** Tie up your walking shoes and hit the sidewalk, the trails at your favorite local park, or the treadmill. You'll burn calories, reduce stress, and energize.

Phase 2a: Days 6–14

◆ **Add 2-pound weights to your yoga routine on alternate days.** Small weights yield muscle-building, metabolism-revving benefits when you combine them with your yoga moves. Use weights on the days you do your steady-paced walks; on days that you do your interval walks, continue to do the routine without weights.

◆ **Take a 20-minute interval walk every other day.** After warming up, you'll alternate 30 seconds of fast walking with 30 seconds of recovery time (still a brisk pace), to burn more calories and fat.

◆ **Continue your 20- to 30-minute steady-paced walks on alternate days.** You may choose to step up the pace a little bit, but keep these to a relatively easy speed. You'll do three or four of these walks each week.

Phase 2b: Days 15–30

◆ **Build more muscle.** If you'd like, now's the time to increase the weight you're using in the yoga-with-weights routine. In moves where you hold your weight in just one hand, try holding both weights instead of only one. Or move up to 3-, 4-, or 5-pound weights. You'll also find new variations on several poses that challenge your muscles a little more.

- ◆ **Walk a little longer.** If you've been taking 20-minute interval walks, now's the time to increase your walking time to 30 minutes. It's always fine to go even longer in both the interval walks and the steady-paced walks, but you don't have to. Test panelists got impressive results in just 20 to 30 minutes, and you can, too.

Important note: While these routines are safe and gentle enough for nearly every woman, lifting weights and working at the higher intensity of an interval walk may not be right for you if you have a chronic medical condition or are more than 20 pounds overweight. Be sure to discuss the workout details with your doctor first if you have arthritis, asthma, diabetes, heart disease, high blood pressure, or osteoporosis (brittle bones). Call now—and continue getting ready so

Is a Morning or an Evening Workout Better?

When Art Mollen, DO, a family and preventive medicine doctor in Phoenix, Arizona, asked 500 patients about their exercise habits, he made a dramatic discovery: Three out of four morning exercisers were still working out a year later, compared with half who exercised at lunchtime and just 25 percent who exercised at the end of the day.

But is morning exercise always better? Maybe not. In a recent Italian study, after 12 weeks of walking, evening walkers shed nearly 4 pounds of fat, seven times more than those who walked in the morning.

So what's best? It's really all about your schedule and your likes and dislikes. If you just can't imagine working out at 6:00 a.m. but are perfectly happy to tie up your walking shoes or roll out your yoga mat at 6:00 p.m., go for it. The best exercise time is the one that suits you best.

that when you get the thumbs-up to do the full routine, or even part of it, you can jump right in.

See pages 168–169 for a day-by-day calendar that shows you how the different components of the exercise program can work together.

THE WALKING PROGRAM

You'll walk 5 to 6 days per week on the Natural Menopause Solution exercise plan. In Phase 1, you start with a simple, steady-paced walk just to get you moving. But keep in mind that this shouldn't just be a stroll around the park! While you don't need to push yourself to walk so fast that you're sweating or panting, you do want to make some effort to keep up a brisk pace. And don't forget to warm up and cool down! Launching into a fast walk without warming up your muscles could lead to an injury. Cooling down helps your heart rate return to normal before you stop exercising. See the chart below for some guidance on how this works.

STEADY-PACED WALK

TIME	ACTIVITY	INTENSITY*	WHAT IT FEELS LIKE
1–2 min	Easy, leisurely stroll	3–5	Light effort, rhythmic breathing; you can sing.
2–3 min	Moderate, purposeful pace	5–6	Some effort, breathing somewhat hard; you can talk in full sentences.
15–25 min	Brisk pace, as if you were in a bit of a hurry	6–7	Hard effort, slightly breathless; you can speak only in brief phrases.
2–5 min	Easy, leisurely stroll	3–5	Light effort, rhythmic breathing; you can sing.

*Intensity is how hard the activity feels for you, with 1 being extremely light and 10 being as hard as you can push yourself.

In Phase 2, you'll alternate between steady-paced walks and interval walking. What's an interval walk? Instead of keeping a steady pace after you warm up, you'll alternate 30 seconds of fast walking with 30 seconds

(continued on page 170)

The Natural Menopause Solution

DAY 1	DAY 2	DAY 3	DAY 4	
Yoga (no weights) Walk (20–30 min at a steady pace)	Yoga (no weights)	Yoga (no weights) Walk (20–30 min at a steady pace)	Yoga (no weights)	
DAY 8	**DAY 9**	**DAY 10**	**DAY 11**	
Interval walk (20 min) Yoga (no weights)	Yoga (with weights) Walk (20–30 min at a steady pace)	Interval walk (20 min) Yoga (no weights)	Yoga (with weights) Walk (20–30 min at a steady pace)—optional	
DAY 15	**DAY 16**	**DAY 17**	**DAY 18**	
Interval walk (20 min) Yoga (no weights)	Yoga (with weights) Walk (20–30 min at a steady pace)	Interval walk (30 min) Yoga (no weights)	Yoga (with weights) Walk (20–30 min at a steady pace)—optional	
DAY 22	**DAY 23**	**DAY 24**	**DAY 25**	
Rest	Yoga (with weights) Walk (20–30 min at a steady pace)	Interval walk (30 min) Yoga (no weights)	Yoga (with weights) Walk (20–30 min at a steady pace)—optional	
DAY 29	**DAY 30**			
Yoga (with weights) Walk (20–30 min at a steady pace)	Interval walk (30 min) Yoga (no weights)			

WORKOUT CALENDAR

DAY 5	DAY 6	DAY 7
Yoga (no weights) Walk (20–30 min at a steady pace)	Rest	Yoga (with weights) Walk (20–30 min at a steady pace)

DAY 12	DAY 13	DAY 14
Interval walk (20 min) Yoga (no weights)	Yoga (with weights) Walk (20–30 min at a steady pace)	Rest

DAY 19	DAY 20	DAY 21
Interval walk (30 min) Yoga (no weights)	Yoga (with weights) Walk (20–30 min at a steady pace)	Interval walk (30 min) Yoga (no weights)

DAY 26	DAY 27	DAY 28
Interval walk (30 min) Yoga (no weights)	Yoga (with weights) Walk (20–30 min at a steady pace)	Interval walk (30 min) Yoga (no weights)

of moderate/easy walking (if you graphed your speed, it would look like a series of peaks and valleys). Research shows that this method can increase your calorie burn by as much as 100 percent during your workout and afterward. The following chart shows how the different segments of the walk fit together:

INTERVAL WALK

TIME	ACTIVITY	INTENSITY*	WHAT IT FEELS LIKE
1–2 min	Easy, leisurely stroll	3–5	Light effort, rhythmic breathing; you can sing.
2–3 min	Moderate, purposeful pace	5–6	Some effort, breathing somewhat hard; you can speak in full sentences.
Intervals: Alternate for 15–25 min depending on the length of your workout			
30 sec	Fast pace, as if you were late for an appointment	7–8	Very hard effort, breathless; yes/no responses are all you can manage.
30 sec	Brisk pace, as if you were in a bit of a hurry	6–7	Hard effort, slightly breathless; you can speak only in short phrases.
2–5 min	Easy, leisurely stroll	3–5	Light effort, rhythmic breathing; you can sing.

*Intensity is how hard the activity feels for you, with 1 being extremely light and 10 being as hard as you can push yourself.

THE YOGA ROUTINE

Remember, in Phase 1, do this workout without weights. After a rest day, you'll start Phase 2 and add 2-pound dumbbells for most moves. On alternate days you'll do the routine with and without the weights—it's important to give your muscles a day off between weight workouts so they can recover and become stronger. The 2-pound weights may feel too light at first, but if you concentrate on doing the repetitions slowly, you'll work plenty hard. On Day 16, you can increase the weights you're using if you feel you're ready for more of a challenge—go from 2 to 3 pounds, for example, but don't jump to a much heavier weight because that could cause injury. You can also add a "Muscle Move" to get even more muscle-building benefit from many poses.

As you become familiar with the poses, start moving from one to the next without stopping so that they flow together like a dance. We've included tips on how to make them flow. Take it slow; you may need a few days or weeks to achieve this connection. You may find some moves are easier to link in a flowing way, and it's perfectly okay to stop between poses and reposition yourself for the next one without flowing at all if you prefer.

Caution: If you have a back, neck, or spinal injury or other problem, or if your knees, hips, shoulders, or other joints are injured or in pain, consult your doctor before doing this routine.

Pose 1: Find Your Focus

Sit cross-legged on a mat. With eyes closed, take three deep breaths—in through your nose and out through your mouth.

Make it more comfortable: If one or both of your knees feel too stiff for you to sit comfortably in a cross-legged pose, place one or more blankets, cushions, or bolsters on the floor under your knee, or knees, for support. You can also sit on the blanket or cushion to lift your torso and allow your hips to open.

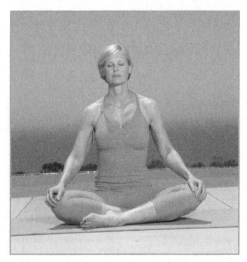

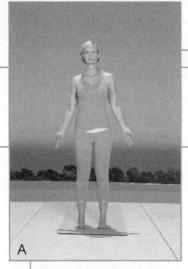

A

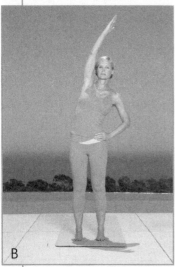

B

Pose 2: Standing Forward Bend

1. Stand at the front of a mat, feet hip-width apart (A). If you're doing the workout with weights, place dumbbells a few inches in front of your feet.

2. Reach your right arm up, stretching your right side, for one breath (B).

3. Repeat on your left side.

4. Hinge forward from your hips, bringing your chest toward your knees (C).

5. Bend your knees slightly. Hold each elbow with the opposite hand (D). Gently shake your head from side to side. Stay bent forward for 45 seconds.

6. Slowly roll up to standing (A). If you're using weights, pick them up as you stand.

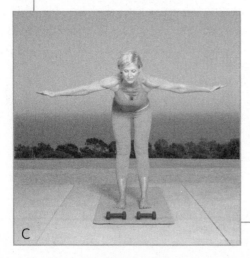

C

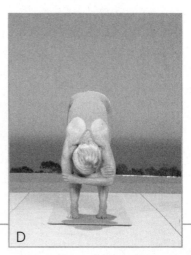

D

Pose 3: Chair Pose with Shoulder Press

1. Step your feet together and reach your arms above your head, palms facing in. If you're using weights, you'll be holding them directly over your shoulders.

2. Bend your knees and sink your hips back, as though you were about to sit in a chair (A).

3. Slowly bend your elbows at right angles, lowering your upper arms to shoulder height and turning palms forward (B). If you're using weights, be sure to keep your wrists straight.

4. Straighten your arms overhead. Repeat 5 times.

5. Bring your hands back to your shoulders and straighten your knees to return to standing position.

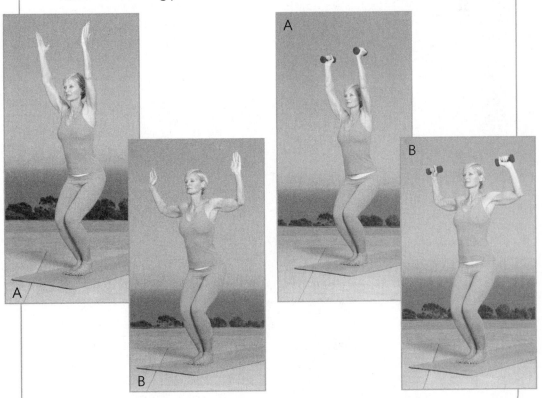

Pose 4: Warrior 2 with Mini Lift

1. From the standing position, step your left leg back 3 to 4 feet and bend your right knee.

2. Straighten your arms, still at shoulder height, with your right arm forward and left arm back and your palms down. If you're using weights, be sure to keep your wrists straight.

3. Lift your arms 4 to 5 inches. Hold for 10 seconds, then lower. Do 5 times.

   Muscle Move: *From the standing position, add 5 slow biceps curls before you begin the mini lift, bending your elbows and bringing your hands toward your shoulders.*

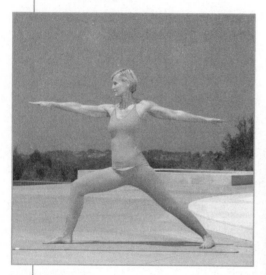

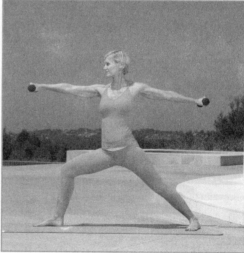

Pose 5: Side-Angle Pose with Lat Row

1. From Warrior 2, bring your right elbow to your right knee. Reach your left hand inside your right shin, your chest facing the floor (A). If you're using weights, keep one dumbbell in your left hand, but place the one in your right hand on the floor in front of you.

2. Slowly bend your left elbow up toward your chest, turning your torso to the side (B). If you're using weights, keep your wrist straight and the dumbbell in front of you. Hold for 10 seconds.

3. Lower your left elbow back to the starting position. Do 5 times.

4. Bring your hands to your shoulders and step forward with your left leg to meet your right. If you're using weights, pick up the dumbbell with your right hand. Repeat Warrior 2 and Side-Angle Pose on the opposite side.

Muscle Move: *At the top of each row, straighten your left arm, extending your hand toward the ceiling.*

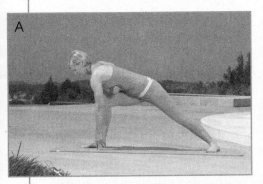

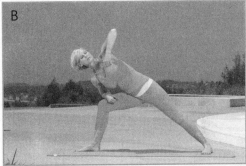

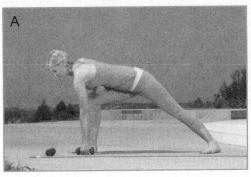

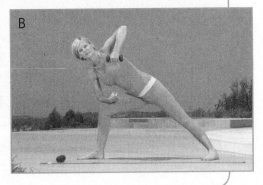

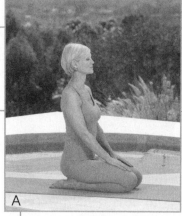

A

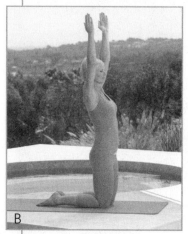

B

Pose 6: Hero Pose with Arm Raise

1. Kneel with your butt resting on your heels, your hands on top of your thighs, palms down (A). If you're using weights, rest them on your thighs.

2. Slowly lift your hips so that your body is in a straight line from your knees to your head. At the same time, raise your hands toward the ceiling with straight arms (B). If you're using weights, keep your palms facing forward.

3. Slowly lower to the starting position. Do 5 times.

Make it more comfortable: Kneel on a folded blanket (placed over your mat). If your knees are stiff and you can't sit comfortably on top of your feet, place a yoga block or a thick book on the floor between your feet (spread your feet and lower legs apart to make room), and sit on that. If your ankles hurt, roll up a towel and slide it under your ankles before you sit.

Tip: Don't swing the weights as you move up and down. Use your quadriceps muscles (the large muscles at the front of your thighs) to pull your body forward and up and to slowly lower your body.

A

B

Pose 7: Seated Wide-Angle Pose

1. Sit on the mat with your legs extended wide, your left hand behind your left hip. If you're using weights, put down the dumbbell in your left hand. Bend your right elbow to shoulder height (A).

2. Reach your right arm overhead and to the left (B). If you're using weights, keep your palm facing in.

3. Return to upright, bending your right elbow to shoulder height. If you're using weights, turn your palm to face forward. Do 5 times. Repeat on opposite side.

   Muscle Move: *Hold both weights in your working hand.*

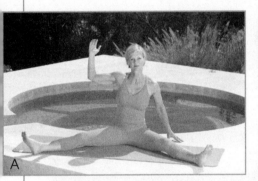

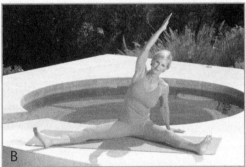

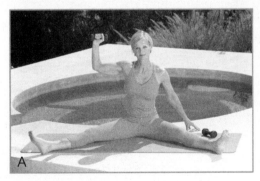

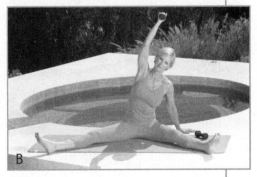

Pose 8: Cobbler Pose with Chest Fly

1. Sit on the mat and bring the soles of your feet together, knees wide.

2. Raise your arms and bend your elbows at right angles in front of your chest, forearms together, palms facing in (A). If you're using weights, hold one in each hand.

3. Keeping the bend in your elbows, open your arms out to the sides (B). If you're using weights, they should be facing forward. Remember to keep your shoulders relaxed and draw your shoulder blades down and together.

4. Hold for 10 seconds, then return to starting position. Do 5 times.

   Muscle Move: *After each rep, lift your hands 2 to 3 inches. Hold for 10 seconds.*

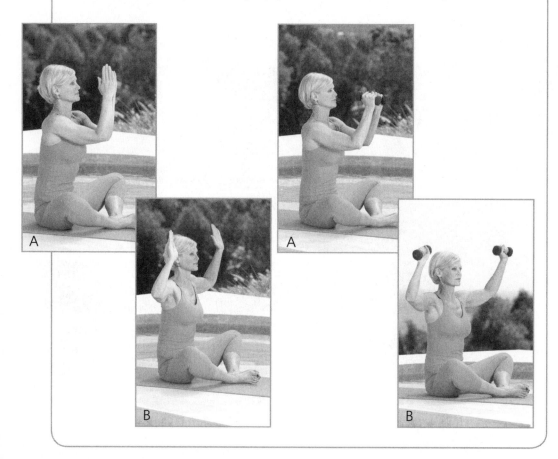

Pose 9: Bridge with Lift

1. Lie on your back with your knees bent and your feet on the mat, hip-width apart.

2. Extend your arms along your hips, palms down (A). If you're using weights, rest the dumbbells on the floor.

3. Raise your hips off the floor.

4. Raise your arms up, then overhead (B). If you're using weights, they will be facing the ceiling.

5. Lower your hips and arms, and return to starting position. Do 3 times.

   Muscle Move: *Lift your arms and hips at the same time.*

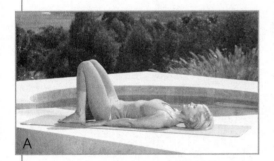

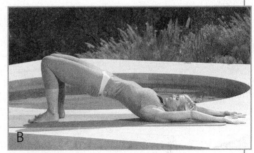

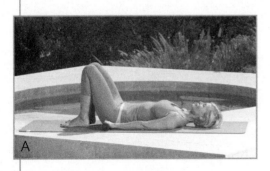

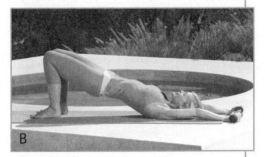

Pose 10: Spine Twist

1. Lie on your back and bend your right knee toward your chest, holding your shin with your left hand, your left leg extended on the mat. If you've been using weights, put them down.

2. Keeping your right shoulder down, twist your hips to the left and bring your right knee toward the floor. Extend your right arm, and turn your head to look over your right shoulder. Hold for 45 seconds. Remember to take deep abdominal breaths while you hold the pose.

3. Return to center. Repeat on opposite side.

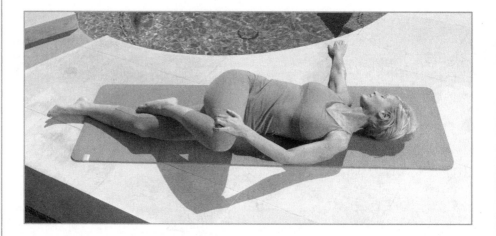

Pose 11: Corpse Pose

1. Lie with your legs extended and arms at your sides, palms up. Take a few deep breaths, then relax all the muscles of your face and body in this position for 2 minutes, breathing naturally.

2. Roll onto your side and gently use your arms to push yourself up to a seated position. Take a second to notice how you feel.

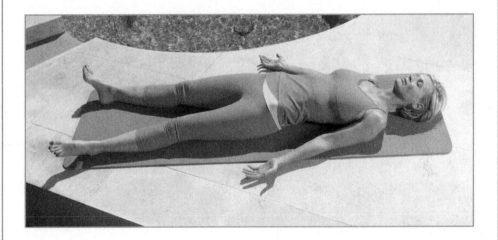

Part III

Natural Menopause Solutions

Chapter 7

Hot Flashes

*F*lushing. Flashing. Power surge. Night sweats. Personal summer. The lexicon for hot flashes is as varied as the women they affect. And while hot flashes *are*, without a doubt, the most troublesome symptom of menopause—and the most common menopause symptom to send women to their doctor's office—they are by no means unavoidable. Some women (the lucky ones!) never feel the first warm tingling. Others spend their days shucking out of sweaty clothes, adding and removing layers, standing in front of fans, and flapping their arms so often you'd think they were ready to take off. Overall, about three out of four women over age 50 will experience hot flashes (or the more scientific term, *vasomotor symptoms*).

What determines whether you experience this milestone of menopause lies partly in your weight (overweight women are more likely to experience hot flashes), your ancestry (African American and Latino women tend to have the most flashes, Asian women the least), and your diet and lifestyle (if you're a yoga aficionada, you may be spared the worst; if you smoke, get ready to sweat). The good news is that their time in your life is limited. Most women suffer with the flashes for just 6 months to a year around the menopausal transition. And only about 10 percent report symptoms for 10 or more years post-menopause.

We wish we could tell you exactly what causes hot flashes and exactly how to banish them. Unfortunately, even the experts in the field still haven't figured out the underlying cause, although they do know that estrogen loss alone doesn't fully explain them. Still, they have lots of theories, including the following:

- **The "shrinking thermometer" theory.** This theory suggests that changes in the amount of hormones like serotonin, norepinephrine, and estrogen "condense" your internal thermometer, so there is less difference between the temperature needed to make you shiver and the one that makes you sweat.

- **The "type of estrogen" theory.** This hypothesis says that changes in the amount of the two primary types of estrogen in your blood—estrone, the weaker form of estrogen, and its stronger sister, estradiol—trigger the flashes. Postmenopausal women have more estrone than estradiol, while premenopausal women have more estradiol than estrone.

- **The "estrogen isn't working right" theory.** In this theory, estrogen simply doesn't bind properly to the cellular receptors, and even when it does, it doesn't have the desired effect on the cell.

But really, does it matter exactly *why* you're flashing? All you really want to know is how to cool yourself, preferably without resorting to hormones (although if hormones are what it takes, we get it; see page 206 for more on what you should know about hormone therapy—and other medications—for hot flashes).

Turns out there are several options that go beyond hormones. Some are lifestyle changes, but some involve complementary and alternative medicine (CAM) such as herbs, vitamins, and mind/body techniques.

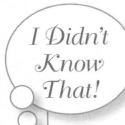

I Didn't Know That!

THE BENEFIT OF HOT FLASHES

Sometimes hot flashes can be more than just an annoyance; sometimes they may serve as an early warning sign that could actually save your life or as a sign that you're on the right track healthwise.

Breast cancer. A study published in the journal *Cancer Epidemiology, Biomarkers & Prevention* found that women who had the most severe hot flashes and other menopausal symptoms like insomnia and mood changes had a 50 percent lower risk for developing two types of breast cancer—invasive ductal carcinoma, the most common form of the disease, and a less common but more dangerous type: invasive lobular cancer. Given that the typical 50-year-old woman's risk of breast cancer is 2 percent, that means the severe hot flashes, vaginal dryness, and so on, drop the risk to 1 percent. The reason? More severe symptoms mean a more abrupt drop in estrogen levels. Since estrogen fuels breast cancer cell growth, less estrogen means less fuel for cancer cells.

That doesn't mean, however, that just because you have hot flashes from hell, you can skip your next mammogram. Your risk of breast cancer increases with age regardless of your midlife symptoms, so get screened! Learn more in Chapter 15.

Heart disease. From the landmark WHI trial comes evidence that women who experience hot flashes at the beginning of menopause have a lower risk of developing heart disease or having a stroke. Conversely, women whose flashes didn't begin until late in menopause had an increased risk of heart disease and death from any cause, while those who had hot

If you've tried such options, you're not alone. Middle-aged women turn to CAM in droves to help manage their menopausal symptoms, particularly hot flashes. In one survey of 423 women, 91 percent used

flashes throughout perimenopause had no increased risk of heart disease, stroke, or death, according to the study published in the journal *Menopause*. The changes in risk weren't huge—about an 11 percent reduced risk in heart disease and a 17 percent reduced risk in stroke for the early-hot-flashes group—but they were still significant.

The reason? Since hot flashes may be the result of dilating blood vessels in response to hormone fluctuations, flashes late in menopause—after hormone levels have adjusted—may signal a problem with your blood vessels that could affect your heart. So if you're a year or more from menopause and still flashing, consider it a warning sign. Make sure you're doing all you can to keep your heart healthy, including maintaining a healthy weight, eating right, and exercising; and talk to your doctor about your risk for heart disease and stroke. For more on postmenopausal heart health, see Chapter 13.

Osteoporosis. A study from Turkish researchers published in the *International Journal of Obstetrics and Gynecology* in late 2009 compared the bone density and menopausal symptoms of 70 perimenopausal women ages 45 to 55. The researchers found that women with hot flashes had far lower bone density regardless of their age, with nearly a third of women who experienced hot flashes having a bone density that put them at significant risk for osteoporosis. Other studies, including one of 5,600 women, found similar results.

The message is that, if you experience hot flashes even before you officially hit menopause, make doubly sure to get enough calcium, vitamin D, and physical activity to maintain the bone you have. Also, have your bone density tested, and ask your doctor if you need bone-building medication. More on maintaining healthy bones in Chapter 16.

CAM—primarily vitamins, relaxation techniques, yoga, meditation, and/ or prayer. A similar survey of 563 menopausal women who stopped taking hormones after the Women's Health Initiative (WHI) results were released found that nearly half used CAM, primarily vitamins and calcium, black cohosh, soy foods and supplements, meditation, relaxation, evening primrose oil, and homeopathy, to handle their hot flashes.

HANDLING HOT FLASHES NOW

Now, on to the most important part of this chapter: finding relief from hot flashes. The suggestions below are all natural, easy changes you can make in your life *right now* to experience the relief you deserve.

Avoid hot flash triggers. These include hot drinks, alcohol, spicy food, and too-warm rooms. Stick to iced coffee for the duration!

Make your own breeze. How did Southern women stay cool before air-conditioning? Why, with handheld fans, of course. We suggest you do the same. Then when a hot flash threatens, you can pull it out, whip it open one-handed, and bat your eyes over the top as you create your own breeze. Another good option? A small electric or battery-operated fan that sits on your desk or attaches to your computer.

Gain control. One thing that seems to help a lot with hot flashes is gaining a sense of control over them rather than feeling as if they are controlling you. It's easy to feel as if you have no control—the flash seems to sneak up on you and take over your entire body. But simply learning more about the flashes themselves and developing coping skills with some of the approaches described here can reduce their impact and help you feel as if they are less severe even if their severity hasn't actually changed.

Check your meds. Certain medications can trigger hot flashes or make existing flashes worse. These include anti-Parkinson's drugs like Sinemet (levodopa); the migraine medication Maxalt (rizatriptan); selective estrogen receptor modulators (SERMs) such as Evista (raloxifene) and tamoxifen; calcium channel blockers such as Norvasc (amlodipine) and Plendil (felodipine); some antibiotics such as Factive (gemifloxacin) and Maxaquin (lomefloxacin); and the antiepileptic drugs Lamictal (lamotrigine) and Topamax (topiramate). If you're taking one of these medications and having hot flashes, talk to your doctor about reducing the dosage or switching to a different drug.

HANDLING NIGHT SWEATS NOW

If you grew up in a household where your mother insisted that the window in your bedroom be cracked at night—even on the most frigid February nights—then you understand the link between temperature and sleep. A cool room really does promote sleep, in part because falling body temperature tells your brain to increase production of the so-called sleep hormone, melatonin. So when hot flashes flare up in the middle of the night, it's obviously not conducive to sleep.

To beat the heat at night, here's what you do.

Sleep in the nude. Or, if you're not the birthday suit kind of gal, make sure your nightgown, sheets, and pillowcases are 100 percent cotton, which breathes and wicks away moisture from your skin. Avoid flannel, satin, and cotton/polyester blends, which trap wetness around your body. Oh, and make the sheets the highest-quality cotton you deserve. It has nothing to do with the temperature; you just deserve the best, especially around this time.

It may also help to keep a light cotton quilt at the foot of your bed. If you get the chills following a nocturnal flash, pull this over you for comfort. Other cottony items to have on hand while fighting night sweats include a short-sleeved, knee-length, all-cotton nightgown; all-cotton underwear; and a small cotton towel to wipe up the sweat. Avoid full-length nightgowns and pj's. They'll only trap heat and make you feel uncomfortable. You can even buy sleepwear made of moisture-wicking materials, the same type used for athletic clothing.

Get a fan. Just as fans help cool your daytime flashes, they can be invaluable at night, too. Whether sitting on the dresser, hanging from the ceiling, or clipped to your headboard, a fan circulates the air, drying sweat and keeping you cool.

Turn on the air conditioner (or at least turn down the heat). If your partner is too cold, sweetly suggest that he sleep in the other room for a bit or pile a blanket on his side of the bed. If you don't want to freeze out the rest of the family, close the vents in your bedroom in the winter and the vents in their rooms in the summer.

Use a "chillow." This special pillow has a foam core surrounding water to dissipate the heat from your head and eliminate the heat trapped between your skin and the pillow. You can make your own chillow with a flexible freezer pack.

PREVENTING HOT FLASHES NATURALLY

The following remedies will need weeks, not hours, to begin working, but over time they should help relieve your hot flashes.

Breathe Slowly and Deeply

Paced breathing, also called diaphragmatic breathing, involves breathing in slowly through your nose for at least 5 seconds and out slowly through your mouth for at least 5 seconds. You'll know you're doing it right if you see your abdomen rise with each breath in and feel your lungs inflate. You'll find it quite a contrast to your normal tight, tense, shallow breathing. Like other mind-body therapies, paced breathing calms the sympathetic nervous system and enhances circulation.

One study of 33 women with frequent hot flashes compared the effects of eight sessions of paced breathing training, muscle relaxation, and biofeedback. Women doing the breathing exercises had half as many hot flashes as those doing biofeedback. They also breathed more slowly overall.

The key to getting benefits from paced breathing is practice. Although the women in this study spent 15 minutes a day, twice a day, practicing paced respiration, we think you can break it into smaller time slots, say, 5 minutes at a time, six times a day. Good times to practice are when you're in the car (particularly if you're stuck in traffic), watching TV, or checking e-mail.

Focus on the Positive

Are you a catastrophic thinker? You are if, for instance, your flight is canceled and you freak out about missed meetings and a destroyed career. Or if, at the first tingle of a hot flash, you immediately focus on how miserable you're going to feel because you know—you just *know*—you're going to be drenched in a few minutes, lose your train of thought, and require an hour or more to return to your "normal" self.

What if, instead of immediately leaping to the worst possible scenario when things go wrong (like hot flashes), you focused on managing the situation? Yes, you might sweat a bit, but if you take off your sweater and pull out the handheld fan you've been carrying for just such an occasion, you can minimize the damage. Or you might silently congratulate yourself for throwing that spare blouse in your briefcase this morning. That type of thinking, British researchers found in several studies, can actually reduce the intensity of the flash. Conversely, thinking of yourself and the flash negatively can make it worse.

For instance, women with low self-esteem who thought of themselves as unattractive or dirty when they had a hot flash tended to have worse flashes. Researchers also found that using coping strategies, such as wearing cotton clothing, isn't enough to minimize the effect of the flash; you have to think positively about the strategy. So if, say, you feel dumpy wearing an all-cotton top instead of a slinky synthetic, you won't reap the potential benefits of the cotton.

So learn to think about the positives of every flush: Your skin looks better when it's flushed; it's one more step on the path to no more periods; you're burning more calories, even if just for a few minutes; and you're saving money on heating bills. If you're having trouble doing this on your own, try cognitive behavioral therapy, which involves learning the facts about your condition, challenging your previous thinking about it, and developing specific steps to handle it.

Relax . . . One Muscle at a Time

Progressive muscle relaxation involves tensing then relaxing each group of muscles in your body. Experts think it works for hot flashes by reducing release of the stress hormone norepinephrine.

British researchers studied progressive muscle relaxation in 150 women being treated for breast cancer. The women had severe hot flashes from their treatments but couldn't take hormones. The researchers assigned the women to either relaxation therapy (in which they met once with a therapist for training in deep breathing, muscle release, and guided imagery) or a discussion session about hot flashes with a nurse. The women in the training session also received audiotapes for at-home practice and did the muscle relaxation exercises at least twice a week for 20 minutes at a time. Both groups tracked their hot flashes for 3 months.

After a month, the women in the relaxation-therapy group had 20 percent fewer—and less severe—hot flashes than those in the comparison group. They also reported less distress over their flashes, which translated into an improved quality of life. By 3 months, however, there was no change in the number or severity of hot flashes between the two groups, possibly because most of the women in the relaxation group had stopped doing the exercises, researchers said.

Although this study was done in women with breast cancer, it should work just as well in menopausal women without cancer. You can learn progressive muscle relaxation through audio recordings, books, or classes. Or just try this: Lie down in a comfortable position, scrunch your forehead muscles together as tightly as you can while breathing in, and then let them all relax while you breathe out. Next, do the same with your nose and cheek muscles. Continue working your way down your body, one muscle group at a time, until you reach your toes.

Try Yoga

Who knew that Child's Pose could help return your body temperature to that of a 12-year-old? Yet a small study in 14 postmenopausal women who were having four or more moderate-to-severe hot flashes per day found that learning eight restorative yoga poses (like Child's Pose) and taking a weekly 90-minute restorative yoga class for 8 weeks led to an average one-third drop in the number of hot flashes and in their severity. Restorative yoga focuses on relaxing the body in restful postures using props such as blankets, bolsters, and straps. The poses are usually sustained for 5 to 10 minutes each, putting you in a deep state of relaxation.

Researchers think one reason for yoga's benefits is the sense of control it provides, a sense you learn to bring to the hot flash itself. As one woman said after finishing the program, "I can see a hot flash coming and say, 'Oh, yeah, I can ride this wave.'" The deep relaxation that occurs with restorative yoga also engages the parasympathetic nervous system, the part of the nervous system that controls unconscious responses such as sweating. Other types of yoga, such as Bikram, have also been shown to have similar benefits. And our Natural Menopause Solution yoga routine is a good place to start!

Mindfulness-Based Stress Reduction

Mindfulness-based stress reduction combines mindfulness meditation with yoga and other movements. It helps you focus on your body and understand how your unconscious thoughts and feelings affect your physical and emotional health. Studies have found that it can calm numerous unconscious processes in your body, such as reducing pain and lowering blood pressure, so it makes sense that it could improve your body's temperature control. Plus, it restores some of that much-needed control we've talked about.

When researchers at the University of Massachusetts Medical School in Worcester had 15 women with frequent hot flashes learn mindfulness-based stress reduction in a weekly class for 8 weeks, the women's quality of life improved overall as the severity of their hot flashes plummeted by 40 percent. It's best to learn mindfulness meditation through a class, however, rather than on your own to make sure you're doing it right. To find a program near you, go to w3.umassmed.edu/MBSR/public/searchmember.aspx.

Look into (Someone's) Eyes

We're talking hypnosis. Forget the hypnosis you've seen magicians and comics perform. The hypnosis we're referring to is performed by specially trained medical professionals, often doctors. The hypnotherapist teaches you to relax and suggests mental images to focus on during a hot flash to make you feel cooler. In other words, you learn to use your mind to control your body's reactions and to handle stress better.

In a Baylor University study of 26 breast cancer survivors who had severe hot flashes after their cancer treatments catapulted them into menopause, five sessions of hypnotherapy with a psychologist led to a 68 percent drop in hot flashes, along with less anxiety and insomnia. Preliminary data suggest hypnosis works just as well for women experiencing natural menopause.

Look for a practitioner trained in "medical hypnosis." A good source is the American Psychotherapy and Medical Hypnosis Association at www.apmha.com.

Lose a Few

It makes intuitive sense that the more excess weight you're hauling around, the hotter you'll feel—with or without menopause! And, in fact, studies have found that overweight women often have more hot flashes than healthy-weight women. This could be because excess fat traps heat, making you sweat more to cool off your body, or because the blood vessels in overweight women dilate more when they encounter heat or stress. That dilation brings more blood to the surface of the skin, making you feel hotter.

The good news, according to a study published in the *Archives of Internal Medicine* in 2010, is that losing weight could help you lose your hot flashes. Researchers at the University of California, San Francisco, put 226 overweight or obese women with an average age of 53 on an intensive weight loss program and compared them with 112 women of similar weight and age. About half the women in each group had bothersome hot flashes.

The women in the weight loss group had 1-hour sessions with nutrition, exercise, and behavioral-change experts; were supposed to get at least 200 minutes a week of physical activity like brisk walking; and were told to follow a 1,200- to 1,500-calorie-a-day diet. After 6 months, the weight loss group dropped an average of 17 pounds, while the control group lost only 4. The more weight the women lost, the more their hot flashes improved. Overall, every 11 pounds lost reduced the number of hot flashes by about a third.

The reality is that, if you're overweight or obese, you should try to lose the weight regardless of your hot flash situation. The 30-Day Slim-Down, Cool-Down Diet, in Chapters 4 and 5, can get you started. In addition to the well-known health benefits of weight loss, a bonus may be fewer hot flashes.

Hit the Gym

Even if the most exercise you've done in the past 20 years was carrying in bags of groceries from the car, it's not too late to start, particularly given the possibility that working out could cool your flashes.

Spanish researchers evaluated 48 women, ages 55 to 72, all of whom suffered similarly from hot flashes. During the study, half of them exercised 3 hours a week for a year, and half continued their couch potato ways. By the end of the study, just a third of the women who worked out still had bad hot flashes, while two-thirds of the nonexercisers still rated their symptoms as severe. The women who exercised on a regular basis also reported that they felt better overall, both physically and mentally.

This is by no means the only study to show benefits from exercise on hot flashes. A study from the American College of Sports Medicine found strength training helped slash hot flashes and headaches by 50 percent, while other studies found that it increased overall health-related quality of life. A study published in 2010 in the journal *Climacteric* evaluated the effect of exercise on 336 healthy women ages 45 to 55 and found that the more physical activity the women got, the fewer and less severe their menopausal symptoms—and half of the women had no symptoms at all! Yet another study found that aerobic exercise (think brisk walking, biking, running, dancing) reduced the severity of hot flashes in 55 percent of postmenopausal women.

Experts think exercise helps stem hot flashes in numerous ways.

◆ By helping you lose weight

◆ By enabling you to focus less on your symptoms

◆ By improving how you feel overall so you're better at handling the flashes

◆ By providing a greater sense of control

In one study of 12 menopausal women who began exercising after menopause, the women told the researchers that they felt their bodies and minds were filled with "continuous power" that would let them overcome discomfort.

As with weight loss, exercising on a regular basis is worth it for the multitude of health benefits that have nothing to do with hot flashes. But maybe the need for relief from your flashes will provide that extra bit of motivation for you to lace up your running shoes. Just make sure you check out our exercise program developed especially for midlife women like you, on page 146.

NATURAL TREATMENTS WORTH TRYING

The evidence behind the following natural treatments is mixed, but we still think these are worth trying if you don't want to move on to medications.

Soy Foods and Supplements

If you like tofu, edamame, and miso; prefer soy milk to cream in your coffee; and sub out ground beef for TSP (textured soy protein), you're in luck. There's a good chance that your love of this low-fat protein may protect you from hot flashes. We say "may" because the studies on soy as a hot flash cooler are all over the place.

The thinking that soy may help with menopausal symptoms came from observations that women in Asian countries—who consume a *lot* of soy—were less likely to have hot flashes. The first study was published in 1995; since then, according to functional-foods expert Mark Messina, PhD, more than 50 clinical trials have been conducted evaluating the vegetable protein's role in menopause. Dr. Messina, who now owns a nutritional consulting company, launched much of the research into the anticancer properties of soy while a program director with the National Cancer Institute.

Soy contains powerful estrogen-like compounds called phytoestrogens, which bind to estrogen receptors and mimic some of estrogen's effects in your body. The most prevalent phytoestrogens in soy are the isoflavones genistein, daidzein, and glycitein. Daidzein is believed to be the one with the greatest impact.

After eating soy, certain bacteria in your gut convert daidzein into an estrogen-like compound called S-equol. Experts believe that this compound binds to receptors on cells that are typically reserved for estrogen. Think of receptors as a lock and estrogen as the key; when estrogen binds to the receptors, it "opens up" the cell for the hormonal activity of estrogen. So if S-equol is able to bind to the cell in place of your now-missing estrogen, it can trigger those same processes. This is all still speculative, of course.

But we do know from studies in Japanese women that those who produce S-equol after eating soy have fewer and milder menopausal symptoms than women whose bodies make less S-equol. How much your body produces depends both on the type of bacteria in your large intestine and on the amount of soy you eat, but researchers estimate that about half of Asians and about a third of people of North American and

European descent can make S-equol. Supplements of equol (the synthetic equivalent to the S-equol your body makes) are even being marketed as an alternative to soy.

In a study presented in October 2010 at the North American Menopause Society (NAMS) annual meeting, equol supplements cut hot flashes by 50 percent or more for up to 42 percent of women who tried them. Equol also relieved muscle and joint pain and showed evidence that it may help maintain bone density.

What about other soy isoflavones? In one review of 14 studies, all of which compared hot flashes in women taking isoflavone supplements with those taking placebos, 3 studies found that the women taking iso-

The Truth about Phytoestrogens and Breast Cancer

For years, doctors warned women with breast cancer or a high risk of the disease to stay away from soy and other foods and supplements with high amounts of phytoestrogens. They worried that the estrogen-like compounds would act like estrogen on cancer cells, triggering their growth and division. But a study presented at the American Association for Cancer Research annual meeting in 2011 found that eating soy foods like soy milk and tofu didn't increase the risk of cancer recurrence in more than 18,000 breast cancer survivors. This study supported earlier research that reported similar results, with at least one concluding that cancer survivors who got about two servings a day of soy foods were *less likely* to have their cancer return.

As the authors of a study published in the *Journal of the American Medical Association* in December 2009 noted: "Patients with breast cancer can be assured that enjoying a soy latte or indulging in pad thai with tofu causes no harm, and, when consumed in plentiful amounts, may reduce the risk of disease recurrence."

flavone supplements had fewer hot flashes; 3 found no difference; and 3 found that hot flashes were less severe in the isoflavone group.

Another analysis, of 13 studies, found that the more frequent a woman's hot flashes, the more likely she was to benefit from isoflavone supplements or soy foods.

Finally, a study that analyzed 19 trials and was published in *Menopause* in 2010 concluded that while it appeared that soy *could* help reduce the number and severity of hot flashes, the studies were so different—with different forms and dosages of soy used in women at different stages of menopause—that it was nearly impossible to draw a single conclusion.

Bottom line: Although the research on soy is decidedly mixed, there's no evidence that increasing soy in your diet or taking over-the-counter soy supplements is harmful (see "The Truth about Phytoestrogens and Breast Cancer"), and there *is* evidence that soy might help with your hot flashes. So you have nothing to lose by giving it a try. Just give it 12 weeks before deciding it doesn't work, and don't add other supplements to the mix, or you'll never know which option is actually helping.

Flaxseed

Like soy, flaxseed is high in estrogen-like phytoestrogens, particularly lignans, which could account for its benefits. Studies are mixed, but when Mayo Clinic researchers had 29 women with annoying hot flashes eat 1.5 ounces of crushed flaxseed daily for 6 weeks, they found the average number of hot flashes dropped by half and their severity fell by 57 percent. The women also said their mood improved and that they had less joint or muscle pain, fewer chills, and less sweating.

However, another small study of 38 women who had been postmenopausal for 1 to 10 years but were still having hot flashes found that eating two slices of bread containing about an ounce of flaxseed daily for 12 weeks had no more effect on hot flashes than eating two slices of bread containing wheat bran. The good news is that the researchers also measured the thickness of the women's uterine lining to see if the estrogen-like hormones in flaxseed triggered lining overgrowth that could lead to cancer. They found no changes in the uterine lining, thus demonstrating that high amounts of flaxseed in the diet appear to be safe.

Bottom line: Flaxseed is a great source of insoluble fiber, which can help control your weight and cholesterol levels. Since there doesn't appear to be any danger from adding flaxseed to your diet, it's worth a try. However, the therapeutic dose of 40 grams, or 4 tablespoons, of ground flaxseeds comes along with 16 grams of fat and about 200 calories. So make sure the flaxseeds are taking the place of unhealthy fats, not being added on. To get the full benefits, crush the flaxseeds before eating. An easy way to do this is with a coffee grinder. Keep the ground seeds in your refrigerator and add a few tablespoons to your oatmeal or yogurt every day. Also, try the Fig 'n' Flax Muffins on page 92.

Vitamin E

While vitamin E is known for its antioxidant properties, it can also help your arteries work better and reduce inflammation—all of which could improve hot flashes. In an Iranian study published in *Gynecological and Obstetrical Investigations* in 2007, 51 women experiencing severe hot flashes took 400 IU of vitamin E every day for 4 weeks or a placebo. After a week without either vitamin E or the placebo, they switched; the vitamin E group took the placebo, and the placebo group took vitamin E. When the women took the vitamin, they had significantly fewer and less severe hot flashes, leading the researchers to conclude that vitamin E was a good option for women with hot flashes.

The only other major study evaluating vitamin E for hot flashes was conducted with breast cancer survivors. In this study, the women took 800 IU a day for 4 weeks before switching to a placebo. Although the women had some improvement in their hot flashes, the researchers concluded that the "clinical magnitude of this reduction was marginal." In other words, it worked but not very well.

Bottom line: If you decide to try vitamin E, stick to a supplement that supplies 400 IU a day; higher amounts could slightly increase your risk of dying early.

Black Cohosh

Black cohosh, a member of the buttercup family, is one of the most researched herbal options for hot flashes. The herb is thought to act like estrogen in the body, decreasing luteinizing hormone (a hormone that's secreted by the pituitary gland and that may play a role in hot flashes) and affecting serotonin receptors, which are also involved in hot flashes.

Nonetheless, the data on this herb are mixed. One study showed that black cohosh reduced hot flashes by 84 percent. In another, it worked just as well as estrogen in reducing hot flashes; still others have found that the herb has little, if any, benefit.

Perhaps the study that got the most attention was the Herbal Alternatives for Menopause Trial (HALT), sponsored by the National Institutes of Health (NIH) and published in 2006. It included 351 women ages 45 to 55 who took either 160 milligrams a day of black cohosh alone; a multiherb pill with black cohosh and nine other ingredients; a multiherb pill plus counseling to increase the amount of soy in their diet; hormone therapy (estrogen with or without progestin); or a placebo. The frequency and severity of the women's menopausal symptoms fell by about a third over a year whether the women took black cohosh or a placebo. Only estrogen therapy significantly improved their hot flashes.

Bottom line: Black cohosh is worth a try. It's safe (the most commonly reported side effect is mild nausea), and it does work in some women. Although there were reports of liver failure in women taking high doses of the herb, a report from the NIH found no evidence that the black cohosh was responsible. Still, make sure to tell your doctor if you take it. Look for products containing the most-studied dose: an extract standardized to contain 1 milligram of triterpene glycosides, calculated as 27-deoxyactein, per 20-milligram tablet. Take 20 milligrams twice daily or 40 milligrams once a day.

Sage

The anecdotal evidence of using sage (*Salvia officinalis*) to reduce sweating and hot flashes is significant, but until recently, there were no studies

NOT WORTH TRYING

The following are often pitched as menopausal remedies, but there's little evidence that they work at all, so skip these.

Dong quai. This herb has been used for thousands of years for a variety of menstrual problems. There is little evidence that it helps with hot flashes, although one study found some benefit in a formulation combined with chamomile. Nonetheless, dong quai is often included in herbal over-the-counter menopausal formulations. Stay away from it if you are taking blood thinners or have had a reproductive cancer, since the herb has some estrogen-like properties and may stimulate cancer cell growth.

Chaste tree (*Vitex agnus-castus*). This herb is often prescribed for various menstrual symptoms and is especially beneficial for premenstrual syndrome. Although it affects a variety of hormones and neurotransmitters in women, with at least one study finding that it improved mood and hot flashes, it is not very effective. It can also interact with oral contraceptives, making them less effective, and its estrogenic properties mean you should avoid it if you have or have had a hormone-sensitive cancer like breast cancer.

Wild yam. This herbal remedy is often mistakenly considered a natural progesterone. However, the only randomized clinical trial conducted with it found no difference between it and a placebo for improving menopausal symptoms, although there were no side effects. There is also no evidence that it is converted to progesterone when taken as a pill or used as a cream.

Evening primrose. Another herb often included in herbal supplements sold for menopausal treatments, evening primrose used alone shows no effect on hot flashes. It should also be avoided by women with hormone-sensitive cancers.

on its benefits. That changed in late 2010, with the publication of a Swiss study evaluating the effects of a once-daily sage tablet on 71 postmenopausal women. The researchers found that the average number of hot flashes dropped by half within 4 weeks and by 64 percent within 8 weeks. Women with severe and very severe hot flashes had even greater benefits, with 79 percent and 100 percent, respectively, seeing improvements.

Bottom line: Brew your own tea with 1 tablespoon of fresh sage leaves or 1 heaping teaspoon of dried sage per cup of boiling water. Let the sage leaves steep for 5 minutes, then strain. You can drink the tea hot or iced, and add some lemon, stevia, honey, or agave nectar to make it more refreshing.

Acupuncture

Seriously? Sticking needles in your body could really improve hot flashes? Possibly. A randomized, controlled trial of 267 women published in the May/June 2009 issue of the journal *Menopause* found that women who had 10 acupuncture treatments over 12 weeks had far fewer hot flashes than those who received a sham procedure. The women getting the acupuncture also reported that they slept better and had less pain. Another study, this one in women with breast cancer treatment–related hot flashes, compared applied relaxation and electroacupuncture (which uses tiny electrical impulses across acupuncture needles). The women received the treatments for 12 weeks and were followed for another 6 months. Those who had either treatment saw their hot flashes slashed in half during treatment and follow-up; their overall sense of well-being also improved.

However, a review of six trials in which real acupuncture was compared with sham acupuncture concluded that there was no evidence that acupuncture was effective, although the authors admitted that more well-designed studies were warranted.

We don't exactly know why acupuncture works when it does work. There's some evidence that needling acupuncture points affects the sympathetic nervous system, as well as the release of hormones such as cortisol, endorphins, and serotonin.

Bottom line: Acupuncture is not harmful and there is some evidence that it may help. As with many of the options listed throughout this chapter, you need to give this treatment time to work. It may take several sessions before you notice any improvement. A good place to find a qualified acupuncturist is the American Association of Acupuncture & Oriental Medicine at www.aaaomonline.org.

WHEN ALL ELSE FAILS . . . MEDICATIONS FOR HOT FLASHES

Sometimes, no matter what you do, you still can't get control of your hot flashes. That's okay. It happens! But if the hot flashes are affecting your quality of life despite your best efforts with nonmedical therapies, it's time to talk to your doctor about the next step—medication. We've listed them here in order from most effective to least effective.

Estrogen

Yes, this book is called *The Natural Menopause Solution*. However, our primary goal is to help you through menopause without losing the best of yourself, physically and emotionally. Sometimes, when all else fails, that means synthetic hormones. Particularly for hot flashes. That's because nothing works better. Study after study show that estrogen or estrogen/progestin therapy (for women who still have a uterus) reduces the severity of hot flashes from 65 to 90 percent, regardless of the type of estrogen used.

But with more than a dozen types of estrogen and estrogen/progestin combinations on the market and even more formulations and dosages, how do you know what's right for you? Follow these basic guidelines:

1. **Choose bioidentical.** Ask for a product made with estradiol, a type of estrogen identical to that produced by your own body rather than conjugated equine estrogens, which are derived from horse urine. The same goes for choosing the type of progestin you take. Bioidentical progesterone comes as either the FDA-approved micronized (meaning "finely ground") Prometrium or as a prescription formulation prepared through a compounding pharmacy. The over-the-counter cream form of progesterone, while helpful for some menopause-

related conditions, is not strong enough to prevent uterine cancer if you're also taking estrogen.

2. **Avoid oral estrogen.** Oral estrogen is metabolized, or broken down, by your liver. The liver is also where most cholesterol is made, so there is some concern that clearing estrogen through the liver contributes to greater production of so-called "bad" cholesterol and may be related to the heart problems seen in the WHI and other studies. Oral estrogens are also associated with an increased risk of blood clots, as the body's clotting factors are manufactured in the liver. So ask your doctor for a different formulation. You have lots of options, including a vaginal ring, vaginal pill or suppository, a cream or lotion, a patch, and even a nasal spray that's currently under development.

3. **Go low dose.** Since the WHI, manufacturers have introduced estrogen products with far lower hormonal doses. The lower doses are thought to be safer than higher doses in terms of heart disease, blood clots, stroke, and breast cancer. They can also reduce side effects such as breast tenderness and irregular bleeding. Start with the lowest dose possible and increase as needed until your hot flashes dissipate.

4. **Go short term.** No longer are women put on hormone therapy for life. Instead, if your goal is to use the hormones only to manage the most severe symptoms around menopause, you should use them for a short time, and then see if you still have symptoms. After 6 months, for instance, work with your doctor to wean yourself off the medication; if your hot flashes return, you can start again. If not, you're done! If you're taking hormones for other health-related benefits, you may decide to keep taking them, but talk with your doctor and make sure you understand the relative risks and benefits.

Here's what else you should know about hormone therapy.

- **Give it time.** It may take 8 to 12 weeks of low-dose estrogen therapy to relieve your hot flashes, so be patient.

- **Take it right.** Some estrogen formulations are taken every day, others applied a few times a week, and others (like the vaginal ring) changed only every 3 months. The progesterone portion may be included daily or prescribed for just 2 weeks a month. Remember that if you have a uterus, taking progesterone regularly is critical to help prevent endometrial cancer.

- **Understand the risks and benefits.** There are benefits (reduced risk of colon cancer, improved bone strength, and more) and risks (including increased risk of gallbladder disease, breast cancer, heart disease, and stroke in some women) to hormone therapy. An in-depth discussion with your doctor is critical so you can make an informed decision about what is right for you. One of the greatest risks is blood clots in your lungs or legs. So if you have a personal or family history of these clots, tell your doctor! Occasional vaginal bleeding may also occur. If the bleeding occurs for more than a year (and you're not taking a cyclical product that induces monthly bleeding), is very heavy, or lasts for more than a couple of days, talk to your doctor.

Bottom line: It's the gold standard.

Potential side effects: Breast pain, headache, back pain, abdominal pain, nausea, and bleeding

Neurontin (Gabapentin)

Two studies show that a daily 900-milligram dose of this antiepileptic drug reduced the number of hot flashes by 45 to 50 percent. Another trial compared a 2,400-milligram dose with estrogen in 60 postmenopausal women. After 12 weeks, both the estrogen and Neurontin groups saw their hot flash scores drop by about 71 percent, compared with 54 percent in the placebo group.

Bottom line: Worth a try

Potential side effects: Headache, dizziness, disorientation

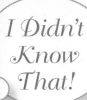

NEW DRUGS FOR HOT FLASHES

Once estrogen therapy became disgraced as a treatment for hot flashes, pharmaceutical scientists realized they had an entirely new market available. To that end, several new drugs are in late-stage clinical trials specifically to help manage hot flashes, including:

Selective estrogen receptor modulators (SERMs). These drugs are designed to mimic estrogen in the body. The beauty of SERMs is that they can be designed to provide only the estrogen-like benefits you want—like temperature regulation—without the ones you don't want, like triggering the growth of uterine and breast tissue. Several companies are testing SERMs for hot flashes. The results of one study from Radius Health presented at a major medical meeting in 2010 found that 28 days of treatment with its drug, known as RAD1901 for now, reduced the frequency and severity of hot flashes by 77 percent, compared with 54 percent for a placebo.

Another SERM-like drug being tested is Menerba, an estrogen receptor beta agonist (ERBA), which activates different estrogen receptors than most SERMs. Results of a study in 217 healthy postmenopausal women with moderate to severe hot flashes found that after 12 weeks of treatment, the women in the Menerba group were more than twice as likely to have a more than 50 percent drop in the number of hot flashes as women in the placebo group.

Ditropan (oxybutynin). This drug is approved for stress incontinence, also known as an overactive bladder. It has shown some benefit with hot flashes in cancer patients, so researchers are now testing it in menopausal women.

Seroquel (quetiapine). This drug is approved to treat major depression, bipolar disorder, and schizophrenia. An ongoing clinical trial is testing it in menopausal women with major depressive disorder to see if it can also improve mood, sleep, and hot flashes.

It Worked for Me!

**Lori Klase, 46, lost 6½ pounds and 3¾ inches—
and her hot flashes have been reduced dramatically.**

When Lori embarked on the Natural Menopause Solution program, she gave her mornings a major makeover. The "before" picture: No breakfast, probably no exercise. The "after": A serene routine that includes yoga and a filling morning meal before she heads out the door to her job as an activities assistant at a retirement community. "I've always heard that breakfast is the most important meal of the day. Well, I've discovered that isn't just hoopla. It's real. This program got me to start eating in the morning, and I feel better all day because of it. I have more energy and am less hungry. Adding breakfast is one reason I lost nearly 7 pounds in a month!"

Her biggest food challenge? "The major adjustment was cutting back on red meat," Lori says. "My husband and I enjoyed the one recipe with steak in it, but most of the meals call for turkey or chicken or fish. They're better for you. Trying out the recipes for things like the seafood chowder got me into eating them. I would definitely make that one again—delicious!"

An early riser, Lori found morning to be the perfect time for yoga. "The routine helped me stretch and wake up. And the yoga-with-weights poses toned my arms and legs. I feel tighter. I think the yoga even helped my sleep!"

Lori is still having regular periods—but is also experiencing perimenopausal hot flashes, night sweats, and disturbed sleep. All of these improved on the Natural Menopause Solution Plan. "I used to have two or three hot flashes a day, but now I get them maybe twice a week," she says. "And my sleep is less restless, maybe because I'm not getting night sweats as often."

Antidepressants

In recent years, researchers have found that several antidepressants, particularly venlafaxine (Effexor), paroxetine (Paxil), and desvenlafaxine (Pristiq), can help with hot flashes. Advantages of the antidepressants are that they work fast and they can help improve your mood if you're also suffering from even minor depression. Some, however, can cause weight gain, and several can reduce libido and make it harder to have an orgasm. As with any drug, herb, or supplement, you need to weigh the potential benefits against the potential risks.

Effexor. This drug is the most studied antidepressant for hot flashes. While most of the studies were conducted in breast cancer survivors, the first trial in menopausal women involved 80 women who were having at least 14 hot flashes a week. They received either Effexor or a placebo. After 12 weeks, the women's hot flash scores had dropped by 51 percent compared with a 15 percent drop in the placebo group. Researchers note that it may take only a week or two on the drug to start to see a benefit.

Bottom line: Worth a try

Potential side effects: Dry mouth, decreased appetite, anxiety, constipation, and nausea, although most should fade after a couple of weeks

Pristiq (desvenlafaxine). A study of 707 healthy menopausal women with no history of breast cancer who had at least seven moderate to severe hot flashes a day found that, by 3 months, the women taking Pristiq had 51 to 64 percent fewer hot flashes (depending on the dosage of the drug) compared with those who received a placebo.

Another evaluation, this one in 365 women, found that after 4 weeks of taking Pristiq, the number of hot flashes decreased by half on average, compared with a 31 percent drop in women taking a placebo. By week 12, the number had dropped by 62 percent in the Pristiq group, compared with a 38 percent drop in the placebo group. The hot flashes were also about 20 percent less severe in the Pristiq group but only 8 percent less severe in the placebo group. As of the summer of 2011, the US Food and Drug Administration was reviewing the drug to see if it should have an indication for hot flash prevention.

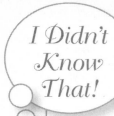

BOTOX FOR HOT FLASHES?

Botox (botulinum toxin A) is well known for its ability to paralyze the muscles in the forehead and to banish frown lines. But did you know that it has also been approved to treat excessive sweating, a condition called hyperhidrosis? And that it has been used to reduce menopausal flushing? All of which begs the question: Could Botox be used to stem hot flashes?

That's just what physiologist Craig Crandall, PhD, of the University of Texas Southwestern Medical Center, has been researching. In a 2011 issue of the journal *Menopause,* he and his team reported on a unique study in which menopausal women who suffered from hot flashes were divided into three groups. One group received Botox in their forearm, another in their forehead. The researchers then compared changes in blood flow and sweating at both the treated site and nearby untreated areas before, during, and after a hot flash. A third group of women were monitored in one foot but didn't receive any Botox injections.

The researchers found that the Botox injections dramatically reduced the expected increases in blood flow and sweating at both sites. At the same time, they noticed that women who didn't get the injections showed significant increased activity in the nerves in the skin of their foot, suggesting an important link between the nervous system and hot flashes. The study also clearly showed that a hot flash affects the entire body, not just the face, neck, or underarms. Researchers also found that the women's blood pressure *dropped* during the hot flash and that there was no major increase in their core body temperature just before the flash, contrary to what other researchers have found.

This doesn't mean Botox should be used to treat hot flashes! You'd need to inject the drug throughout your entire body, which is not only painful but dangerous. Instead, the new findings could help researchers in their quest to find other medical options to cool the flashes.

Bottom line: Worth a try

Potential side effects: Nausea, dry mouth, fatigue, constipation, diarrhea, and sleepiness

Paxil (paroxetine). In a study involving 151 menopausal women, 80 percent of whom were breast cancer survivors, both 10- and 20-milligram doses of Paxil reduced the frequency of hot flashes about 25 percent and the severity of the flashes about 30 percent.

Bottom line: Worth a try

Potential side effects: Headache, nausea, sleepiness, insomnia, and dry mouth. It may interact with tamoxifen, so if you're taking that drug, make sure that your doctor knows before starting you on Paxil.

Lexapro (escitalopram). A study published in the *Journal of the American Medical Association* in 2011 randomly assigned 254 postmenopausal women with at least 14 bothersome hot flashes a week to receive either 10 to 20 milligrams of the drug each day or a placebo. After 8 weeks, more than half of the women receiving Lexapro (55 percent) reported that their hot flashes had dropped by at least 50 percent, compared with 36 percent of the women in the placebo group. The Lexapro group also reported that their hot flashes were far less severe. However, 3 weeks after the women stopped taking Lexapro, their hot flashes returned with greater frequency than those of women in the placebo group.

Bottom line: Worth a try

Potential side effects: Nausea, insomnia, fatigue and drowsiness, increased sweating, decreased libido, and difficulty achieving orgasm

Prozac (fluoxetine). This antidepressant flunked a trial comparing it with black cohosh. The black cohosh not only had fewer side effects but reduced hot flash scores by 85 percent, compared with 62 percent for those taking Prozac. Another study comparing it with Celexa (citalopram) or a placebo in 150 healthy menopausal women found no significant differences among the three groups in the number or severity of hot flashes during the trial's 9 months.

Bottom line: Not worth trying for hot flash relief

Zoloft (sertraline). Two studies evaluating Zoloft in healthy menopausal women compared with women taking a placebo found that the drug worked significantly better than the placebo at reducing the number and severity of hot flashes, lowering the average number of hot flashes by five and the hot flash score by 48 percent, as compared with a 30 percent drop in the placebo group. However, another study of 99 women who took the drug or a placebo for 6 weeks found no difference between them.

Bottom line: Not worth trying for hot flash relief

Cymbalta (duloxetine). Just one small trial involving 20 women was done with this drug, and the researchers never reported the results. The drug also was not compared with a placebo.

Bottom line: Not worth trying for hot flash relief

Given the length of this chapter, by now you may be thinking that nothing in menopause can be as important as hot flashes. That's not the case. Menopause itself is just a phase in your life, as you know, and hot flashes are just a symptom of the changing levels of hormones in your body. What is most important, as you will learn throughout the rest of the book, is maintaining your overall health as you move from the pre- to peri- to postmenopausal life. The hot flashes will fade, but your risk of heart disease, diabetes, and osteoporosis only increases.

Having said that, we also want to help you cope with other menopause-related symptoms, including sleep issues; variations in your sexual desire, mood, and energy levels; and changes in your skin, hair, and nails. Read on to learn how to cope with whatever the meno-goddesses throw at you.

Chapter 8

Sleep

When is the last time you had a good night's sleep? We're talking about the kind of night in which you dropped off to sleep just minutes after turning out your light, slept through the night, and woke in the morning before your alarm feeling refreshed and ready to face the day.

If you're like many women your age, the answer is probably "Not in a long time." Studies find that younger women sleep better than men; however, once we hit perimenopause, the gender benefit ends. Then we have a harder time falling asleep *and* staying asleep.

The evidence is compelling. For instance, a survey of 1,500 British women age 47 found that postmenopausal women were more than twice as likely as pre- and perimenopausal women to report trouble sleeping. The large Study of Women's Health Across the Nation (SWAN) found a

30 to 60 percent increased likelihood that peri- and postmenopausal women would have trouble sleeping, with 40 percent of women waking throughout the night, 16 percent of them frequently.

Meanwhile, the National Sleep Foundation found that 61 percent of menopausal women experience insomnia symptoms, while a 2010 survey of 982 women ages 35 to 65 from the Red Hot Mamas group found that a third of premenopausal women had insomnia compared with half of peri- and postmenopausal women. The International Classification of Sleep Disorders even classifies menopausal insomnia as a "menstrual-associated sleep disorder," defining it as a "disorder of unknown cause, characterized by a complaint of either insomnia or excessive sleepiness, that is temporally related to the menses or menopause."

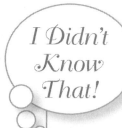

I Didn't Know That!

YOUNGER WOMEN SLEEP BETTER THAN MEN OF THE SAME AGE

Researchers don't know for sure but suspect the reason for this gender diversity may be an evolutionary development designed to help us cope with the sleepless nights that go hand in hand with young children. In fact, not only do younger women sleep better than men of the same age (when they *can* sleep), but they also seem better able to cope with less sleep. Their bodies release fewer inflammatory chemicals and stress hormones than do those of men who get too little sleep, and women are able to get the benefits of even fractionated sleep (the 2 to 3 hours you get before you hear a cry for feeding, water, or soothing after a bad dream). Scientists speculate that this could be one reason women live longer and have lower rates of heart disease than men (at least prior to menopause). All these benefits, alas, fade along with our skinny jeans as we age.

And yet, in a pivotal study published in the journal *Sleep* in 2003, researchers from the University of Wisconsin found no difference in sleep *quality* between peri- and postmenopausal women, as compared with that of premenopausal women. The researchers evaluated the women overnight, measuring their brain waves and electrical activity while they slept. They found that postmenopausal women had more deep sleep and slept longer than premenopausal women. However, peri- and postmenopausal women were twice as likely to *complain* about the quality of their sleep.

Whether your sleep problems are real or all in your head is not really the issue. The issue is the effect they can have on your life because we're not talking about an occasional lost night of sleep that can be solved with an afternoon nap. The Red Hot Mamas survey found that 76 percent of menopausal women surveyed said that their insomnia moderately to significantly impacted their overall quality of life. They had significant daytime sleepiness and problems concentrating. Even their personal and romantic relationships suffered, with nearly a third saying they had less sex with their husbands because they were too tired.

Lack of sleep can also contribute to that midlife weight gain we're all trying to avoid. Harvard researchers evaluating sleep and weight in 68,000 women followed for 16 years found that those who slept 5 hours or fewer a night weighed an average of 5.4 pounds more than those who got just 2 hours more of shut-eye. They were also 15 percent more likely to become obese. Turns out that when you don't get enough sleep, the hormones that signal hunger or fullness go haywire.

With inadequate sleep, the satiety (fullness) hormone, leptin, drops, while the appetite hormone, ghrelin, increases. Other hormones affected include orexin, which also helps regulate how you eat. The end result is that not only do you feel hungrier, but it takes more calories before you feel full. Plus, of course, when you're tired from lack of sleep, exercising falls off your radar, as does finding the time and energy to shop for and cook healthy meals.

Waking up several times during the night, the most common form of insomnia in menopausal women, also disrupts your REM sleep, the type required for memory and mood. That could be part of the reason many women complain that they just don't feel as mentally sharp at this time of life (more on mental fuzziness on page 256).

Poor sleep also plays havoc with your appearance. In a study published in the *British Medical Journal*, Swedish and Dutch researchers found that observers ranked 23 sleep-deprived men and women as looking more tired, less attractive, and unhealthier than they did after a full night's sleep.

There's no reason for you to lose sleep during menopause. The key is identifying the underlying cause of your sleep problems, whether it's hot flashes, hormonal changes, run-of-the-mill stress-related insomnia, or one of the handful of sleep disorders that often affect women during this time of life. You may not be able to identify the cause yourself; that's where your doctor comes in. But you can certainly identify some of the components of your insomnia and then find remedies within this chapter. For instance, if hot flashes are keeping you up at night, flip back to Chapter 7 for our advice on battling night sweats. If you're lying awake at 4:00 a.m., worrying about your shrinking bank account, you need to read the section on stress-induced insomnia more closely. And if you've tried our natural remedies for hot flashes, hormonal changes, and stress-induced insomnia and you're still haggard with lack of sleep, it's time to see your doctor.

IS IT HOT FLASHES OR JUST HORMONES?

For years, doctors blamed our midlife insomnia on the hot flashes of menopause that would strike with the suddenness of a tornado, leaving us drenched in sweat in their wake. Who wouldn't lose sleep when you had to get up and change the sheets and your pajamas once or twice a night? And, sure, nocturnal hot flashes, aka night sweats, can wake you just as dependably as a fire alarm.

But even if you don't have hot flashes, your sleep may suffer. Here we can blame hormonal effects beyond temperature changes. In a small but important study, researchers at Weill Cornell Medical School in White Plains, New York, assessed the levels of reproductive hormones and sleep quality in 10 women between the ages of 57 and 71, all of whom were at least 5 years past menopause. They found that lower estrogen and higher levels of luteinizing hormone (which stimulates the ovary to pop out a monthly egg and increases during perimenopause) led to poorer sleep quality. They found, too, that higher body temperature before and during sleep was also related to worse sleep, particularly waking up too early and not being able to go back to sleep.

Here's what you need to know about hormones and sleep.

Progesterone. This hormone acts as a sedative in your body, stimulating the same parts of your brain that many sleeping pills and anti-anxiety medications target. That's why you may have found yourself having problems sleeping just before your period, when progesterone levels plummet. In fact, a small study in 21 women showed that micronized progesterone (Prometrium) improved the quality of women's sleep by 8 percent.

Progesterone also helps you breathe. That's why researchers think pregnant women and premenopausal women, whose progesterone levels are high, are far less likely than postmenopausal women to experience sleep apnea (a breathing-related disorder that disrupts your sleep numerous times throughout the night). More on sleep apnea on page 220.

Estrogen. Estrogen increases REM cycles and is linked to the release of several chemicals related to sleep, including serotonin. When estrogen levels are high, you tend to fall asleep more quickly, wake up less often during sleep, and sleep longer overall. Plus, you know that estrogen affects body temperature, particularly core temperature, while you sleep. The higher estrogen levels you experience premenopausally keep your body's thermostat working better, which means you're cooler at night. This low body temperature is important in maintaining sleep, so even if you're not suffering from hot flashes that wake you up, you might have a higher core body temperature that does. High estrogen levels in the first couple of weeks after your period are one reason you sleep better during this time of the month.

Cortisol. Estrogen also affects levels of the stress hormone cortisol, which is supposed to begin rising early in the morning. During menopause, however, cortisol peaks tend to occur earlier in the night, so you wake earlier. They also rise higher even when you're dealing only with mild stressors.

Melatonin. Melatonin is, quite simply, the sleep hormone. It is produced by the pineal gland, a pea-size structure in the center of your brain

Five Signs That You're Sleep Deprived

You know you have a problem when:

1. **You can't make a simple decision to save your life.** Bursting into tears when the bagger asks if you want paper or plastic is a clue. That's because it's harder to differentiate between important and innocuous decisions when you're tired.

2. **You're always hungry—even though you're not dieting.** Recall the effect that sleep deprivation has on hunger and fullness hormones.

3. **You seem to catch every bug in the office.** Blame it on a worn-down immune system. Sleep is critical to maintaining a strong immune system.

4. **You wear your emotions on your sleeve.** The other day you saw a cardinal and started crying. Inconsolably. Blame changes in your brain that shift activity to the parts of your brain involved in anxiety and fear, while it's communicating less with the parts that determine the appropriate emotional responses to situations.

5. **You keep spilling your coffee.** When you're sleep deprived, your motor skills go on hiatus. You may also have problems with depth perception and balance.

behind your eyes that is often called the third eye. The pineal gland reacts to light and darkness, producing melatonin as the sky darkens and switching off the melatonin faucet as day approaches. Both the pineal gland and the hormone it produces are critical to maintaining normal circadian rhythms. That's why, if you work the night shift or fly through several time zones, you feel so tired. The changing light and darkness throw your circadian rhythms all out of whack.

Melatonin levels drop just before menopause and then increase for several years following menopause. However, postmenopausal women who have insomnia typically have lower levels of melatonin than post-menopausal women who don't suffer from insomnia.

If your insomnia continues despite trying the various remedies throughout this chapter, it might be time to consider a brief bout of hormone therapy. Numerous studies have found that women taking supplemental estrogen and progesterone report less insomnia. A Brazilian study found that supplementing with estrogen and progesterone also reduced limb movements, hot flashes, and teeth grinding at night, as well as daytime sleepiness and fatigue.

THE SLEEP STEALERS

Plummeting hormone levels are just one thing going on in your life in middle age. Health-related issues, pain, depression, anxiety—all can affect your sleep, as can medically related sleep disorders like sleep apnea and restless legs syndrome. For instance, a study published in 2007 in the journal *Menopause* found that 53 percent of women over 44 who had trouble sleeping also had restless legs syndrome or sleep apnea. We also know that rates of restless legs syndrome and thyroid disorders increase with age and that dropping estrogen levels may play a role in sleep apnea. Depression is another contributor to sleep problems, and the incidence of depression in perimenopausal and early-postmenopausal women is more than twice that of younger women.

The only way to know for sure what's going on is to talk to your doctor. Yet 62 percent of women questioned during the Red Hot Mamas survey about sleep problems said that they hadn't talked to their health-care provider about their sleep issues. Of those who did, 92 percent said they had to start the conversation. The takeaway? Don't wait for your doctor or nurse practitioner to ask how you're sleeping. If you're having sleep problems, make an appointment specifically to discuss them.

Among the health conditions that may be stealing your sleep are:

Depression. When you're depressed, it feels like someone painted the world gray. No color, no light, no joy. It's as if you were going through your days covered in cotton batting. But depression is also a sleep killer. In fact, one way that doctors diagnose depression is by asking patients how they're sleeping. Some people with depression sleep all the time. For others, however, depression is marked by problems sleeping, particularly falling asleep and staying asleep. And they don't get that all-important deep REM sleep so they wake unrefreshed.

What's menopause got to do with it? In the SWAN study, researchers found that women had the highest risk of depression in the early or late stages of perimenopause, as well as just after menopause occurred. Women with stressful issues in their lives, such as divorce, job loss, or financial problems, as well as those with intense hot flashes and little social support in the form of family or friends were most likely to be depressed.

Symptoms, please. In addition to sleep-related problems, other signs of depression include a loss of interest in those things that normally interest you, feelings of sadness, lack of energy, irritability or anger, and changes in appetite.

What do I do about it? There's more on depression in Chapter 9, along with our recommendations for treatment. The first step, however, is an appointment with your doctor. Who knows? You might finally get a good night's sleep out of it!

Sleep apnea. This is a condition in which you stop breathing during sleep, sometimes hundreds of times a night. When this happens, your brain kicks into gear, waking you just long enough to get you breathing again but not so much that you'd know you'd stopped or had even woken.

What's menopause got to do with it? Although the condition is more common in men, particularly overweight men, we now know that it's also common in women during menopause because that's when we tend to gain weight and lose estrogen. One study found that postmenopausal women were more than twice as likely as premenopausal women to have sleep apnea or some other form of sleep-disordered breathing. However, the risk was halved in women who used hormone therapy.

Symptoms, please. The trickiest thing about sleep apnea is that you may not even be aware that you're waking up many times in the night. Your body is, though, so over time you get more and more tired. People with sleep apnea run other risks as well, including a higher risk of high blood pressure, stroke, and heart disease. Ask your partner if you've been snoring, snuffling, gasping, or choking in your sleep. Or if you sleep alone, set up a digital tape recorder. One clue? You're always tired, even after a good 10 hours of sleep, and often wake with a morning headache.

What do I do about it? Start with a visit to your primary care physician, who may then refer you to a sleep specialist. Sleep apnea is typically diagnosed after a night spent in a sleep lab in which your sleep, heart rate, brain waves, and breathing patterns are monitored. Treatment is pretty effective, beginning with a device that pushes air through your nasal passages called a continuous positive airway pressure (CPAP) machine. These days, CPAPs come in all sizes and shapes and can even travel with you. Another option is an oral appliance to keep your throat open (see your dentist about this).

Quitting smoking and losing weight can also reduce the severity of the condition. If none of these options works, surgery to remove excess tissue blocking your upper air passages may be the next step.

Restless legs syndrome (RLS). This is a neurological condition in which throbbing, pulling, creeping, or other sensations in your legs lead to an uncontrollable urge to move them.

What's menopause got to do with it? Although the condition is more common in women as they age, the link is likely related to aging, not menopause per se.

Symptoms, please. As you can imagine, RLS can make it difficult to fall asleep—just as you are relaxing, something jars you out of the doze.

Many people with the condition also have periodic limb movements of sleep (PLMS), jerking every 20 to 30 seconds on and off throughout the night, even while asleep.

What do I do about it? Talk to your doctor. You will likely need a referral to a sleep specialist or a neurologist. Tests include a physical exam and checking your medical and family history, but no diagnostic test will conclusively tell if you have RLS. It's more likely that tests will rule out other potential conditions, like low iron levels, that can cause the symptoms.

Treatment depends on the underlying cause. If your symptoms are the result of a vitamin or mineral deficiency, you may only need supplemental iron, magnesium, folate, or vitamin B_{12}. Avoiding caffeine and alcohol can also help.

For more severe RLS, you may need a prescription for one of the following medications.

- **Dopaminergic agonists.** These drugs include Requip (ropinirole) and Mirapex (pramipexole). Originally developed for Parkinson's disease, they work by activating brain receptors for the neurotransmitter dopamine, which helps regulate movement and mood. Side effects include nausea, light-headedness, drowsiness, and low blood pressure when you stand up, which can cause dizziness.

- **Benzodiazepines.** These are usually used as sleeping pills or as anti-anxiety medications and include Klonopin (clonazepam), Restoril (temazepam), and Xanax (alprazolam). Major side effects of these drugs are daytime drowsiness, confusion, unsteadiness, falls, and worsening of sleep apnea.

- **Pain relievers.** Narcotics such as codeine or more potent medications like oxycodone, methadone, or levorphanol can help if your condition doesn't respond to other medications. Make sure that your doctor follows you closely, since side effects include tolerance and potential addiction. Other side effects include dizziness, sedation, nausea, vomiting, and constipation.

◆ **Anticonvulsants.** Typically used to treat epilepsy, these drugs include Tegretol (carbamazepine), Neurontin (gabapentin), and Depacon (sustained-release valproate). Side effects include dizziness, drowsiness, unsteadiness, nausea, and vomiting.

Chronic pain. Chronic pain is a notorious sleep stealer. The most common culprits are lower-back pain, arthritis, and fibromyalgia, all of which become more common as we age. But autoimmune conditions such as rheumatoid arthritis and lupus, both of which occur primarily in women, are also to blame.

What's menopause got to do with it? One of the most common types of chronic pain is fibromyalgia, which is characterized by fatigue, chronic pain in the muscles and soft tissues surrounding joints, and tenderness at specific sites in the body. It typically occurs at the same time as menopause and is seven times more common in women than men. In addition, there is evidence that women who enter menopause before age 45 are far more likely to develop fibromyalgia than those who start menopause later. Besides pain, the most common symptom is sleep problems; conversely, the more your sleep improves, the less pain you have.

Joint pain is also more prevalent in midlife women, affecting more than half of women around menopause. It's not clear, however, if menopause itself is responsible for the pain or if it's just related to the higher risk of joint conditions like osteoarthritis during this time of life and beyond. Still, it is likely that lower estrogen levels play *some* role, given the effects of estrogen on pain perception and the benefits of hormone therapy in relieving joint pain.

Symptoms, please. You hurt. Whether in a specific place, like your knee or lower back, or all over, as with fibromyalgia. And that pain keeps you from falling asleep or staying asleep throughout the night.

What do I do about it? Make sure your doctor knows that pain is interfering with your sleep, and don't accept the sleep problems as a "normal" part of your disease.

Treatment depends on the underlying disorder causing your pain. But if it's fibromyalgia, talk to your doctor about trying a course of Xyrem (sodium oxybate), a drug used to treat narcolepsy. A study of women with fibromyalgia found that it significantly improved symptoms of pain and fatigue, as well as sleep quality.

END STRESS-INDUCED INSOMNIA NOW

Diminishing estrogen levels, researchers say, can raise stress levels—so when you wake up at 4:00 a.m. to use the bathroom, your mind starts spinning with plans and solving problems before you can stop it. Bye-bye, sleep. Here's what to do.

Quick Tip
CHECK YOUR MEDS

Several medications can affect melatonin levels, including beta-blockers and nonsteroidal anti-inflammatory drugs (NSAIDs), particularly in people 55 and older. So if you take either of these medications on a regular basis, talk to your doctor about the possibility of melatonin supplementation.

In addition, several medications can contribute to insomnia, including Dexedrine (dextroamphetamine), Concerta/Ritalin (methylphenidate), Adderall (mixed amphetamine salts), Cylert (pemoline), alpha-blockers, beta-blockers, methyldopa, reserpine, albuterol, theophylline, Acutrim (phenylpropanolamine), phenylephrine, pseudoephedrine, corticosteroids, thyroid medications, monoamine oxidase inhibitors, selective serotonin reuptake inhibitors, anticholinesterase inhibitors, Lodosyn (carbidopa, levodopa), and Dilantin (phenytoin).

If you're taking any of these drugs and experiencing insomnia, talk to your doctor about alternatives. Also, cut out all caffeine (including the caffeine in over-the-counter medications like certain pain relievers and in chocolate), nicotine (which is a stimulant), and alcohol (as your body metabolizes the alcohol, it wakes you up).

Start a worry journal. Write in it before you go to bed. Make a list of things you need to remember for the next day, and jot down any worries stressing you out now. You can even go an extra step and rank the likelihood of any of them actually occurring so you can see how silly most of them are (do you *really* think your 14-year-old is going to marry the goth girl he's dating?). Keep the journal by your bed; if you find yourself obsessing about another worry or another item for your to-do list, turn the light on low and write it down.

Practice progressive muscle relaxation. We told you about this technique for quelling hot flashes in Chapter 7, but it can also help relax you enough to sleep. Progressive muscle relaxation involves tensing a group of muscles, like those in your forehead, as you breathe in and then relaxing the muscles as you breathe out. You usually start at your toes and work your way up or at your head and work down. Numerous studies have found that it helps ease anxiety-related insomnia.

Get up when you can't sleep. It sounds counterintuitive, but lying there wide awake in the dark worrying about the sleep you're missing will actually keep you up *longer* than if you just turned on a dim light and read for a few minutes or got up and went to the bathroom or even made yourself a soothing cup of chamomile tea. This approach is called sleep restriction. The goal is to stay in bed only when you're asleep. Eventually, your sleep deprivation will lead to longer and longer time in bed—asleep.

Prepare your bedroom for sleep. Researchers have found that environmental changes like the ones described here are often just as effective as sleeping pills.

- **Get rid of the electronics.** We're talking computer, television, cell phone, iPad, iPod. Anything that connects you to the outside world (i.e., the Internet) should be banned. You can keep an electronic book reader—but only if you promise not to check your e-mail while using it.

- **Put the alarm clock across the room.** You need the alarm to wake you in the morning, but keeping it on your bedside table sabotages your sleep in two ways: The light from the radium dial can be awfully bright, and the minutes clicking by just remind you that you're *still* not asleep. Plus, there is some concern that the electromagnetic field emitted by the clock and its cord may disrupt sleep.

- **Block the light.** We're talking blackout curtains or shades *and* an eye mask. Even the ambient light from streetlights can interfere with appropriate melatonin release.

- **Soundproof your room.** Move your bed away from any outside walls, turn on a white noise machine (or even a ceiling fan), and/or wear earplugs.

- **Spray some lavender.** Around the room, on your pillow, on the sheets: The scent is known for inducing relaxation.

PREVENTING INSOMNIA

If the options above don't work for your stress-induced insomnia, bump it up a bit with the following strategies, which work over a longer term. The mind/body strategies work by reducing the activity of your sympathetic nervous system (responsible for the fight-or-flight response) and increasing activity of the parasympathetic function (responsible for rest and sleep), while the herbs and supplements apparently boost the hormones and the neurotransmitters associated with sleep.

Yoga/Tai Chi

Both yoga and tai chi are Eastern exercises that incorporate meditation in movement. Both help relieve anxiety and induce relaxation, which is why they've been researched for stress-related insomnia.

A small study of Hatha yoga had 12 peri- and postmenopausal women take weekly yoga classes for 10 weeks and practice every day for at least 15 minutes. Although the women's hot flashes didn't improve, their sleep did.

In a larger study, during which women did 75 minutes of yoga per day (60 minutes during the day plus 15 minutes at night), 6 days a week, yoga participants were generally sleeping an hour longer than women in a control group. That's yet another reason to try the yoga routine that's part of our 30-Day Slim-Down, Cool-Down Diet.

When 118 older people did 60 minutes of tai chi three times a week for 6 months, they slept an average of an hour longer a night than they had before. Plus, they were less sleepy during the day and reported an overall improved health–related quality of life.

Mindfulness-Based Stress Reduction

This form of stress reduction involves sitting quietly and simply being in the moment, letting thoughts come and go in your head as you try to focus on your breathing. Don't do anything with the thoughts; just note them and let them pass through as you continue to focus on breathing. One study of 30 people with chronic insomnia compared the effect on them of eight weekly meditation classes and a daylong retreat, along with home practice over a 3-month follow-up period, with that of a control group that took the drug Lunesta (eszopiclone) nightly for 8 weeks, followed by as-needed use during the next 3 months. Both groups showed similar improvements in all parameters of sleep.

Another study, of 151 people, found that after 8 weeks of mindfulness-based stress-reduction training, sleep quality had improved by 26 percent; daytime sleepiness symptoms dropped by nearly a third; middle-of-the-night awakenings fell by 16 percent; and participants slashed their use of sleep medication by a quarter. As a lead researcher of that study noted in an interview: "When people become more mindful, they learn to look at life through a new lens. They learn how to accept the presence of thoughts and feelings that may keep them up at night. They begin to understand that they don't have to react to them. As a result, they experience greater emotional balance and less sleep disturbances."

Even better is that a review of studies involving mindfulness meditation for insomnia found that participants slept better for up to a year after the studies ended.

Biofeedback

Biofeedback involves consciously managing typically unconscious physiological processes, like slowing your heartbeat, lowering blood pressure, increasing blood flow to a certain part of your body (like your temples, to prevent migraines), and reducing muscle tension. You typically learn biofeedback with some kind of device so you can "see" your unconscious physical reactions. Over time you learn to control these reactions on your own, no device needed (although several portable bio-/neurofeedback devices are available for home use, including StressEraser, HeartMath/emWave2, and RESPeRATE).

In one study, participants learned to control changes in their heart rate with a portable device. After 3 weeks, their anxiety and anger had dropped significantly, and they were falling asleep faster and staying asleep longer. Participants told researchers that they found the device helped them more than other relaxation techniques they'd tried, including meditation, yoga, and breathing exercises. In fact, one side effect was sleepiness!

In another study, 17 people with insomnia were randomized to use either neurofeedback (a form of biofeedback that focuses on controlling brain waves) or regular biofeedback (which focuses on controlling processes elsewhere in the body). The total amount of time that participants spent asleep improved far more in the neurofeedback group than in the biofeedback group, but both groups fell asleep much faster than they had before beginning the treatments.

Massage Therapy

You may think of massage as a self-indulgent experience reserved for high-priced spas. But it can make a big difference in stress-related disorders like insomnia. In one small study, seven postmenopausal women who had insomnia at least three times a week received twice-weekly massages for 8 weeks. They also completed detailed questionnaires about their sleep quality and quality of life and underwent a sleep study before the study began, after the last massage, and again a year later. The researchers found that the women had less anxiety and depression after their massages, fell asleep faster, had improved sleep quality, and woke feeling better. The sleep study, which measured brain waves during sleep, also showed significant improvements in sleep quality. Meanwhile, a larger study, of 166 people, compared the effect of daily massages for 15 days on half of the participants with that of those in the other half, who took a placebo (a pill they thought was a sleep aid). Sixty-seven people in the massage group were "cured" of their insomnia as compared with just 10 in the placebo group. Researchers suspect the ability of massage to reduce stress hormones and pain likely contributed to the sleep improvements.

Acupressure/Acupuncture

In one Taiwanese study, 45 postmenopausal women who had suffered with insomnia for an average of 5 years received auricular acupressure— stimulating specific points on the ear with the fingers rather than needles—nightly for 4 weeks. Researchers found that the women slept longer and better and fell asleep much faster. Studies using acupuncture also found improved sleep, with one study finding increased melatonin secretion at night and reduced anxiety/stress scores after the treatments.

Isoflavones

The evidence is pretty solid on the ability of isoflavones—plant-based estrogen-like chemicals—to help with insomnia. In one study in 38 postmenopausal women, one group of women took 80 milligrams of isoflavone supplements daily for 4 months, while the second group took a placebo. Brain-wave studies found that the women taking the isoflavones slept far better than those getting the placebo. Not only did the isoflavones reduce the women's hot flashes, but by the end of the study, just 37 percent of the women taking isoflavones still had insomnia, down from 90 percent. Meanwhile, 63 percent of the placebo group still had insomnia, down from 95 percent.

Researchers aren't sure how isoflavones work for insomnia but believe that their estrogen-like effects could improve melatonin release.

St. John's Wort

St. John's wort is used primarily to relieve depression. Because depression and insomnia are so tightly linked, it has been shown to improve sleep in a few studies. You can read more about St. John's wort in Chapter 9.

Valerian

Valerian is an herb that works on various brain cell receptors for neurotransmitters associated with sleep. Study results vary depending on the dosage used and the sleep parameters measured, but in general valerian seems most effective at helping you fall asleep faster. It can also help

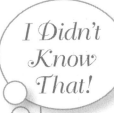

I Didn't Know That!

PERSONALITY MATTERS IN INSOMNIA THERAPY

Are you an extrovert or an introvert? The answer could make a difference in terms of which relaxation therapy works best for your insomnia. A study comparing the effects of music relaxation and progressive muscular relaxation in 15 older adults found greater improvements in sleep, including lower anxiety, after music relaxation in introverts. Extroverts, however, benefited from either option.

wean you off prescription or over-the-counter sleeping pills, particularly antianxiety medications like Ativan. In fact, valerian was just as effective in one study as the benzodiazepine Serax (oxazepam).

Just make sure that you choose a high-quality valerian product from a trusted manufacturer and that includes appropriate levels of a standardized form of the herb. A 2010 ConsumerLab.com investigation of valerian supplements found that just one in five passed quality controls; the rest were either contaminated with ingredients not on the label or had lower levels of valeric acid than expected. Three that passed muster were Solgar, Shaklee, and Bluebonnet Herbals. Also, don't take any other sleep aids, muscle relaxers, or antianxiety medications while taking valerian.

You can take valerian 1 to 2 hours before bedtime. But give it time—as in several days or even weeks—to get the full effect on your insomnia. In addition to the standard capsules, you can also try it in one of these forms.

- Tea: Pour 1 cup of boiling water over 1 teaspoonful (2–3 grams) of dried valerian root and steep for 5 to 20 minutes.

- Tincture (1:5): 1–1½ teaspoons

- Fluid extract (1:1): ½–1 teaspoon (1–2 milliliters)

Once you're sleeping better, continue the valerian for 2 to 6 weeks to maintain the benefits.

NATURAL TREATMENTS WORTH TRYING FOR INSOMNIA

If none of the remedies listed above works for your stress-induced insomnia, try the following. They may not work immediately and they may not work for you at all, but they are safe and certainly worth a try.

Melatonin

Although melatonin supplements are very effective at treating circadian rhythm disorders, including jet lag, the overall evidence on melatonin for run-of-the-mill insomnia is mixed. One study of 334 people ages 55 and older found that they fell asleep faster, slept better, were more alert in the morning, and had an overall improved quality of life when they took sustained-release melatonin supplements. Yet a large analysis of several studies on melatonin and insomnia found that while people taking the supplement fell asleep about 8 minutes faster, the quality of their sleep wasn't any better than that of those taking a placebo. However, people with a condition called delayed sleep phase syndrome, in which they weren't even tired until late in the evening, did have a greater benefit, falling asleep nearly 40 minutes faster. Other studies have found that the lower your natural melatonin levels, the more benefit you get from supplements.

Bottom line: Worth a try. Melatonin is pretty safe, with no evidence that it's addictive or leads to increased tolerance like some prescription or over-the-counter sleep medications. Doses range from 0.1 milligram to 10 milligrams. As with all medications and supplements, start with the lowest dose and work your way up until you get the relief you need. Also, remember that melatonin works much like a sleeping pill; don't take it and then go for a drive. The effects can last up to 7 hours in your brain. Take it and go to bed!

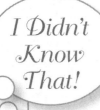

I Didn't Know That!

MELATONIN FOR CHOLESTEROL

There's some evidence that supplemental melatonin can both reduce levels of the so-called "bad" LDL cholesterol and increase levels of "good" HDL cholesterol. A study of 36 peri- and postmenopausal women found that higher nighttime levels of melatonin were associated with lower LDL levels and higher HDL levels. When researchers gave 10 of the women a month of melatonin supplements (1 milligram/day), they found that the women's blood levels of HDL cholesterol increased significantly.

Chamomile

Chamomile is an age-old herb used for anxiety and insomnia. Its benefits are likely related to a plant-based chemical called apigenin that binds to the same receptors as antianxiety medications like Valium.

There are few clinical studies on chamomile. One small study in 10 heart patients reported that participants fell into a deep sleep 1½ hours after drinking chamomile tea. Other studies have found that it reduces levels of stress hormones, which could help you sleep.

Bottom line: Worth a try. We recommend the tea; the very process of brewing and sipping the warm tea can have a relaxing, soothing effect.

WHEN ALL ELSE FAILS . . . INSOMNIA MEDICATIONS

While several medications are approved specifically for insomnia, many drugs are used off-label, meaning that they are approved for other conditions, but doctors can still prescribe them for insomnia. Here's what you should know about available options . . . if nothing else works.

Antidepressants. The antidepressants Elavil (amitriptyline) and Desyrel (trazodone) are often prescribed for insomnia. Although they work pretty well, their sedating effects can last through the next day. Desyrel can also cause dizziness and low blood pressure if you sit or stand too quickly, as well as some sexual side effects. Make sure that you don't take Desyrel with other drugs that affect serotonin levels.

Bottom line: There are better prescription options available.

Antihistamines. Most over-the-counter sleeping medications contain the antihistamine diphenhydramine (aka Benadryl) with or without pain relievers. Potential side effects include confusion, problems urinating, and a "hungover" feeling the next day. Plus, you may eventually become tolerant to its effects and need more and more to get to sleep.

Bottom line: Okay for occasional insomnia only

Benzodiazepines. These drugs bind to receptors for the brain chemical GABA. When GABA fits into these cellular receptors, it triggers sleep. Benzodiazepines are divided into long, intermediate, and short acting based on how long they remain in your body. Dalmane (flurazepam) and Doral (quazepam) are the longest acting, remaining in the body for more than 2 days. They are not a good option for occasional insomnia.

ProSom (estazolam), Restoril (temazepam), and Ativan (lorazepam) are intermediate acting and can take up to a day to leave your body; they're best used if you have trouble staying asleep. Halcion (triazolam), the shortest-acting benzodiazepine, still shouldn't be used as a first-line option for insomnia because it can lead to anxiety and has other serious side effects. In fact, none of these drugs is an ideal sleeping aid, in part because extensive use can lead to tolerance and even physical addiction as well as rebound insomnia once you stop taking it.

Bottom line: These may be helpful for short-term or situational insomnia, but it's not a good idea to take them on a nightly basis.

Nonbenzodiazepines. These drugs—Lunesta (eszopiclone), Sonata (zaleplon), and Ambien (zolpidem)—work similarly to benzodiazepines in that they also bind to GABA receptors. However, these drugs are gradually replacing benzodiazepines for insomnia because they have fewer next-day effects and a lower risk of tolerance and addiction. Lunesta is best if you have trouble staying asleep, Sonata and Ambien for falling asleep; yet both Sonata and a long-acting formulation of Ambien can also help with staying asleep.

In one study, women with breast cancer or a high risk of breast cancer who also had nightly hot flashes were assigned to either take 10 milligrams daily of Ambien or a placebo each night for 5 weeks. Forty percent of the women taking Ambien slept through their hot flashes compared with just 14 percent of those getting the placebo. Meanwhile, a study of Lunesta in 59 peri- and postmenopausal women who had problems falling asleep and/or staying asleep, as well as hot flashes, depression, and/or anxiety, found that 3 milligrams per day of Lunesta over 11 weeks not only improved all aspects of their sleep but also their symptoms of depression and anxiety and of nighttime hot flashes. It didn't help with daytime hot flashes, however.

Bottom line: Okay for short-term use. Side effects include a nearly doubled risk of depression, a risk of withdrawal symptoms if you've been taking them for a few weeks, amnesia, hallucinations, and, more rarely, sleepwalking.

Rozerem (ramelteon). This drug acts like melatonin in the body but is 17 times more potent. It is the only FDA-approved insomnia drug indicated for long-term use (more than 6 weeks).

A study published in *Menopause International* in 2009 compared the effects of 6 weeks of Rozerem on 20 healthy peri- and postmenopausal women. Researchers found significant improvements in the time it took the women to fall asleep, the total time they stayed asleep, and their overall sleep quality. The women also reported improved quality of life, daytime functioning, and mood. One caveat is that there was no placebo used in this study. Another is that 40 percent of the women reported side effects, particularly headaches, daytime fatigue/fogginess, dry mouth, light-headedness, and dizziness, although most were mild and improved within a few days of taking the drug.

Bottom line: Okay to use if you need something for more than a few nights

---

If there's one thing we want you to take away from this chapter, it's that hot flashes are probably *not* the only reason for your sleep problems. Anxiety, changing hormones, and underlying medical problems are more likely the cause. The only way to know for sure, however, is to talk to your health-care provider about it. Once you identify what's going on, you can then pick and choose from the plethora of options described in this chapter.

Happier and Healthier…
THE NATURAL MENOPAUSE SOLUTION WAY

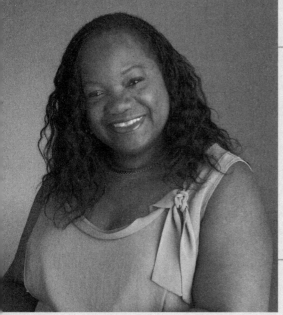

CHERYLYN RUSH

Age: 51

Pounds lost: 3½

Inches lost: 7

Major changes: Fewer hot flashes, very few night sweats, sounder sleep. Total cholesterol fell 41 points.

"I Thought I Just Wasn't a Good Sleeper"

"Is that new?" A week or two into the Natural Menopause Solution, Cherylyn's colleagues at the college where she works noticed something different about her. "They thought I was wearing a new outfit," she says. "But my clothes were fitting better because I was losing pounds and inches. Between Thursday afternoon, when I left work, and Monday morning, when I returned, they could see that I'd lost weight in my figure and in my face."

Logging her menopausal symptoms helped her spot another good thing: Her hot flashes were reduced to just three per day, and her night sweats all but disappeared as she followed the program. "Keeping track helped me realize how much the night sweats had disrupted my sleep in the past," Cherylyn recalls. "I thought I just wasn't a good sleeper, but I found out that most nights I was really sweating—sometimes it was so severe that I threw off the blankets and stood in front of the air conditioner to get relief. I would have to wipe the sweat off my forehead and neck."

Before the program, Cherylyn woke up two to three times a night almost every night. The alarm clock seemed to taunt her. "I always woke up at exactly 3:33 in the morning; it was so odd," she says. Now that she's having fewer night sweats—from nearly every night to just two or three times a week—she's sleeping more soundly. Goodbye, 3:33 a.m. wake-ups!

Cherylyn says that her commitment to healthy eating on the 30-Day Slim-Down, Cool-Down Diet retrained her tastebuds and her digestive system so both became more finely attuned to the difference between good-for-you and not-so-good-for-you foods. "I'm much more aware now. I ordered a salad the other day, and it came with fried chicken fingers. Right away I realized that the fried part didn't taste right. My stomach wasn't too happy with it, either. The fat, the salt—I could feel how heavy it was."

Keeping a food journal has helped Cherylyn celebrate great choices and see the consequences of slipups. "I don't get down on myself, because that's not productive," she says. "But I really try to keep track of what I'm eating. I try to write even when I don't make really good choices, because I include how I feel physically and emotionally so I can learn from it."

Cherylyn says she and her husband really enjoyed the Beef 'n' Broccoli Pasta Salad. "I took the leftovers for lunch the next day, and when I got home I found out that my husband had been looking for it in the refrigerator," she says. "And I liked trying new ingredients. I'm not usually a tomato lover, but once I found dried tomatoes in the supermarket and added them to recipes—wow, this food was a party in my mouth!"

And she found that doing interval walks on her treadmill kept her on track on days when it was too hot or rainy to hit the pavement. "On the treadmill I could keep track of the fast bursts and slower-paced sections of the walk. It worked better for me," she says. "And I could see that I was working hard, so it kept me motivated. And that paid off in so many ways."

Chapter 9

Mood, Memory, and Energy

*H*ow are you feeling these days? No, we're not talking about hot flashes or that ache in your knee. We're talking about emotionally. Do you find yourself snapping at people over the littlest things? Crying like your dog just died simply because your flight got canceled? Feeling as if your heart is going to jump out of your chest whenever there's a full moon? Maybe you feel as if you're fighting your way through quicksand just to make it through the day without a nap, and the idea of anything more energetic than channel surfing only makes you feel even more tired.

Rest assured that you're not alone. In an Internet survey of 961 members of the National Association of Female Executives, most of whom were either within or past the menopausal transition, 79 percent reported emotional symptoms during that transition, and 40 percent said the

238

symptoms were troublesome. Another survey, of 100 women who visited a menopause clinic, found that about 65 percent had significant emotional symptoms, primarily depression. But depression is just one of the mood-related effects of menopause. Studies have also found that anxiety and fatigue can increase during this transitional time.

None of this has to occur, however. In fact, the Melbourne Women's Midlife Health Project in Australia found that women reported that their sense of well-being had *improved* as they moved through perimenopause. And a study of 541 women in Pennsylvania's Allegheny County found that women who experienced a natural menopause rather than having had their ovaries removed had no significant differences in anxiety or depression levels compared to younger women.

To make sure that your menopausal transition mimics those of the women in Australia and Pennsylvania, flip back to the 30-Day Slim-Down, Cool-Down Diet in Part II, then return to this chapter to read more about how to maximize your overall physical health. And follow our advice throughout this chapter to improve your mental health and prevent or, if necessary, manage any mood-related symptoms.

IS IT DEPRESSION?

Signs that your low mood is more than just the blues include feeling hopeless, losing interest in activities you previously enjoyed, lack of energy, problems sleeping (or sleeping too much), changes in your appetite, and irritability or anger. Clinical depression is nothing to fool around with. It is *not* simply a case of the blues, and it can be deadly—as deadly as diabetes or heart disease. In fact, it may even contribute to heart disease. Researchers in SWAN, or the Study of Women's Health Across the Nation, evaluated 346 women for coronary artery calcification, a major risk factor for heart disease. They found that the more depressed the women, the higher their calcification scores. Depression, the researchers concluded, posed the same risk for heart disease as did being overweight or having high blood pressure.

Unfortunately, midlife is a time when the risk of depression increases dramatically. The following are among the causes:

Hormones. SWAN, which followed women for more than 10 years, found that women in perimenopause with no prior history of depression were still four times more likely to have symptoms of depression and 2½ times more likely to be diagnosed with depression than women who weren't entering menopause. The greater their hormonal fluctuations, the greater the risk of depression.

Hot flashes. Hormones are not the only contributor to the rise in midlife depression, however. One study found that, regardless of whether they had any history of depression, perimenopausal women with hot flashes were four times as likely to be depressed as those who hadn't experienced hot flashes.

Life changes. And don't forget what else occurs during this time: major life changes. For many women, this is when the kids go off to college, careers change, parents get ill or die, and the reality of their own mortality looms. Medical problems, many associated with depression, also begin to creep in. So maybe we shouldn't ask why so many women get depressed during midlife but why any woman doesn't!

The good news is, depression is very treatable. Lifestyle changes, therapy, medication, supplements, herbs, and other complementary approaches can help. The first step is to make an appointment with your doctor for a complete physical (certain medical conditions can mimic the symptoms of depression or even cause it, such as thyroid disease). The next step is to take action.

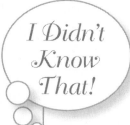

I Didn't Know That!

PMS AND DEPRESSION

Your risk of depression during the menopausal transition is much higher if you had severe premenstrual syndrome (PMS) symptoms. Other risk factors include sleep disorders and a high variation in reproductive-hormone levels.

Because it appears that midlife depression may be related to hormonal fluctuations as well as lifestyle issues and changes in brain chemicals that control mood, clinicians have begun looking at which treatments work best for menopausal women versus women in general. They're beginning to get some answers.

Natural remedies are a good place to start. A recent study showed that 40 percent of people with depression turned to natural remedies like herbs and supplements to treat their disease. That's great; just make sure to tell your doctor if you're taking any herbs or supplements.

LIFTING YOUR MOOD NOW

Before you reach for a pill bottle, give the following natural remedies a try. You may find that they work unexpectedly well and fast.

Exercise. The mood-boosting effects of exercise have been known for decades, and they don't discriminate based on age. A study published in 2010 in the journal *Obstetrics and Gynecology International* evaluated the effects of exercise on mood in 46 women ages 45 to 60. They worked out 3 days a week for 8 weeks; half of the women did aerobic exercise on a bike, while the other half did resistance training. Both groups showed significant drops in depressive symptoms and just as significant improvements in all menopausal symptoms and in overall quality of life. Another study, of 648 middle-aged Korean women, found that the women who exercised regularly were less depressed and had fewer depressive symptoms than those who didn't exercise.

Distraction. One symptom and cause of depression is rumination— when you find yourself unable to shift your thinking away from specific thoughts that contribute to your mood, like certain worries. Distraction can help. When you find your mind getting into that spiral, give yourself a mental shake and shift both your thinking and your actions. Physical activity is a great distraction, especially something that requires mental focus and puts you around other people, like a Zumba class or a tennis match. Other good distractions include watching a funny movie, going shopping, cooking a gourmet meal, or simply having coffee with a friend. Just limit the conversation to positive topics.

REMEDIES THAT MAY RELIEVE DEPRESSION

The research on the following treatments and supplements is mixed, but while they may take time to work, they may be worth a try.

St. John's wort. This herb has been used for centuries to treat everything from depression to pain and wounds. A chemical called hypericin, which provides the red coloring for parts of the herb, interferes with a brain enzyme called monoamine oxidase (MAO), which destroys various "feel good" neurotransmitters like serotonin, epinephrine, and dopamine. St. John's wort can also help with insomnia, a common problem in women who are depressed. At least eight studies have found that St. John's wort works just as well as antidepressants, particularly for people coping with their first bout of the disorder, though not as well for those with chronic severe depression. In one study of 301 menopausal women, those taking St. John's wort plus black cohosh for 12 weeks showed improvements not only in depression but also in other menopausal symptoms.

Bottom line: A good natural option. Make sure that the product you buy has at least 0.3 percent of hypericin. Take 300 milligrams up to three times a day, and, as with most herbs, give it time. It may take 4 to 6 weeks to have much effect, about the same as many antidepressants. St. John's wort interacts with numerous medications, including antidepressants, birth control pills, and blood thinners, so tell your doctor if you decide to start taking it.

Omega-3 fatty acids. You might know these healthy fats more for their heart health benefits than for their effect on the brain, but in recent years we've come to realize that they can have a tremendous impact on mood, thanks to their support of brain and nerve function. The first study that looked at omega-3 fatty acids for menopausal depression was published in March 2011 in the journal *Menopause.* Twenty women experiencing depression were treated with capsules containing 2 grams of

EHA and DHA (two types of omega-3 fatty acids) a day. After 8 weeks, the women's scores on a depression test had dropped by half, and, as a bonus, those with hot flashes at the beginning of the study had far fewer at the end. Plus, the flashes that remained were far less annoying.

Bottom line: A good natural option. Although eating more fatty fish is the best way to increase your consumption of omega-3 fatty acids, these fish (particularly tilefish, swordfish, and mackerel) can also be high in mercury. Stick with wild salmon and tuna, and limit consumption to no more than twice a week. (You can get a wallet-size card that lists the mercury levels in fish at www.nrdc.org/health/effects/mercury/walletcard.pdf.)

For a real boost in omega-3s, opt for mercury-free supplements. It is safe to take them with all antidepressants, but they can have some blood-thinning effects, so talk to your doctor if you're also taking a blood thinner like Coumadin (warfarin).

SAMe. Short for S-adenosyl methionine, SAMe is a naturally occurring compound in your body that boosts levels of the feel-good neurotransmitters serotonin and dopamine. At least three studies have found that SAMe is as effective for depression as tricyclic antidepressants, with far fewer side effects. Two other studies found SAMe to be superior to a placebo in relieving depression. It may even help with memory. A study of 46 people with major depressive disorder who didn't get any benefit from traditional antidepressants found that 6 weeks of SAMe not only helped with their depression but also improved their ability to remember things, as compared with the placebo.

Bottom line: A good natural option. The effective dose for depression in most studies is 800 to 1,600 milligrams daily in divided doses. This dosage can be expensive, up to $80 a month. SAMe can also interact with certain antidepressants and may cause some nausea or stomach upset, anxiety, and sleep problems. If you have bipolar disease, avoid this supplement, as it can trigger a manic episode.

Psychotherapy. We consider talk therapy a natural remedy because it doesn't involve swallowing a pill. There's also plenty of evidence of its benefits for treating those with depression, particularly for preventing relapses. The form of therapy that works best is cognitive behavioral therapy, which teaches you to shift your thinking away from negative thoughts and toward more positive ones; and interpersonal therapy, in which you learn to handle stress better and improve how you relate to others.

Bottom line: Definitely worth a try, whether alone or in conjunction with natural remedies or even medication.

Hypnotherapy. It you think hypnosis is only good for stand-up comics, think again. Medical hypnotherapy, which focuses on changing thought patterns, is gaining credence in treating numerous disorders, including depression. In one study, 84 people with depression received 16 weeks of either hypnotherapy or cognitive behavioral therapy. Both groups improved significantly, with the hypnotherapy group scoring slightly better on tests that measured depression and anxiety. The best news is the benefits for the hypnotherapy group lasted for at least a year after the study ended.

Bottom line: Definitely worth a try.

5-HTP (5-hydroxytryptophan). This naturally occurring amino acid is converted to serotonin, which helps explain its mood-boosting benefits. Good-quality studies are limited, but they do show that the supplement (called oxitriptan) works better than a placebo to relieve depression.

Bottom line: Worth a try. Typical doses range from 50 to 300 milligrams (start low and increase as tolerated/needed). Take 5-HTP about an hour before bed to help you relax. If you take a dose at the higher end of the range, you can take it throughout the day. The side effects are similar to those of many prescription antidepressants, including nausea and heart palpitations. Some women also report vivid dreams—so keep your dream diary near the bed! 5-HTP may interact with other supplements or medications that raise serotonin and should be used only with medical supervision.

Folate. Folate is a B vitamin required to make dopamine, norepinephrine, and serotonin, all of which are important players in mood and depression. Too little folate can lead to brain changes related to dementia, Parkinson's disease, and stroke. In fact, people who are low in folate are much more likely to suffer from depression and have more severe and longer-lasting depression. They are also less likely to benefit from antidepressants and more likely to relapse.

Folate has only been evaluated as an add-on to antidepressant medications. One study involved 24 people with depression and low levels of folate who took either 15 milligrams of the vitamin or a placebo, in addition to antidepressant medication. Researchers reported that the vitamin group's depression improved more than the placebo group's. Another study—this one involving 127 people who were already taking Prozac (fluoxetine) for depression and then added 0.5 milligram of folic acid a day for 10 weeks—found that scores on a depression test had improved more for the vitamin group than for those taking Prozac only.

Bottom line: Worth a try as an add-on to antidepressants. Folate occurs naturally in foods such as whole grains and green leafy vegetables; folic acid is the synthetic form of the vitamin. However, more than half the population, and about 70 percent of women with depression, have a gene variation that slows their ability to convert folic acid into the active form of folate. These individuals need a prescription form of active folic acid, either an intermediate form called methylenetetrahydrofolate or the active form called Deplin (L-methylfolate). You won't know if you fall into this category without a genetic test, but folate is a safe supplement to take. Try it and see if you feel better! Typical dosages: 500 micrograms of folic acid, 15 to 50 milligrams of methylene tetrahydrofolate, or 7.5 milligrams of Deplin daily.

DHEA. Dehydroepiandrosterone (DHEA) is an important reproductive hormone that affects levels of dopamine, a brain hormone that plays a role in mood. As with so many other reproductive hormones, the levels decline with age. There is some evidence that supplementing with DHEA can help with mood and overall well-being, although the studies are mixed. Because it is transformed into androgens and estrogen in the body, however, don't use DHEA without physician oversight.

Your doctor can prescribe oral DHEA supplements. There are few side effects with either type when taken in recommended doses, although too-high doses can affect cholesterol levels and lead to androgen-related side effects such as acne, hair growth, and a deepening voice.

Bottom line: Only use DHEA if you're found to be deficient on testing by your doctor (using a blood test for DHEA-Sulfate) and your doctor feels you are a good candidate for supplementation. Also make sure you consult your doctor for the right dosage: Doses for women are much lower than for men, and over-the-counter DHEA supplements are often too strong.

WHEN ALL ELSE FAILS ... MEDICATIONS FOR DEPRESSION

If you've tried the natural remedies and still feel rotten, it's time to talk to your doctor about prescription medication. Here's what you need to know.

Antidepressants

Most antidepressants work by affecting levels of various neurotransmitters in the brain, particularly serotonin, norepinephrine, and dopamine. Studies conducted in peri- and postmenopausal women have found that Celexa (citalopram) and Lexapro (escitalopram) are especially effective for depression in this age group. They also improve hot flashes, night sweats, and problems like headaches and aches and pains. In addition, an analysis of eight studies found that Effexor (venlafaxine), which impacts both serotonin and norepinephrine levels, was much more effective than selective serotonin reuptake inhibitors (SSRIs) such as Prozac and Zoloft (sertraline), particularly in women who were not using hormone therapy.

Common side effects of antidepressants, especially when you first start taking them, include gastrointestinal discomfort or nausea, reduced sex drive, problems reaching orgasm, fatigue, sleep disturbances, and, in some instances, weight change. Most improve after a few weeks, but some may continue long term.

Antidepressants may also have some benefits for hot flashes, which you read about in Chapter 7.

Bottom line: Definitely worth a try if natural remedies don't work. Choosing which antidepressant to start with is a decision for you and your doctor. Make sure that you give each medication at least 4 weeks before trying another, however; it takes this long for the drug to reach its maximal effect.

Estrogen

Estrogen, particularly estradiol, acts as a kind of CEO for various chemical systems related to mood and behavior, especially those in your brain that involve the production and transmission of the mood-related chemicals serotonin and norepinephrine. Estrogen also reduces the activity of enzymes that break down serotonin and ups the activity of enzymes that help produce it. These actions help increase the amount of serotonin available for transmission. So you can imagine what happens when natural levels of estrogen begin fluctuating more than the stock market. Thus, it makes sense to suspect that adding back estradiol might help with midlife depression.

One study, of 50 perimenopausal women with depression, assigned the women to two groups: One was given estrogen patches, and the other, placebo patches, which they wore for 12 weeks. Depression improved in nearly 70 percent of the women who received estrogen patches, compared with just 20 percent of those in the placebo group, no matter how severe the initial depression. And the benefits for the first group continued even 4 weeks after they stopped using the estrogen patches.

For more on estrogen therapy, see Chapter 18. The goal should be to take the smallest dose possible for the shortest amount of time and to use the form most like your body's own estrogen: estradiol.

Bottom line: Unless you want to use estrogen therapy for other menopausal symptoms like hot flashes, it should be a final medical option only if antidepressants don't work.

ALL ABOUT MIDLIFE ANXIETY

You know that feeling you sometimes get when you feel like you can't breathe or there's a weight on your chest or your heart starts beating like crazy? You may think you're having a heart attack—and you should definitely have your symptoms checked—but you are just as likely to be having a panic attack or, at the very least, a bout with anxiety.

Yup, you guessed it, our anxiety levels increase as our hormones decline. Here the main culprit is progesterone, which, as you learned in Chapter 8, is the calming hormone. It's the first reproductive hormone to decline in perimenopause, says Melinda Ring, MD, medical advisor for *The Natural Menopause Solution.* "That's one reason why a lot of women heading into perimenopause note more anxiety and palpitations," she explains. The decline in progesterone leaves more estrogen—the stimulating hormone—hanging around. The result? That "I'm-going-to-jump-out-of-my-skin" feeling.

Don't believe us? Answer this question: Did you notice (or are you noticing) that your PMS got worse as menopause drew closer? Or that you, who never had PMS, now find yourself bursting into tears and throwing something like a temper tantrum the day before your period? Uh-huh, we thought so.

Another reason for the anxiety? Hot flashes. In one study in which 436 women ages 35 to 47 were followed for up to 6 years, researchers found a strong link between hot flashes and anxiety. Women with moderate anxiety were nearly three times as likely to report hot flashes—and women with high anxiety were nearly five times as likely to report them—as those with fewer or no hot flashes.

And, of course, the same life changes that can trigger depression, not to mention the seemingly never-ending flood of bad news these days, can also contribute to anxiety.

SOOTHING MIDLIFE ANXIETY NOW

To manage anxiety naturally, follow these tips:

Make a worry chart. Divide a sheet of paper into three columns. In the first column, write down all your worries. In the second, write the worst thing that could possibly happen as a result of those worries. And in the third, list two ways in which you would handle the worst if it happened.

Visualize the situation. No matter how horrible a situation, something positive always eventually occurs. You wouldn't have your current job, which you love, if you hadn't been fired from the job you hated. You wouldn't be married to your current husband if you hadn't divorced the previous one (who turned out to be a lying, cheating jerk, but you're done concerning yourself with him). So on your worry list, consider the positives that might occur if the worst happened. And if the worst *does* happen, take a minute to consider where it might lead—on the positive side.

Focus on the here and now. It might sound like a cliché, but today really *is* all that we can control. A good way to integrate this into your life is with mindfulness meditation (described on page 227), mindful eating (in other words, turn off the television and put away the book), and mindful walks (forget the iPod).

Break the issue into pieces. Instead of obsessing that your son will never get into college, sit down and make a list of all the steps he and you have to take to even get a letter of acceptance or denial, then methodically work your way through each, focusing on the next task, not the end result.

Be gentle with yourself. Calling yourself a fat slob for not making it to the gym today does nobody any good. Reminding yourself how great it was that you got to the gym yesterday (and promising that you'll take a long walk tomorrow) goes much further toward reducing your anxiety over your weight than the negative self-talk.

Distract yourself. When you're feeling so anxious you think you might just jump out of your skin, it's time to switch gears. Do something else that totally engages your mind, whether it's reading a book, writing in your journal, going to the gym for a Zumba class (keeping up with the moves requires that you focus only on the instructor), or watching a movie you love.

CALMING ANXIETY IN THE LONG TERM

The following remedies will take a bit more time to begin working but are definitely worth the effort.

Applied relaxation. Learning to relax and calm your body's fight-or-flight response (think pounding heart, adrenaline rush) can be a very effective way to reduce and prevent anxiety. We're talking about things like deep breathing, progressive muscle relaxation, and guided imagery, in which you close your eyes and picture a scene that relaxes you (beach and piña colada, anyone?). In one 5-month study, relaxation techniques worked just as well as antidepressants at relieving anxiety.

Bottom line: Worth a try.

Yoga and tai chi. Numerous studies attest to the anxiety-reducing benefits of Eastern practices like yoga and tai chi. They work by changing the way your body responds to stress, thus you're less likely to get anxious when confronted with a stressful event or worry. In a study published in 2005, German researchers assigned 24 women who were "emotionally distressed" to take two 90-minute yoga classes a week for 3 months or to maintain their normal activities (the control group). After 3 months, the yoga group had significantly fewer symptoms of anxiety and depression. They also reported having more energy and feeling better overall.

Bottom line: Definitely worth a try. Start with the yoga-with-weights routine in the 30-Day Slim-Down, Cool-Down Diet.

Cognitive behavioral therapy (CBT). This therapy, described on page 243 for depression, can also work well for anxiety. It takes time, however; you'll need weekly 1- to 2-hour sessions for about 4 months before you'll see significant improvements.

Bottom line: Worth a try, but make sure that you find a therapist specifically trained in CBT.

Kava. This herbal remedy contains kavapyrones, natural muscle

Don't Bother with Estrogen Therapy for Anxiety

If you're considering trying hormone therapy for your anxiety, skip it. Three good-quality studies that evaluated estrogen therapy for anxiety in peri- and postmenopausal women found no benefit from estrogen for that condition.

relaxants that work like narcotics in your brain. Although kava relieves anxiety, it usually doesn't make you tired or woozy like prescription anti-anxiety medications can (though you should not drive or mix with other medications just in case). Numerous studies have been conducted over the past 20 years with this herb, most of which have shown benefits.

There has been some concern about kava's link to liver problems; though reports aren't conclusive, it's best to avoid if you have any liver problems and use only for a few days at a time even if you don't.

Bottom line: May be worth a try for short-term use. Limit the dose to no more than 400 milligrams daily of a standard kava extract. However, the risk of liver damage is idiosyncratic and not dose related, so use caution.

Passionflower (*Passiflora incarnata*). This herb has been used for centuries to calm anxiety. In studies, it works as well as prescription anti-anxiety drugs in improving symptoms. Potential side effects include dizziness, drowsiness, and confusion, but those occurred in only one study.

Bottom line: Worth a try. You can purchase passionflower extract and pills in health food stores.

Lysine. This amino acid is thought to influence brain chemicals involved in anxiety. In one study of men with high-anxiety traits, lysine improved their ability to handle stress better than a placebo. In another study, of Japanese men and women, it lowered levels of the stress hormone cortisol in men but not women, though it reduced anxiety in both genders.

Bottom line: Worth a try. Use the supplement and follow the recommended dosage on the label.

Magnesium. Low levels of this mineral have been linked to anxiety-related disorders, likely because of the vital role it plays in various hormonal systems. Most studies have evaluated magnesium's benefits in combination with other vitamins or minerals, such as calcium, zinc, and vitamin B_6, and all have shown significant benefits. In a study of women who had menstruation-related anxiety, a 300-milligram supplement reduced all of their symptoms; it worked even better when combined with B_6.

Bottom line: Worth a try if nothing else works. Magnesium is one of our Flash-Fighting Four, so you'll get plenty if you're following our 30-Day Slim-Down, Cool-Down Diet. But you may also need to add supplements in order to get the full 300-milligram dosage used in the studies. Magnesium comes in different forms: Magnesium citrate is more likely to cause loose stool (good if you have constipation!), while magnesium glycinate, gluconate, and lactate are less prone to have that effect.

St. John's wort. This herb is officially licensed in Germany for treating anxiety, although it's known more for its antidepressive effects. It works on similar brain receptors as kava. Most studies have assessed its use in people with depression and anxiety, which occur together in as many as 85 percent of people who have either condition; it also works on receptors in the brain involved in anxiety. Research on it is mixed.

Bottom line: Start with other herbal remedies, though it may be worth a try, especially if you also suffer from depression. Remember to be cautious about herb–drug interactions.

WHEN ALL ELSE FAILS . . . MEDICATIONS FOR ANXIETY

If our natural remedies don't help and your anxiety is interfering with your quality of life, it might be time to step it up a notch. The following medications can help:

Benzodiazepines. These include lorazepam (Ativan), clonazepam (Klonopin), alprazolam (Xanax), and diazepam (Valium).

Bottom line: Approved for use with anxiety and shown to be quite effective, benzodiazepines should be taken for only a few days or a couple of weeks because they are habit-forming, leading to withdrawal symptoms when you try to stop taking them. They also have a strong sedative effect, so don't drive after taking one.

Beta-blockers. These drugs include propranolol (Inderal) and metoprolol (Lopressor). They are typically prescribed for high blood pressure and angina (chest pain). They block the effects of stress hormones on blood pressure and heart rate and slow the heart rate.

Bottom line: Worth a try, but don't take them if you have asthma or circulatory problems. And don't stop taking them abruptly; work with your doctor to taper off.

Antidepressants. Antidepressants, particularly the selective serotonin reuptake inhibitors (SSRIs) like sertraline (Zoloft), are often prescribed in low doses for anxiety.

Bottom line: Studies of midlife women have found antianxiety benefits with trazodone (Desyrel), paroxetine (Paxil), citalopram (Celexa), venlafaxine (Effexor), and duloxetine (Cymbalta). They are safe to use over the long term.

Heart Palpitations? Breathe!

A classic sign of anxiety is feeling like your heart is beating so fast that it will fly right out of your chest. This rapid heartbeat is also known as heart palpitations. They can be so bad that they send some people to the emergency room, certain that they're having a heart attack. If your palpitations are caused by anxiety (because when you thought you were having a heart attack, your doctor assured you that it was an anxiety attack), try the natural remedies suggested here. If they don't help, check with your doctor about other options. You should also

- **Cut back on caffeine.** Caffeine is a stimulant, which can increase heart rate.

- **Practice paced breathing.** You can read more about paced breathing on page 190.

- **Keep a record.** Write down what you were doing when you had the palpitations; you should be able to see a pattern.

If, however, you feel lots of extra heartbeats during palpitations; have heart disease or a risk factor like diabetes, high blood pressure, or high cholesterol; or the palpitations suddenly feel different, or your pulse is more than 100 beats per minute and you haven't been exercising, call your doctor immediately. You may be experiencing a potentially dangerous heart-rhythm abnormality.

Happier and Healthier...
THE NATURAL MENOPAUSE SOLUTION WAY

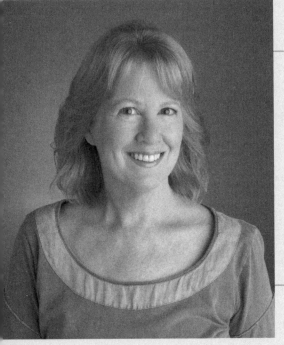

EILEEN FEHR

Age: 58

Pounds lost: 7

Inches lost: 6¼

Major changes: Lowered fasting blood sugar, blood pressure, and total cholesterol. Feels less stressed and is tapering off HRT.

"I Don't Spazz Out about Things the Way I Used To"

"At this age, it's harder and harder to lose weight, so losing 6 pounds in just 30 days was pretty exciting," says Eileen. "Most of my clothes are getting big, but so far I'm resisting the urge to shop for more—I'm planning to stick with this program and see how much more weight I can lose. I do have a pair of favorite cutoff shorts that had gotten really tight. I fit into them easily now. And I can tuck my shirt in instead of wearing a big top to hide the tight waistband."

Eileen has been having hot flashes since she was 44, has been on and off birth control pills, and recently started hormone replacement therapy to help regulate them. "I was getting about 20 hot flashes a day, and I had to do something. I weighed the pros and cons and decided that short-term HRT would be beneficial. It has helped me, but I don't want to stay on it long term. I am working with my doctor to taper off now and hope that this eating plan and all the exercise will help control my symptoms."

One midlife—and possibly menopausal—symptom that's already improved? She feels less stressed out, more relaxed, and peaceful. "I have a tendency to explode when things go crazy," she admits. "That's almost completely under control now. . . . I think the serenity of the yoga routine has made a big difference there."

A longtime fan of yoga, Eileen says she was skeptical about the apparent simplicity and ease of the Natural Menopause Solution yoga-with-weights routine. "I thought those little 2-pound weights wouldn't make a difference, but they definitely did. It gives some oomph to the yoga routine, and I can feel that I'm more toned; I feel stronger in my legs and arms."

During a physical last year for Eileen's job, her doctor noticed that her blood pressure was creeping up into the prehypertensive range—a risk for developing high blood pressure. "Now it's down to 118/80, just about in the healthy range," she notes. "I suspect that high blood pressure runs in my family, and I'd like to avoid it if at all possible. I was pretty excited to see that my cholesterol and my blood sugar were lower, too."

One of Eileen's favorite foods on the program was the daily Slimming, Cooling Smoothie. "I loved it," she says. "Sometimes I varied the fruit, but the combination of the pineapple, almond butter, and vanilla soy milk was so incredible and excellent that it really didn't need to be improved upon. And it stored well in the refrigerator. I would make up the full recipe, have one serving, and have three left over: Just stir it up and it was ready to drink. It was so filling, I would wait until I got to work to eat the rest of my breakfast."

WHAT WAS YOUR NAME AGAIN?

If you find yourself calling your teenage son by the dog's name, using the word "thingy" as a noun in every other sentence, and getting a late notice from the mortgage company for the first time in your life, blame it on hormones. One study found that 60 percent of perimenopausal women experience short-term memory loss and have a hard time concentrating. Meanwhile, SWAN found significant changes in how long it took menopausal women to process information and get words from their brain to their mouth. The good news is that the effect appears to be temporary. A couple of years after menopause, you should get your brain back.

Researchers aren't sure what causes the cognitive problems at this time of life, but they suspect that it's strongly related to sleep problems and sudden shifts in hormones. Researchers on the SWAN project also found that women with more medical problems, such as depression and metabolic syndrome (a constellation of conditions including high blood pressure, high triglycerides, abdominal obesity, and insulin resistance), were more likely to have memory and learning problems in midlife. Yet another reason to follow our advice throughout this book on healthy living through menopause and beyond!

When to Worry

If you forget your kid's name, lose your keys, or forget to pick up the dry cleaning, you're having midlife memory problems. But if you look at your son and for a minute don't remember who he is; lose your keys on a daily basis or find them in odd places, like the freezer; or forget how to get to the dry cleaner you've been going to every week for 10 years, see your doctor. These types of significant memory problems may suggest an underlying medical problem or the beginnings of dementia.

IMPROVE YOUR MEMORY NOW

Some simple changes in your daily routine, like those listed below, should improve your memory now—or, at the very least, reduce the things you forget to do!

Stop multitasking. There's good evidence that multitasking wreaks havoc on your concentration, making it harder to get memories from the short-term part of your brain to the long-term part. Instead, try to be mindful of what you're doing when you're doing it. So instead of walking into the house while reading the mail, petting the dog, calling for the kids to get ready for soccer, and checking your cell phone—and later having no memory of where you put your keys, purse, or the mail—just walk in and hang your keys on a hook—the same one every time. *Then* you can read the mail, greet the dog, etc., etc.

Use Post-its. Stick them everywhere. For instance, if you need to remember to get gas in the morning, put a Post-it on your bathroom mirror. When you brush your teeth, you'll see it, remember, and get out of the house 15 minutes earlier.

Do it now. If you're doing the dishes and suddenly remember that you need to drop off the dry cleaning tomorrow or mail a package, stop, get the clothes or package, and put it in your car—on the front seat so that you'll see it first thing in the morning. Then make a note on a Post-it and stick it on the door so you'll see it when you leave the house. Or, if it's best not to leave valuables in your car, put your clothes or packages in front of your door so you're sure to remember them.

Embrace technology. Use the calendar and the alarm on your cell phone and computer to remind you of tasks. You can even sync the two, so what you record on one shows up on the other. Put everything on one calendar—even a reminder to pick up the dog from the groomer. Leave nothing to chance.

Have a place for everything and everything in its place. Now is the time to really declutter. Assign locations for items like your purse, your cell phone, the charger, the mail, the grocery list. And remember, the less stuff you have, the less stuff you have to lose.

NATURAL REMEDIES THAT MAY HELP PREVENT MEMORY LOSS

The best thing you can do to prevent memory loss and the dementia of aging is to live a healthy life. A growing body of evidence suggests that high cholesterol and diabetes are both significant contributors to dementia, likely because of their effects on blood flow in the brain. Follow the 30-Day Slim-Down, Cool-Down Diet in Part II for a healthier you, and also check out the prevention strategies in Chapter 13 to keep your arteries clear and Chapter 14 to keep your blood sugar levels normal. You might also try the following:

Ginseng. This herb has been used for centuries as a cognition booster and, indeed, studies suggest that both Asian and American ginseng can improve memory and alertness. However, there are no published studies on its use in midlife women or any evidence that it helps people who have already begun to lose memory.

Ginkgo biloba. Another herb often touted for its memory-enhancing benefits, ginkgo was found to improve memory and thinking speed in 20 young, healthy volunteers better than a product that combined ginkgo and ginseng, according to a study published in 2002. However, there are no published studies on its use in midlife women.

Fish oil supplements. Fish oil contains essential fatty acids like

NOT WORTH TRYING

Phosphatidylserine (lecithin). This naturally occurring substance is thought to increase levels of certain chemicals in the brain that help with memory. Although early studies were positive, most of those were conducted with a form of the supplement derived from cow brains. Given the fear of disease, that source is no longer used. Instead, today's supplements are made from soy, and there is little evidence of their effectiveness.

DHA that form important components of brain cells. Researchers from the Rhode Island Hospital Alzheimer's Disease and Memory Disorders Center followed older adults using brain MRIs and regular testing for 3 years, and found that those who took daily fish oil supplements had far better cognitive function and less brain shrinkage than those who didn't take the supplements.

Bacopa monnieri. This Aryuvedic herb has memory-enhancing properties. In one well-designed Australian study published in 2010 in the *Journal of Alternative and Complementary Medicine,* 98 healthy people ages 56 and older received either 300 milligrams per day of an extract of *Bacopa monnieri* called BacoMind or a placebo. The participants had their memory and ability to learn screened at the beginning of the study and 12 weeks later. Those getting the supplement showed significant improvements in several areas of memory, including their ability to acquire new information and remember it later. Two earlier studies of the supplement published in 2008 also found those receiving the drug had significant improvements in various areas of learning and memory.

Learning a foreign language. People who speak more than one language have a lower risk of memory problems, reported researchers at the American Academy of Neurology's annual meeting in 2011. The finding fits with a large body of research showing that the more you challenge your brain and continue to learn throughout your life, the lower your risk of developing cognitive problems or even Alzheimer's disease. You can accomplish this with a variety of things beyond learning a new language, including doing crossword puzzles and brain teasers, reading literature, taking college courses, and acquiring any new skill or hobby.

Hitting the gym. A review of more than 100 studies on the brain-protecting benefits of exercise published in the *Journal of Applied Physiology* in July 2011 found that both aerobic exercise (think walking and tennis) and strength training are vital for maintaining brain health and memory throughout your lifetime.

The bottom line when it comes to midlife mood and memory is this: Both are interconnected with other issues going on in your life and your body right now. So if you're not sleeping well, you're more likely to be depressed and have memory problems, and if you're having a lot of hot flashes, your anxiety levels are likely to be higher. And if you're not getting enough exercise, you're more vulnerable to depression and anxiety. The reality is that you can't focus on just one symptom of your midlife transition and try to fix it. You need to focus on your entire self—emotionally, nutritionally, physically, and even sexually—in order to feel your best and have a terrific menopause!

Chapter 10

Sex

*I*f the idea of having sex these days is about as appealing as changing your furnace filter, you're not alone. A survey of 3,167 women in the Study of Women's Health Across the Nation (SWAN) found that one in four postmenopausal women said they never felt desire, while 41 percent said they rarely felt it. However, nearly all said they *could* be aroused, and only 13 percent said sex wasn't important.

This study was important for several reasons, particularly because it addressed the fact that desire and arousal were two different things in women, regardless of age. We now know that women are *not* built like men when it comes to sex.

Men, as you probably already know, can get turned on by the least little thing. Once aroused, they want sex, they have sex, they go to sleep (usually). Women come to sex in a more roundabout way. We might not even be aroused when things start or even feel like having sex in the first place! Instead, we decide to have sex for reasons that may have nothing to do with desire. Maybe it's a simple yearning to feel closer to your husband, a way of thanking him for cleaning the kitchen, or wanting to squelch that guilty feeling you have because it's been 2 weeks since you last made love.

So you may not have any feelings of desire (aka emotional arousal) or even wetness and warmth (aka physical arousal) when sex starts. Quite often, those feelings start *after* the process begins. Sometimes desire never arrives and yet you still get aroused.

Men and women also view sex differently. The 2004 AARP Sexuality at Midlife and Beyond study of 1,682 men and women ages 45 and older found that only about 3 percent of men surveyed said they didn't really enjoy sex, as compared with 15 percent of women. In addition, the survey found that men thought about sex and engaged in sexual activities far more than women. For instance, men were more likely to watch adult films, go to strip clubs, have sex in a public place, take erotic photos and videos, and have affairs.

The survey also found that age matters when it comes to sex. Those 45 to 59 years old (men *and* women) tended to be more sexual than those 60 and older, to say that sex plays an important role in their relationship, and to highlight the impact of sex on their quality of life. They also had more sexual thoughts and, perhaps not coincidentally, more sex.

Make no mistake—sex is important to a relationship's health. A study of 30 postmenopausal Portuguese women found a direct link between the frequency of sex and their satisfaction with the relationship, intimacy with their partner, trust, passion, and love. And the AARP survey found that people who were in committed relationships were more likely than those who weren't to say that sex played a critical role in their relationship and quality of life—regardless of age.

One thing we know for sure: The better you feel and the better you feel about yourself, the sexier you will feel (and look). So the path to a good sex life begins by following the Natural Menopause Solution, starting with the 30-Day Slim-Down, Cool-Down Diet in Part II.

You're Not Too Old . . .

To get pregnant. Remember that you aren't considered postmenopausal until you've gone 12 consecutive months without a period. Even 7 months period free doesn't make you safe. Which may be why about half of all pregnancies in women ages 40 and older are unintended, with many ending in abortion. In fact, rates of unintended pregnancy ending in abortion are highest for women 40 and older.

Another thing to watch out for: sexually transmitted infections (STIs), particularly if you're embarking on new relationships at this time in your life. Vaginal thinning and dryness increase your risk of an STI because the vaginal walls are more likely to become irritated and inflamed, giving bacteria and viruses a toehold.

So in addition to insisting that your partner use a condom, you need to use birth control. You can still take oral contraceptives containing estrogen if you don't smoke and have no history of heart disease or blood clots. In fact, you can safely take oral contraceptives until age 50. The main reason to stop then? To find out if you're in menopause, something that oral contraception can mask.

Other estrogen-based birth control options include NuvaRing, which is inserted into the vagina like a diaphragm and works for 3 weeks at a time, and the skin patch Ortho Evra, which is replaced weekly. As with the Pill, neither of these devices should be used by women who smoke or have a history of blood clots.

Nonestrogen options for perimenopausal women include Mirena, an IUD that can be worn for 5 years. An added bonus? It may reduce menstrual bleeding and cramps and even eliminate periods. You can also get a progestin-only pill or have progestin-only rods inserted in your upper arm, where they can remain for up to 3 years.

The other thing we know is that the amount of sex you think is normal is probably not. The reality is that, on average, women in their twenties through their forties are having sex between 1 and 11 times a month—an average of about three times a week for those getting it most often. And if you think you have to have mind-blowing sex every time, consider this: A Pennsylvania State University survey of 34 of the country's leading sex experts who had treated thousands of couples found that just 7 to 13 minutes of lovemaking is considered "desirable" by both

Painful Sex

Here's a commandment to live by: Sex should not hurt. Any level of pain is a sign that something is wrong and a warning that you should see a doctor. In addition to the vaginal changes that occur with menopause, other conditions can cause painful sex. If sex hurts, chances are you don't want it or anything remotely resembling it. Consequently, your libido dries up like a flower in the desert.

Painful sex can occur at any age. Coupled with other midlife issues like vaginal dryness, a changing body, and boredom with a long-term partner, however, they can kill off your sex life faster than having your teenager walk in on you. Unfortunately, doctors usually won't ask about this, so you need to become your own advocate and force the issue. Here are some of the most common causes.

Provoked vestibulodynia (PVD) or vulvar vestibulitis syndrome. Symptoms of this condition (actually, it includes many separate conditions) include pain at the entrance to the vagina, sometimes so severe that even lightly brushing the area with a cotton swab can make you scream in agony.

Treatment: Physical therapy (particularly with a growing specialty known as pelvic floor therapy), medication, and, sometimes, surgery

Hypertonic pelvic floor muscle dysfunction. Women with this condition involuntarily clench their pelvic and vaginal muscles whenever anything comes near those areas. Sometimes the muscles involuntarily spasm. As you might expect, this makes intercourse nearly impossible.

Treatment: Physical therapy, biofeedback, and counseling

men and women, and even shorter sessions of 3 to 7 minutes were considered "adequate."

And the third thing we know for sure? If you're having sex once a month, and you and your partner are fine with that, then you don't have a problem. Only if the state of your sex life bothers you or it's negatively affecting your quality of life and your relationship do you need to read on.

Vulvar and vaginal skin disorders. These dermatologic conditions cause blistering, ulcers, and scarring of the vagina and the tissue around it, called the vulva, and include lichen sclerosus and erosive lichen planus.

Treatment: Medication

Interstitial cystitis. If it seems like you always have to pee (but only a dribble comes out), you have a lot of pain in your pelvic area, and trying to have sex gives new meaning to the word *painful*, you may have this condition. It is also called painful bladder syndrome, and it occurs when the bladder lining becomes severely irritated.

Treatment: Dietary changes, therapy, medication, pain management

Irritable bowel syndrome. This condition is diagnosed based on the symptoms: abdominal pain, constipation and/or diarrhea, gas. Along with other gastrointestinal symptoms, IBS can lead to painful sex.

Treatment. Dietary changes, hypnosis, supplements to address gut health, therapy, medication

Infection. You know about sexually transmitted infections such as herpes, gonorrhea, and chlamydia, but did you know that they can also cause pain during sex? While they're relatively rare as the cause of sexual pain, you should still get checked out.

Treatment: Depends on the infection, but generally antibiotics and antiviral medications (to prevent flare-ups of genital herpes)

Pudendal neuralgia. The pudendal nerve carries sensations from your vulval area (including the clitoris), lower rectum, and perineum (the area between your vagina and rectum). If the nerve gets damaged or trapped, it can cause excruciating burning pain.

Treatment: Physical therapy, surgery

Beyond the relationship benefits of sex, there are health benefits to a good sex life, including the following:

- **Better mental health.** Numerous studies have found that the more often women (and men) have intercourse, the less likely they are to be depressed. There's some thought that semen may have some sort of antidepressant effect, since women who have intercourse without using a condom are even *less* likely to get depressed than women who have sex about the same amount but whose partners use condoms.

- **A healthier vagina and pelvis.** A review of several studies found that having vaginal intercourse helps maintain the health of your vagina and pelvis. The thrusting and other movements of intercourse give a boost to the muscles "down there," while prostaglandin, a chemical messenger found in semen, helps get more oxygen and blood to the vaginal area.

- **Better blood pressure.** The more often you have sex, the less your blood pressure spikes when you get anxious. This only works, however, if you're having intercourse. Masturbation or other sexual activities (think oral sex) don't have the same effect.

- **Calmer heart rate.** Heart rate variability describes the time between heartbeats. The more inconsistent your heart rate, the healthier you are. This heart rate variability is also linked to improved mood, attention, and reaction to stress, and, researchers have found, more frequent sex. Researchers don't know if the heart rate variability leads to increased sexual desire or vice versa, but either way, it's a nice bonus.

- **Fewer hot flashes.** Yes, it's true, having sex could stem the heat. African researchers instructed a group of 43 menopausal women to have sex once a week with their husbands and another group of 42 women to refrain from sex for 6 months. At the end of the study, the sexually active women were having an average of 37 hot flashes a week, as compared with 120 for those in the celibate group. The sexually active women also had higher levels of natural estrogen.

So let's recap. We know that sex is important for a healthy relationship and a healthy you. We also know that many midlife women are about as interested in sex as they are in shaving their heads. What's going on?

CAUSES OF A LOW LIBIDO

There are numerous reasons for your loss of desire, ranging from medical conditions to relationship factors. They don't work in isolation; if sex is painful for you due to vaginal dryness, for instance, and your husband isn't supportive, then solving the vaginal dryness may not solve your libido issues if you're too angry with him to feel loving. So we urge you to take a holistic approach to resolving your sexual issues, picking and choosing the options that you think will work best for *you*, given your specific situation.

Physically, though, the primary culprit behind low libido around menopause is vaginal atrophy. Your vagina depends on estrogen to help maintain moistness and flexibility. As estrogen dries up, so can your vagina. The tissue thins and shrinks even as less blood flows to the area, drying up secretions. So when your partner tries to enter you, it can feel like sandpaper.

Another physical issue related to hormonal changes has to do with the entrance to the vagina called, appropriately enough, the vestibule. Although contiguous to the vagina, the vestibule is actually composed of different tissue. Besides estrogen, this tissue depends on testosterone to keep it healthy. Recall that testosterone levels begin falling in our late twenties! Without enough estrogen or testosterone, vestibular tissue becomes dry and thin, so penile entry hurts.

Symptoms of vaginal atrophy, as it's called, include the dryness we just discussed as well as a burning feeling. You may also have some bleeding with intercourse, discharge, and itching. You don't have to live with it, however.

RELIEVING VAGINAL DRYNESS NOW

If your problem is the pain and dryness of vaginal atrophy, you're in luck. You can find relief tonight with the following:

Over-the-counter lubricants and moisturizers. You can buy them in drugstores or online. The most studied vaginal moisturizer is Replens, which contains oils, glycerin, and polycarbophil. It works by binding to vaginal tissue, releasing water, and creating a thin film over the tissue like a layer of greased plastic wrap. You need to apply the moisturizer every 2 or 3 days, not just before intercourse. Similar products include K-Y Long Lasting Moisturizer, Vagisil Feminine Moisturizer, and Feminease. More natural options include Sylk and Good Clean Love lubricants. Zestra is an "arousal fluid" made with botanical oils that stimulates nerves and blood vessels to increase arousal. In a study published in the *Journal of Sex & Marital Therapy*, women ages 31 to 57 who used Zestra five times over 2 to 3 weeks reported that their sexual pleasure increased significantly.

You can also use a water-based moisturizer such as Astroglide or K-Y Personal Lubricant. Other products use silicone to create a slippery feel. If one product doesn't work, don't despair. Simply try another.

Vitamin E. Just open a capsule and apply the oil daily inside your vagina.

PREVENTING VAGINAL ATROPHY NATURALLY

Once you've figured out which moisturizer or lubricant works best, put it to work in the bedroom. Turns out that sexual intercourse, masturbating, and using a vaginal dilator (various-sized, penis-shaped objects that you insert into your vagina to gently stretch the tissue) can all help reduce dryness by increasing blood flow (which means more oxygen) to the tissues.

WHEN ALL ELSE FAILS . . . MEDICATIONS FOR VAGINAL ATROPHY

If lubricants and additional sex don't help, you may need to talk to your doctor about estrogen therapy. The beauty of estrogen for vaginal atrophy is that you put the drug right where you need it—in your vagina.

NOT WORTH TRYING

Wild yam. Search the phrase "wild yam and vaginal dryness" on the Internet and you'll get dozens of sites claiming the supplement works. Don't believe it. There is no medical evidence that wild yam alleviates vaginal dryness or even that it has any estrogen- or progesterone-like effects in women.

Black cohosh. While there is some mixed evidence as to the benefits of black cohosh for hot flashes (see page 201), there is no evidence that it has any effect on vaginal dryness.

Studies have found that estrogen products such as rings, creams, and vaginal suppositories are the best options for treating this problem. They restore normal tissue health and blood flow, increase vaginal secretions, help thicken the lining of the vagina, and restore normal vaginal pH balance to reduce the risk of yeast and urinary tract infections.

You and your doctor need to decide on the appropriate dosage and, if local forms of estrogen don't work, whether or not you'll try systemic estrogen (a patch or cream). Otherwise, in a study of 4,000 women, creams, tablets, and rings all worked just as well at improving vaginal atrophy. Here are some local estrogen options.

- ◆ **Ring (Estring).** This estradiol ring is worn for 3 months at a time. Studies suggest that just 10 percent of the estrogen released is absorbed throughout your body; the majority stays in your vaginal area.

- ◆ **Tablet (Vagifem).** You insert the estradiol tablet in your vagina every day for 2 weeks, then twice a week thereafter.

- ◆ **Cream (Premarin, Estrace).** These estrogen creams are typically inserted in your vagina every day for 3 weeks, then twice a week thereafter. Studies have found that the creams return the vagina to its premenopausal state with no significant increase in blood levels of estrogen.

Premarin is a synthetic conjugated estrogen, while Estrace is bioidentical estradiol. You may also want to look for Estriol creams and suppositories, which are widely available in Europe but can also be found in some U.S. pharmacies.

OTHER HEALTH-RELATED ISSUES FOR LAGGING LIBIDO

Other medical conditions can also affect your desire, including:

Depression. Face it, when you're depressed, you don't want to get out of bed. But when you're in bed, the last thing on your mind is sex. If nothing else gets you to a doctor for your depression, maybe the desire to get your love life back will.

What does menopause have to do with it? As we discussed in Chapter 9, midlife women have a strikingly high risk of depression as they travel through the menopausal transition.

Symptoms, please. You may experience loss of interest in activities you usually enjoy (like sex), changes in sleep and appetite, chronic sadness, and irritability.

What do I do about it? Check out our recommendations on page 241 in Chapter 9.

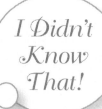

I Didn't Know That!

NO PROGESTERONE NEEDED

The good news about local estrogen options for vaginal atrophy is that you don't need to use progesterone unless you're using high doses (above 0.3 milligram of conjugated estrogen or 50 micrograms of estradiol). Local estrogen treatment can be used by women who have had breast cancer, but you should always consult your doctor before using.

Diabetes. When a man has problems getting an erection, he's usually tested for diabetes. So if you're having problems getting aroused, ask your doctor to test your blood sugar levels. Diabetes can damage small blood vessels like those feeding the vaginal area. Without a healthy supply of blood and the oxygen it brings, you can have trouble getting aroused. Diabetes can also make midlife vaginal dryness worse.

What does menopause have to do with it? Midlife is when insulin resistance, a diabetes precursor, rises sharply. The shift could be related to the increased weight many of us gain during this time of life, but shifting hormones also play a role, possibly with your body's ability to obey insulin's signals.

Symptoms, please. You may not even have any symptoms in the earlier stages. But if your waist measures more than 35 inches; you have high blood pressure and high fasting blood glucose levels; low levels of the "good" form of cholesterol, HDL cholesterol; and high triglyceride levels, your risk for diabetes or prediabetes is dramatically higher than the risk of a woman your age without any of these indicators.

What do I do about it? If you're in the early stages of diabetes or you only have insulin resistance, diet and exercise may be enough to restore you to health. Start with the 30-Day Slim-Down, Cool-Down Diet in Part II, and read more about other diabetes prevention strategies in Chapter 14.

Hypothyroidism. Low thyroid hormone levels can lead to a low libido.

What does menopause have to do with it? Hypothyroidism is quite common in midlife women, so ask your doctor to check your levels.

Symptoms, please. The symptoms of hypothyroidism actually often mimic those of menopause, including weight gain, hot flashes, fatigue, and depression.

What do I do about it? If you have a sluggish thyroid, you will need thyroid hormone replacement, which your doctor can prescribe.

Overactive bladder (urge incontinence). If you have this condition, you never leave the house without knowing the location of every toilet on the way to, at, and from your destination. You go to the bathroom more often than you apply lipstick, and there are times when you don't quite make it. One study of 34 women found that just 50 percent of those who had problems with urinary incontinence had had sex at least once during the previous month, compared with 91 percent of women who had no such problem.

What does menopause have to do with it? Urge incontinence becomes more common in midlife. In fact, one-third of the women in the Women's Health Initiative experienced urge incontinence in the year prior to joining the study.

Symptoms, please. Overactive bladder syndrome is simply a constellation of incontinence symptoms, including urge incontinence, urinary urgency and frequency, and urinating throughout the night.

What do I do about it? We tackle the often hidden condition of urinary incontinence in Chapter 11, where we offer numerous options for staying dry.

WHEN YOU'RE SIMPLY NOT INTERESTED

For all the focus on physical changes that occur at midlife and their supposed effect on desire, the reality is that much of the falloff in a woman's desire at this time of life has nothing to do with hormones and everything to do with relationships. If the problem with your relationship has to do with the fact that you've fallen out of love, he had an affair, you had an affair, you simply don't like the guy anymore . . . well, there are other books you need to be reading (and, possibly, lawyers to be calling). But if the problem is that the sex has simply become predictable, we may be able to help.

Let's face it: If you've been having sex with the same man (or woman) for 20 years or more, it's almost inevitable that no matter how much you love your partner, the sex can get, well, dull. He always touches your breast *there.* You know that 3 minutes and four kisses later, he will enter you. Missionary style. Always missionary style. As one woman told researchers when they interviewed her about changes in her sex life, including fewer orgasms: "I don't think it's down to the menopause. I think it's down to my partner being a bit lazy. It's true what they say, as they get older, you might as well put something in the microwave and 3 minutes later you've finished but the microwave's not 'pinged.' It's over more quickly for him, so consequently it's over more quickly for me."

PERK UP YOUR SEX LIFE NOW

Listen up, girlfriend, you are too young to become a microwaved snack. It's time to shake up your sex life. Before you try any of our suggestions below, however, sit down and have "the talk." Remind him how much you love him, tell him how you're feeling (in a nonconfrontational, non-judgmental manner), and then ask for his ideas on how to liven up the marital bed. Once you're both in agreement that a little variety is in order, suggest some of the following:

Make yourself feel sexy. Remember sexy? Pre-kids, stretch marks, mortgage? That woman is still within you somewhere, so take a day to find her. Start with a lingering bath in sandalwood or musk oil, followed by a new haircut, a professional makeup job, lingerie, and even a new perfume. Then text your partner and tell him to meet you at the bar at one of the nicest hotels in town. Who knows what could happen?

Play with toys. Sex toys may sound kind of silly—until you try them with someone you love. Then they can bring out a side of him—or you—that you didn't even know existed. Suggestions include a vibrator, a blindfold, and handcuffs. Oh, and don't forget flavored, scented gels for a more *tingly* feeling down there.

Find your fantasies. Come on . . . we all have them. Pour a glass of wine for each of you, and then ask him if there's a sex fantasy he has that you can bring to life. After he tells you (men *always* have sex fantasies), share one of your own. Then figure out how you can each make the other's fantasies come true.

Change your environment. If the only place you have sex is your bedroom, it's time to switch settings. Try other rooms in your house (after all, the kids are either gone or rarely there anymore, right?). How about pitching a tent if you have a private backyard? Or going camping (just bring an air mattress)? And if you have a minivan or a large four-wheel drive, maybe it's time for a return to those days of necking in the car—which brings us to our next piece of advice:

Kiss and touch only. Sex therapists use this exercise quite a lot. They'll tell you to spend an hour a day only kissing and touching—no sex allowed. Trust us, within a couple of days, you'll be sexting *him*.

Have vacation sex. You know what we're talking about: feeling as if you just got a shot of some female Viagra the minute the suitcase-jammed car left the driveway; the turn-on you felt as you checked into the hotel, your husband by your side, his fingers barely grazing that slight indentation in the curve of your back. Well, you can have vacation sex more than 2 weeks a year. Stay at a hotel in your town for the weekend, offer to swap houses with a friend, or take a 3-day cruise to nowhere. All are affordable (and maybe even free); and all are guaranteed to get the juices running again.

Rent a movie. One of our favorites is *9½ Weeks*. But straight porn can be kinda fun, too. Remember the women in the study at the beginning of the chapter? The ones who got turned on physically even if they weren't turned on emotionally? Imagine if they'd been watching that porn with someone they loved.

Can Food Turn You On?

For centuries, foods like oysters, chocolate, and hot peppers have been touted as aphrodisiacs. Too bad there's no medical evidence for these claims. That doesn't mean you shouldn't start a romantic dinner with oysters; the very act of slurping one from its shell while staring into your partner's eyes can be a turn-on. And there are things you can do with chocolate to improve your sex life that we can't go into here; suffice it to say that chocolate sauce works best. Really, though, we think the best way to use food to increase desire is to eat a healthy diet so you feel better about yourself and your body. *That*, in our estimation, is sexy.

Don't underestimate the benefits of a long-term marriage. You know how to handle the wet spot (switch sides with him so he sleeps in it), are okay telling him "This is a quickie—go for it" when you're not really interested but just want to make him happy, and know which positions will leave you crooked in the morning. Sometimes you may need to just cherish the boredom and the routine sex if you are in an otherwise healthy relationship, because men and women really *do* have different sexual desires.

PERK UP YOUR SEX LIFE OVER TIME

While you're trying out our right-now tips above, don't forget the importance of maintaining your libido over the long term. That's where the following remedies come in.

Strive for a healthy weight. The more body fat you have, the lower the levels of two hormones important in desire: testosterone and dopamine. In addition, a German study found that the more often women had intercourse, the slimmer their waist and hips. This happens even in the animal kingdom—researchers found that slim and obese male rats will lick the vaginal area of slim female rats, but the obese male rats were much less likely to get lucky and the obese female rats less likely to get licked. And a study of 161 women and 26 men found that losing an average of 13 percent of their body weight (26 pounds in a 200-pound woman) greatly improved their sex lives. Within 3 months of the weight loss, the women reported feeling more sexually attractive, having more sexual desire, and enjoying sex more. They were also more comfortable being seen naked and were less likely to avoid sex. The 30-Day Slim-Down, Cool-Down Diet in Part II will help you lose the weight you want to lose and keep off the weight you don't want to gain.

Up your vitamin C. Did you know that vitamin C plays an important role in blood flow (even to the vagina!), stress and anxiety reduction, and the release of several hormones associated with desire, including prolactin, oxytocin, and dopamine? In one study, German researchers gave 81 healthy men and women either 3,000 milligrams of vitamin C or a placebo every day for 2 weeks. The group getting the vitamin had more frequent intercourse than the group getting the placebo. They also scored lower on a depression test. Good food sources of vitamin C include citrus fruits and red and orange vegetables. (If you decide to supplement, take your vitamin in divided doses throughout the day; if you take it all at once, you'll just wind up peeing away the extra.)

Follow a Mediterranean diet. This type of "diet" is not really a diet at all, but a way of eating that includes large amounts of vegetables, fruits, and whole grains; fish and small amounts of animal protein; and a large helping of heart-healthy monounsaturated fats like olive oil. A study of 33 women with metabolic syndrome and sexual problems found that following a Mediterranean-style diet for 2 years not only improved the women's blood sugar, insulin, triglyceride, and blood pressure levels but also their scores on a test that measured female sexual dysfunction. Oh, and by the way, this way of eating is quite similar to our 30-Day Slim-Down, Cool-Down Diet.

Exercise. The benefits of exercise are too numerous to list here. Suffice it to say, however, that many of them—including increased blood flow, greater energy, and weight loss—can improve your libido, too. But the links between exercise and a great sex life go even further. Exercise is the *only* "treatment" that addresses all of the components of metabolic syndrome and can actually cure the condition. It is also critical for improving insulin sensitivity in people with diabetes or other blood sugar issues. Both conditions—metabolic syndrome and diabetes—are linked to much higher rates of sexual problems in women. Plus, exercise can lead to a short-term increase in testosterone levels. The Natural Menopause Solution exercise plan is a great place to start.

Do the Downward Dog. Not only can yoga quell hot flashes and soothe anxiety but it can improve your sex life. In a study published in the *Journal of Sexual Medicine*, researchers enrolled 40 healthy married women ages 22 to 55 in a yoga program and taught them 22 yoga poses to improve abdominal and pelvic muscle tone, digestion, joint function, and mood. The women were tested on their sexual function at the beginning of the study and again after practicing the poses for an hour a day, followed by breathing and relaxation exercises. After 12 weeks, they had all significantly improved their scores on the sexual function test. They were more aroused (and had greater lubrication), were more likely to have an orgasm, and had less pain during intercourse. The benefits were greatest in the women 46 and older, although three out of four said that they were more satisfied with their sex life after the yoga training than before, regardless of their age. For more on yoga and its benefits, check out the Natural Menopause Solution exercise plan on page 151.

NATURAL REMEDIES WORTH TRYING

The following supplements have less science behind them but may still be worth a try for a flagging libido:

ArginMax for Women. This nutritional supplement contains ginseng, ginkgo, multivitamins, and minerals. It also contains L-arginine, an amino acid that helps increase circulation (more circulation to your vagina means more lubrication). Several studies have found that women who took the supplement had increased sexual desire, including clitoral sensation and orgasm. In another study, women taking ArginMax daily for 4 weeks reported a 74 percent improvement in satisfaction with their sex lives.

Maca (*Lepidium meyenii*). This Andean herb is a member of the mustard family and has been used for centuries to improve sex. A review of four clinical trials found half suggested benefits in healthy menopausal women. You can find maca supplements in health food stores.

WHEN ALL ELSE FAILS . . . MEDICATIONS FOR LOW LIBIDO

Unfortunately, we still don't have a female Viagra. So if the natural remedies aren't working and the lack of loving is bothering you, talk to your doctor about the following:

Testosterone. This sex hormone is more commonly associated with men, but as women we make a fair amount of it ourselves, primarily through our ovaries and adrenal glands. Good thing, too, because the hormone plays a fairly significant role in women's desire. That's why some health-care practitioners prescribe low doses of testosterone to women whose sexual desire has flagged (and for which no physical reason for the flagging can be found). Since there is no testosterone-only product approved in the United States for women, you have to use products meant for men, such as a testosterone gel or patch, albeit in far lower doses. (There is a drug prescription called Estratest that combines oral synthetic esterified estrogens and methyltestosterone available.) Your doctor can also order an appropriate dose of testosterone for you through a compounding pharmacy. Other options include pellets inserted in your arm and swapped out every 3 months.

In one study, 36 healthy menopausal women in stable relationships used an estrogen gel for 2 weeks, then added either a testosterone or a placebo cream that they applied to their forearm every day for 12 weeks. After 3 months, the women's blood testosterone levels had risen significantly, as did the quality of their sex lives. More specifically, they had sex more often, initiated sex more often, and their petting and foreplay increased by a third. Before the study, about 6 percent of the women receiving the cream said that they had foreplay two or three times a week; after the study, 25 percent of the women did. In addition, 9 percent of the testosterone group reported having had sex two or three times before the study began, and by the end that number had jumped to 31 percent. Finally, while 3 percent of the placebo group were having sex that often when the study began, just 9 percent were when it ended. There were no side effects in the testosterone group.

Another study of women who had their ovaries removed and who had little desire for sex, a condition called hypoactive sexual desire disorder, found that twice-weekly testosterone patches for 6 months resulted in a significant increase in the number of satisfying sexual activities and orgasms compared with those of women who were given a placebo patch.

Bottom line: If none of the remedies in this chapter works for you and you really want your sex life back, talk to your doctor about supplemental testosterone. Blood levels need to be monitored to ensure that you stay in a safe range.

Potential side effects: Side effects of too-high doses of testosterone include hair growth and acne. There is also conflicting data on whether testosterone affects breast cancer risk like other sex hormones. Some testosterone is converted into estrogen in the body, so women who have a history of breast or ovarian cancer should likely avoid supplemental testosterone for now. Testosterone can also lead to increased liver enzymes and increased blood pressure, so make sure you have regular follow-ups with your doctor.

DHEA. Dehydroepiandrosterone, or DHEA, is the most prevalent reproductive hormone in women and serves as an important precursor to estrogen and testosterone production outside of the ovaries. DHEA also affects levels of dopamine, the "reward" hormone that can contribute to desire. As with so many other reproductive hormones, levels decline with age.

There is some evidence that supplementing with DHEA can help with libido, mood, and overall well-being, although the evidence is mixed. One study published in the *Journal of Women's Health & Gender-Based Medicine* found that women taking 300 milligrams of DHEA an hour before watching an erotic video were more mentally and physically aroused than women who took a placebo.

Bottom line: Worth a try. Your doctor can prescribe oral DHEA supplements and vaginal suppositories prepared by a compounding pharmacy. Some preliminary data suggest that vaginal suppositories may be even more effective than oral supplements on the libido. Most women need only 5 to 15 milligrams of DHEA daily to keep their DHEA–sulfate levels in the optimal range. Ask your doctor about testing your levels if you are considering DHEA supplements.

Potential side effects: There are few side effects with either type when taken in recommended doses, although too-high doses can affect cholesterol levels and lead to androgen-related side effects such as acne, hair growth, and a deepening voice.

It Worked for Me!

Malissa Kuzma, 44, lost 2½ pounds and 6¼ inches, including 1½ from her hips—and she has more energy for her kids and her husband.

It seems counterintuitive at first, but Malissa has discovered that the secret to having more energy is to expend more energy. "I was so inspired by the exercise elements of this plan," says this stay-at-home mom of two children. "Before I had my children, I used to walk for exercise, but I'd become very inactive. Finding time for myself for exercise was a big challenge, but the 20-minute walks fit in. Sometimes I'd take my son, or the dog, or even push my mother in her wheelchair. I tried hard to make it happen."

The results have thrilled Malissa and her children. "Because I have more energy, I've been able to spend more time with them when they go outside and play," she explains. "I've taken them to lakes and parks—one day I even took them to two different parks. And they're enjoying the fact that I can keep up with them now."

The benefits have spilled over into her home and her marriage. "If you saw the difference in my house, you'd be amazed," Malissa says. "I've gotten rid of clutter. I dust and vacuum more often. The trash goes out to the trash can outside more often. And I'm able to do more to help my husband, who travels quite often for business. We help each other and feel closer—when he's home, I can take a few quiet minutes to fit in a walk."

At 44, Malissa suspects that the hormonal changes of perimenopause are beginning. "I still have my menstrual cycle, but I'm also experiencing

---

In the end, only you can decide what you want out of your sex life. If you're happy with the way things are—including not being all that interested—and it isn't negatively affecting your relationship, then fine. You don't have a problem. But if you would like to feel sexier and have heat flashes and night sweats. In the past year, something definitely changed with my sleep patterns. I used to be a very sound sleeper who had trouble waking up in the morning. Then, even on weekends, I found myself awake at 5 in the morning—even if I got to bed late. I felt more tired."

She's noticed a big improvement since starting the program. "I haven't had any night sweats, and I've been sleeping better and longer," Malissa says. "I only have hot flashes in the morning now."

The stress relief that walking and yoga bring has helped calm her food cravings, too. "I'm definitely an emotional eater," she notes. "But if I can walk and get some alone time to think about things, the cravings are less intense. And walking has another advantage for me. It doesn't make me hungry like other forms of exercise do, so my food intake doesn't go up when I burn calories this way."

The yoga-with-weights routine was a new concept that she loved. "I felt I was breathing better, and I knew I was doing something really good for myself. You get the best of two worlds with that routine—more strength plus the calming yoga poses." Moving through the routine was sometimes a challenge in her household. "I'd go into a pose and end up with two dogs on the mat with me or my daughter wanting to do it along with me," she says with a laugh. "But I still looked forward to doing it."

more (and better) sex, take some action. Talk to your partner and to your doctor. Try some of the tips in this chapter, and see where it all takes you. Remember, menopause is only the end of periods and reproduction. It should not be the end of an active, healthy, fun, and satisfying sex life.

Chapter 11

Incontinence

Menopause is amazing, isn't it? Twenty years ago, you'd never even heard of overactive bladder syndrome and stress incontinence; 10 years ago, you were convinced they had been invented by some pharmaceutical company; and today you list them on medical forms without giving it a second thought. Or, if you're like most women, you suffer silently, too embarrassed to tell your doctor or even your best friend about the Depend package that you sneak into your grocery cart and hide under the frozen pizza.

It's time for the suffering and secrecy to end.

There are two main types of urinary incontinence: stress incontinence, in which a bit of urine is released involuntarily when you laugh, cough, sneeze, or even jump up and down; and urge incontinence, in which the urge to go to the bathroom comes on suddenly, and before you can make it to a bathroom, you've leaked a bit (or a lot). Then there's mixed incontinence, in which you have both. Overactive bladder syndrome is simply a constellation of incontinence symptoms, including urge incontinence, urinary urgency and frequency, and urinating throughout the night.

If you're experiencing either type (or both), you're not alone. The Women's Health Initiative, a study of 161,800 postmenopausal women, found that 23 percent of women had urge incontinence, 25 percent stress incontinence, and 16 percent mixed incontinence in the year before the trial began.

WHY SOMETIMES YOU JUST GOTTA GO

Which brings us back to menopause. Not surprisingly, menopause plays a role in incontinence. Lower estrogen levels weaken the tissue and muscles that make up your pelvic floor. This can lead to a weakening of the sphincter, the muscle that keeps the urethra closed and prevents urine leakage. Other causes include pelvic prolapse, in which the organs in your pelvic area drop because the ligaments and muscles that support them weaken or stretch, often due to pregnancy, childbirth, or (wait for it!) lower estrogen levels.

Urge incontinence is often caused by abnormal bladder contractions or nerve signals. It can be triggered by high-caffeine liquids, certain medications, or even high anxiety, hyperthyroidism, and diabetes. It is also related to estrogen loss, which can lead to a smaller flow of urine, leaving more urine in the bladder even as the bladder is unable to hold as much urine as it used to. At the same time, it takes less urine in the bladder to trigger the urge to pee. Add up all these changes and it becomes a perfect storm of incontinence.

AVOIDING "ACCIDENTS" NOW

No single approach will solve any type of incontinence, however; you need a multicomponent line of attack. Depending on the type of incontinence you're experiencing, one or more of the following should help:

Drink less. In particular, nix alcohol and carbonated and caffeinated drinks, all of which have a diuretic effect (i.e., making you urinate more). In one study of 259 women, half with incontinence and half without, those who consumed the most caffeine had the greatest risk of incontinence. In addition to its diuretic effects, caffeine triggers bladder muscle contractions; over time, too much caffeine can even permanently damage the bladder muscle.

Best for: Urge, stress, and mixed incontinence

Wear a pad. Use a menstrual pad to catch the overflow when you exercise or when you're in a situation that could cause leakage, such as going to a comedy club or hitting the gym.

Best for: Occasional stress incontinence

RELIEVING INCONTINENCE OVER TIME

The natural remedies below may take more time before you see results, but they are still worth a try, even if you're also trying the remedies that work immediately.

Drop a few. As with so many issues related to menopause and middle age, losing a few pounds can make a big difference. One study of 338 overweight middle-aged women found that losing just 8 percent of their body weight (an average of 17½ pounds) over 6 months slashed by half the number of times they leaked.

Best for: Stress and mixed incontinence

Pee more (and on schedule). This approach is known as bladder retraining. The goal is twofold: to limit the amount of urine in your bladder at any one time, and to train your involuntary nervous system and pelvic muscles to urinate at specific times. You typically start by going to the bathroom every 2 hours while you're awake, even if you don't think you have to go. Set an alarm on your cell phone, computer, or watch as a reminder.

In the intervening 2 hours, work on addressing the urge to pee when it occurs by sitting down, breathing deeply, and clenching your pelvic muscles as you visualize the urge as a "wave" that peaks and then dissipates. Once you feel in control, you can go to the bathroom.

After a couple of days with no accidents, gradually increase the time between scheduled voids by 30 to 60 minutes until you are able to go on your own, when you want, without running to the bathroom. One study found bladder retraining can reduce the number of incontinence episodes by a third.

Best for: Urge and mixed incontinence

Train yourself. Biofeedback, in which you learn to control involuntary actions like urinating, can work even better than medication for urge incontinence. In one study of nearly 200 women ages 55 to 92 with urge or mixed incontinence, those who had four sessions of biofeedback over 8 weeks reduced the number of incontinence episodes by 80 percent. That compared with a 70 percent reduction in women taking the incontinence drug oxybutynin (Ditropan) and 40 percent in women taking a placebo. Perhaps most compelling is that just 14 percent of the women undergoing biofeedback wanted to switch to another treatment, versus 75 percent of the women in the other two groups.

Best for: Urge and mixed incontinence

Exercise your muscles. Your pelvic muscles, that is. You've likely been told before that you should be doing Kegel exercises to maintain pelvic floor strength. Well, it's time to listen. Kegels involve clenching the muscles that control the flow of urine. You can find these muscles the next time you pee; just try to stop the flow of urine midstream. You'll likely discover that your pelvic muscles are too weak to do much good; use this as your benchmark to track your progress as you practice.

Ideally, you should do 3 sets of 8 to 12 clenches (clenching for 6 to 8 seconds at a time) three or four times a week minimum, for at least 3 to 4 months. But there's no danger in doing more. Kegels shouldn't be your only approach, however (studies find they can reduce incontinence episodes by an average of one a day), but they should be part of your overall management plan. If you want more bang for your Kegel buck, consider physical therapy involving weighted cones that you insert in your vagina and hold in place during activities.

(continued on page 288)

Watch Out for Urinary Tract Infections

There's barely a woman around who doesn't know the signs of a urinary tract infection (UTI). The sudden urge to urinate, only to have a few drops dribble out. The itching, burning, and pain. In addition to the pain, UTIs may also increase your risk of urinary incontinence, with women who have UTIs experiencing twice as many leaking episodes. Worse yet is if the infection travels from the bladder to the kidneys. Get a kidney infection and not only can the pain rival that of childbirth, but it may land you in the hospital for intravenous antibiotics.

One reason women tend to get more UTIs after menopause is because of changes that make the vagina more hospitable to bacteria. From the vagina it's an easy hop over to the urethra and up into your bladder. Taking antibiotics or fungicides for other infections also increases the risk. Another reason for the increased risk of UTIs is loss of estrogen, which thins urethral walls, making it easier for bacteria to adhere.

To keep from getting a UTI:

- **Wash carefully before and after sex.** And urinate after sex. A large study published in *Archives of Internal Medicine* in 2004 found that sexually active women were more than three times as likely to have a history of UTIs as women who were not having sex. Bacteria can enter the urethra during intercourse and make their way into the bladder.

- **Choose your positions carefully.** You're more likely to get an infection if you are on top of him. Try missionary or side positions for a while.

- **Prevent diabetes.** Women with diabetes are twice as likely to have UTIs as women without because of immune system changes and blood sugar levels. More on preventing diabetes in Chapter 14.

- **Drink up.** The more water you drink, the more you urinate, reducing the chance that any bacteria will hang around your bladder long enough to make you sick.

- **Wipe the right way.** Your mother taught you this, but always wipe from front to back so that bacteria in the anal region don't get into your vagina or urethra.

- **Stay away from douches and sprays.** They can irritate the urethra.

- **Try cranberries.** Cranberries, whether as juice, a capsule, or a tablet, change the molecular structure of the bladder lining so that bacteria don't adhere well. If you hate the taste of cranberries, you can also try bilberry or blueberry juices or supplements, which may offer some of the same benefits.

- **Sweeten up.** Dr. Ring uses the natural sugar D-mannose to prevent UTIs in her patients. Like cranberries, it prevents certain bacteria (*E. coli*) from sticking to the bladder wall. You can find D-mannose in health food stores.

- **Change your diet.** If you're prone to UTIs, try adding more fresh fruit and live-culture, sugar-free yogurt or other fermented dairy products (like kefir), which studies have found reduce the risk of infection. Also, cut back on meat and poultry, since women who eat a lot of either are more likely to have antibiotic-resistant UTIs. The link could be the antibiotics used in the animals or because they serve as sources of the *E. coli* bacteria that cause most infections.

- **Insert probiotics.** Studies have shown that probiotic suppositories inserted in the vagina can help prevent UTIs by improving the pH balance of the vagina so it can better fight off bacteria.

- **Consider estrogen.** But make it local estrogen, like the ring or creams; there's no evidence that systemic estrogen like pills or patches helps with UTIs.

If you get frequent UTIs, talk to your doctor about using antibiotics to prevent the infection. Studies have found that taking antibiotics daily for 6 months or longer—particularly at night when the drug remains in your bladder longer—can prevent UTIs, as can a single dose taken just after having sex.

Best for: Stress, urge, and mixed incontinence

Use a pessary. These are devices, often rings, that you insert in your vagina. They have a knob that sits under your urethra, and when you cough, sneeze, laugh, or jump, the urethra closes on the knob, preventing leaks.

Best for: Stress incontinence

WORTH TRYING

The evidence for the natural remedies below is mixed, but there's no harm in trying one of them if nothing else works.

Acupuncture. A study at Oregon Health & Science University, in which 74 women got either real or placebo acupuncture for their incontinence, found that after four weekly sessions, the group getting the real thing had a third fewer incontinence episodes, as compared with just a 3 percent decrease in the placebo group.

Chondroitin sulphate. This supplement is often used to treat arthritis; preliminary evidence suggests that it may also be effective for incontinence. A study of 41 women with overactive bladder and interstitial cystitis assigned half to Detrol (tolterodine), an overactive bladder treatment, and half to a branded chondroitin supplement (Uropol S) for a year. While 43 percent of those in the Detrol group reported improvement, 72 percent in the chondroitin group said they had improved.

WHEN ALL ELSE FAILS . . . MEDICATIONS AND MEDICAL TREATMENTS FOR INCONTINENCE

If none of the natural remedies listed above help, it's time to turn to traditional medicine. From pills to shots to electrical current, there are several that you and your doctor may want to try.

Incontinence medications. These medications work by increasing the amount of urine that your bladder can hold while reducing the sensation that you have to go. They include Ditropan, Vesicare (solifenacin), Sanctura (trospium), and Detrol. All appear equally effective, decreasing the number of incontinence episodes and the times you have to go to the bathroom by about one per day. However, a study of 29,000 women who had been taking the drugs found that most stopped taking them by 6 months, possibly due to side effects.

Bottom line: Worth trying for urge incontinence

Potential side effects: Side effects include dry mouth, blurred vision, rapid heartbeat, sleepiness, and constipation, as well as some fuzzy thinking.

Preventing Incontinence

If you haven't experienced any leaking yet, great! Let's keep it that way. A 2007 National Institutes of Health Science Conference on Incontinence recommended the following to prevent urinary incontinence:

- Lose weight, quit smoking, increase your physical activity, and improve your diet.

- Strengthen your pelvic floor muscles with Kegels. One study of 394 women age 55 and older, half of whom practiced Kegels and learned about incontinence and proper urination and half of whom did not, found that, after a year, the Kegels women were twice as likely to remain or become continent as were the placebo women.

- Prevent or manage conditions associated with incontinence, such as diabetes, stroke, depression, and constipation.

- Avoid medications associated with incontinence. These include certain high blood pressure medications such as Cardura (doxazosin), Minipress (prazosin), and Hytrin (terazosin), as well as some antidepressants, diuretics, and sedatives.

Botox injections. Although not approved for this use, for patients with overactive bladder syndrome who didn't respond to other treatments, Botox injected directly into the bladder wall improved symptoms by an average of 69 percent. In participants with urge incontinence only, an average of 58 percent were completely cured, with a single treatment lasting about 6 months.

Bottom line: Worth trying for urge incontinence if nothing else works

Potential side effects: The paralyzing effects of the drug on bladder muscles could keep you from knowing when you need to go or that your bladder is empty. This, in turn, could lead to serious bladder and kidney infections.

Electrical and sacral nerve stimulation. In this therapy, removable devices are placed in the vagina or the anus to stimulate nerves and muscles associated with urination. They may also be surgically implanted in your butt to stimulate the sacral nerve, which runs through your lower back and affects the bladder, pelvic floor, and urinary sphincter (the part that keeps urine in) muscles. These and similar treatments are typically provided by specialists such as urogynecologists and pelvic floor therapists.

Bottom line: Worth trying if nothing else works

Potential side effects: Side effects are rare but include infection after the device is implanted or failure of the device, which requires reprogramming or reimplantation.

Percutaneous nerve stimulation. This approach uses needles inserted in your calf just above your ankle to deliver mild electrical shocks to the percutaneous nerve, which also controls sensations to the bladder and the pelvic floor. You undergo weekly 30-minute sessions for 10 to 12 weeks, although some doctors do more sessions per week for fewer weeks. In one study of 100 people with overactive bladder (most of them women), the treatment worked about as well as medication at improving symptoms.

Bottom line: Best for urge or mixed incontinence

Potential side effects: Rare. You may have some bleeding at the needle site or a slight tingling in your foot.

Extracorporeal magnetic stimulation. With this treatment you sit in a special chair and receive electromagnetic pulses to contract your pelvic floor muscles. At the same time, a magnet on your back stimulates sacral nerve roots.

Bottom line: There isn't a lot of data on this treatment, although it appears to help in the short term. It works best for urge or mixed incontinence.

Potential side effects: None, though some reports warn that the incontinence may get worse or return after treatment.

Bulking injections. In this procedure, a doctor injects compounds such as collagen or carbon spheres in your bladder neck and urethra to thicken the tissue and prevent leaking. You'll need repeat injections, as the material is slowly eliminated from your body. The procedure is performed under a local anesthetic on an outpatient basis.

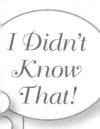

I Didn't Know That!

ORAL ESTROGEN THERAPY MAKES INCONTINENCE WORSE

Hormone therapy is often prescribed to help menopausal and postmenopausal women with urinary incontinence. Yet the Women's Health Initiative showed that women without incontinence who took oral estrogen with or without progestin for a year were $2\frac{1}{2}$ times as likely to have daily stress incontinence than women who took a placebo. The risk of daily urge incontinence was also significantly higher in women who took estrogen only (36 percent), while the risk of mixed incontinence was nearly doubled in women who took estrogen, with or without progestin. However, local estrogen delivered vaginally through rings, creams, or pills *can* improve incontinence by strengthening urethral muscles.

Bottom line: Best for stress incontinence

Potential side effects: Rare, but may include some bruising, urinary retention, and urinary tract infection. May also urinate more frequently or feel a stronger urge to go.

Surgery. Surgery is more commonly used for stress incontinence. One procedure involves placing a sling, or narrow strap, under the urethra to take pressure off the sphincter. The procedure is performed on an outpatient basis, often through a vaginal incision.

The other procedure, colposuspension, basically puts your internal organs back in place with a few stitches. This surgery is done on an inpatient basis through an abdominal incision or laparoscopically through tiny openings in the abdomen. Studies have found that about 2 years after surgery, two-thirds of women getting a sling and half of women undergoing colposcopy are cured of stress incontinence. However, women with the sling have a greater risk of urinary tract infections and problems urinating and may trade their stress incontinence for urge incontinence.

Bottom line: Should be used as a last resort

Potential side effects: These include the risks typical of any surgical procedure, such as a reaction to the anesthesia, bleeding, and infection, as well as potential injury to the urethra or bladder from the surgery itself; urinary retention; and an overactive bladder.

Chapter 12

Beauty

With everything else going on in your life around menopause, it may seem kind of silly to devote an entire chapter to your skin, nails, and hair. But as women, how we look often influences how we feel. Numerous studies have found that how we feel about our bodies and our overall attractiveness has a direct impact on our mood. And that holds true as you transition through menopause—you want to feel good, look good, and live well.

The Natural Menopause Solution will not only benefit your physical and emotional health but will also improve your looks. It's true; studies have shown that diets high in vegetables and lean protein (like the 30-Day Slim-Down, Cool-Down Diet) can improve the appearance of your skin. The exercise plan, meanwhile, will increase blood flow to your skin, bringing all-important oxygen and nutrients to maintain healthy, young-looking skin.

Bottom line: Just because our hormones are going haywire doesn't mean our appearance has to. Here's how to cope and remain beautiful.

CARING FOR MIDLIFE SKIN

The changes in your skin as you approach 50 and beyond are due partly to estrogen loss and partly to gravity. After menopause, women lose about a quarter of their body's collagen, a protein that not only provides scaffolding for our bones but also is behind the elasticity and firmness of our skin. The result? Thin, stiff skin and brittle nails. Estrogen helps prevent this loss, with studies finding that topical and systemic estrogen can actually increase collagen and help maintain strong, elastic, moist skin. So when estrogen fades, many women find that their skin becomes dry and thin and looks lifeless.

Then gravity kicks in. After 50 years, the tendons and muscles holding up your face (and the rest of you) begin to sag, particularly around the neck, jaw, and eyes. Add in the sun damage from our misspent youth (worse if you also smoked), and you get the wrinkles, brown spots, and drooping of middle age.

IMPROVING SKIN APPEARANCE NOW

By this stage of life you've likely read hundreds if not thousands of articles about skin care, skin health, and skin in general, all saying the same thing: Stay out of the sun, cover up, use sunscreen. Well, that's nice to hear *now*, and yes, we're all slathering on the SPF 30 moisturizer, makeup, and sunscreen, but there's not a whole lot we can do about the damage we did sunning in our adolescent youth. Or is there?

Pick the right makeup. This might be the time to ask for help at a department store cosmetics counter. For some women, a powder covers wrinkles and age spots best; for others, a liquid or a cream foundation. The key is to make sure that whatever product you choose doesn't emphasize your wrinkles by sinking or caking into them. You can even find makeup today with ingredients designed to enhance skin health, like those described on page 296.

Add a new product. It's called a makeup primer, and it works just like paint primer or drywall spackle to smooth and prepare your face prior to applying makeup.

REVERSING SKIN DAMAGE OVER TIME

It will take some time before you see the benefits of the following, but once you start, don't stop!

Hit the gym. Studies find that women who exercise regularly have firmer skin than those who don't. Why? Exercise boosts blood flow throughout your body, bringing nutrients to your skin and carrying away waste products like free radicals.

Eat right. A diet high in antioxidants and low in saturated fat works best for healthy skin. Even smokers who eat a lot of vegetables have fewer wrinkles than nonsmokers who eat fewer vegetables. One study out of the United Kingdom found that women who consumed foods rich in vitamin C had fewer wrinkles and moister skin than those who didn't get enough of the vitamin. Good sources include all citrus fruits, as well as red and orange vegetables. So chop up a red pepper for your salad tonight!

Other skin-friendly foods include olive oil, fish, legumes (peas, beans, lentils, and peanuts), and nuts and seeds (such as walnuts, flaxseed, and chia). These contain monounsaturated fats and omega-3 fatty acids, which reduce dryness to keep skin soft, smooth, and supple. They also reduce inflammation, a culprit in skin problems like rosacea and psoriasis. You'll discover that the 30-Day Slim-Down, Cool-Down Diet already includes these beauty-boosting nutrients.

Skip the cookies and crackers. Most important on the food side is cutting out high-sugar, low-fiber carbohydrates (the kind found in most processed foods). They trigger blood glucose spikes that in turn lead to the production of advanced glycation end products, or AGEs, free radicals that destroy the collagen and elastin in your skin. Refined foods like white bread and rice also increase production of androgens, hormones that ramp up the production of facial oil and trigger breakouts.

Lose weight. The AGEs we just mentioned? They're more likely to develop in people who are overweight or obese and in those with diabetes. You can learn more about preventing diabetes in Chapter 14, and follow the 30-Day Slim-Down, Cool-Down Diet in Part II to remain at your target weight.

Wash only once a day. As you've probably noticed, aging skin = drier skin, so you don't need to wash with a cleanser more than once a day. In the morning, just splash your face with water before applying moisturizer; save the full cleansing for just before bed.

Use the right products at the right time. Products containing antiaging ingredients such as vitamins C and E and retinoids are best used at night; sunlight can break down these ingredients, reducing their effectiveness.

Sleep on your back. Studies find that sleeping on your stomach or side with your face smushed into the pillow contributes to wrinkles.

NATURAL MEDICINE FOR YOUR SKIN

They are called cosmeceuticals—creams, lotions, toners, and even makeup packed with antioxidants, enzymes, vitamins, and minerals designed to fight the ravages of time and aging. Here are some of the major antiaging ingredients that may be in your skin products these days.

Antioxidants. Some skin products are so filled with antioxidants (primarily from various vitamins) that smoothing on a skin cream is kind of like giving your face a multivitamin. Ingredients include the B vitamins panthenol and niacinamide; vitamins C and E; lipoic acid; ubiquinone, also called coenzyme Q10; dimethylaminoethanol (DMAE); melatonin; catalase; glutathione; superoxide dismutase; peroxidase; glucopyranosides; polyphenols; uric acid; and cysteine.

Best for: Protecting your skin from sun and the ravages of daily life

Depigmenting agents. These are the products you turn to if you want to fade that brown patch on your cheek or that freckle on your nose. Specific ingredients include hydroquinone, tretinoin, corticosteroids, and N-acetylcysteine. Some products contain acids, such as glycolic acid, resorcinol, and salicylic acid, that trigger the peeling of the top layer of your skin.

Best for: Minimizing the appearance of sun damage and age spots

Hydroxy acids. You'll see these listed on product labels as glycolic acid, lactic acid, citric acid, mandelic acid, malic acid, and tartaric acid. They are natural enzymes derived primarily from fruit and that work by speeding up the rate at which your skin sheds dead cells, uncovering the smoother, brighter skin underneath.

Best for: Reducing signs of aging

Retinoids. Retinoids are powerful antioxidants derived from vitamin A. They are also ubiquitous in today's antiaging products.

Best for: Reversing sun damage, preventing and minimizing wrinkles and thinning skin

COSMETIC PROCEDURES

Office-based procedures to reduce the appearance of wrinkles and skin-smoothing methods that can leave your skin as soft as a baby's bottom have increased exponentially in the past 10 years. They're not cheap, and your health insurance won't cover them, but if you're looking for a personal boost to get you through this time of life, they can certainly help provide it. And many women, it turns out, are looking for exactly that. The American Society for Aesthetic Plastic Surgery reports that these "lunchtime face-lifts" are among the most popular plastic surgery procedures performed today.

Cosmetic injectables. Think Botox (or its cousin Reloxin). These injections paralyze facial muscles to reduce the look of wrinkles. They cost about $400 per session and need to be repeated every 4 to 6 months.

Facial fillers. These include collagen injections; hyaluronic acid (Hylaform, Juvéderm, Perlane, Restylane, Puragen, Prevelle Silk); microspheres (Artefill); calcium hydroxylapatite (Radiesse); and poly-L-lactic acid (Sculptra). The filler is injected directly into your wrinkles, facial folds, and lips to plump them. Prices range from about $550 for hyaluronic acid injections to $2,300 for Sculptra, and the injections will need to be repeated every 3 to 6 months.

Laser skin resurfacing. In this procedure, a laser is used to destroy the top or middle layers of your skin to allow new skin to grow. Laser resurfacing reduces wrinkles, brown spots, and even acne scars. It costs between $950 and $2,500, depending on the procedure, but the more extensive (and expensive) resurfacing procedures can last for years.

Chemical peel. This treatment involves having an acid-based solution painted onto your face, making the top layers of skin blister and peel, revealing fresher, younger skin beneath. A chemical peel can reduce the appearance of wrinkles, sun spots, acne scars, and freckles. The cost depends on the type of peel; mild peels can cost about $100 a session,

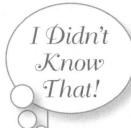

I Didn't Know That!

WRINKLES AND YOUR BONES

Those worry lines that worry you should worry your doctor, too. Seems that women with more wrinkles are also more likely to have lower bone mineral density, according to a study presented at the 2011 Endocrine Society meeting. Bone and skin share several structures, including collagen. In fact, most of bone is composed of collagen. Researchers from Yale Medical School assessed the facial wrinkles of 114 postmenopausal women and their bone mineral density at the lower spine, the hips, and throughout their bodies. The researchers found a significant link between higher levels of skin wrinkling and lower levels of bone density, while fewer wrinkles on the face and forehead were tied to stronger bones at the hip and spine. So if your face is beginning to resemble a cracked plate, it might be a good idea to check out your bone strength. For more on bone health, see Chapter 16.

while intensive peels can run several thousand dollars. The extra cost may be worth it; while a mild peel refreshes your face for only a few months, an intensive one can last for up to 10 years.

NOT YOUR TEENAGER'S ACNE

Is anything more annoying than waking up the morning before a big presentation, peering into the mirror, and finding a huge pimple on your chin? How about two huge zits?

Just as your teens were the years of the dermatologist and acne pads, so too are your forties bound to be the decade of the breakout. Greater stress is likely one culprit. Stress can trigger production of androgens such as testosterone, which contribute to the production of the skin oil sebum. There's also more testosterone available as estrogen levels fall. The overproduction of sebum can attract dirt and bacteria that gets clogged in pores, eventually leading to pimples and blackheads. One study published in the *Journal of the National Academy of Medicine* found that up to one in four women in their forties struggled with acne.

NATURAL REMEDIES FOR TREATING ACNE

Before you hit the drugstore, head to the health food store and try one or more of the following. Don't expect immediate results; it may take a couple of weeks before you see clearer skin.

Azelaic acid. This natural compound is derived from grains and is often found in over-the-counter and prescription acne treatments. It has antimicrobial properties, so it kills bacteria on your skin. Studies have shown that it is just as effective as benzoyl peroxide, tretinoin (Retin-A), and erythromycin ointments, with fewer side effects. Use it twice a day and expect to see benefits in about 4 weeks.

Nicotinamide gel. This gel form of niacin has significant anti-inflammatory benefits. In one study in people with inflammatory acne (when you have large pustules as well as regular pimples), the gel was as

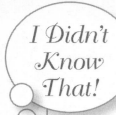

THE MYTH OF FOOD TRIGGERS

If you've been avoiding chocolate and french fries because you're worried about skin breakouts, stop. While a healthy diet definitely helps maintain healthier skin overall, there is no evidence that what you put in your mouth affects the number or severity of zits on your face. Acne is caused by hormones, primarily androgens, and bacteria—not a Dove candy bar.

effective as prescription clindamycin (Cleocin), with no antibiotic resistance and just some mild burning sensation on the face.

Oral zinc. Several studies have found that supplementing with zinc can improve acne, possibly because it helps maintain higher levels of vitamin A, which contains skin-improving retinoids. The evidence is mixed, however. In one study involving 37 people with severe acne who took 200 milligrams of zinc or 250 milligrams of tetracycline three times a day for 12 weeks, both groups noted a 70 percent improvement. A later study comparing the two, however, found tetracycline worked much better. Check with your doctor if you plan to use zinc. Melinda Ring, MD, our medical advisor, recommends just 20 to 50 milligrams once a day. When used for more than 3 months, she also has her patients take a low dose of copper. Excessive intake of zinc can interfere with the absorption of copper, leading to copper deficiency.

Tea tree oil. This essential oil is often used as an antiseptic since it has antibacterial and antifungal properties. One study comparing it with benzoyl peroxide found that although it was less effective and took longer to work on people with mild to moderate acne, after 3 months those using it had far fewer side effects. The researchers determined that using a concentration higher than the 5 percent used in the study may have improved the outcome.

Witch hazel bark. Brew 5 to 10 grams of the herb in 1 cup of hot water and cool. Soak a cotton ball in the concoction, and use it to clean your face twice a day. Witch hazel is naturally astringent, so it works well at clearing away oil and bacteria.

PREVENTING ACNE

Once you've cleared up your latest breakout, take these steps to avoid future flare-ups of this no-longer-adolescent scourge.

Cleanse daily. As we noted before, you only need to clean your face once a day. Wiping off the day's sweat, dirt, and makeup before you lay your head on the pillow keeps pores clean and pimples away. And don't rush it; gently rub the cleanser into your face for a minute or two to loosen dirt and grime before rinsing.

Sweat it out! Exercising and sweating open up pores and flush out impurities that can contribute to acne.

Use the right products. From moisturizers to makeup to sunscreen, look on the label for the word *noncomedogenic*, which means it won't get clogged in your pores and contribute to acne.

WHEN ALL ELSE FAILS . . . MEDICAL OPTIONS FOR ACNE

If the natural options don't work for you, try these.

Over-the-counter options. Look for acne products that contain salicylic acid, which helps slough off the top layer of skin, and benzoyl peroxide, which gets into the lower skin layers to reduce bacteria and clear out pores. Start with the lowest concentration of each, and gradually increase it if your acne doesn't improve. Watch out, however; benzoyl peroxide is very drying.

Bottom line: Best for mild acne and preventing acne

Antibiotics. If over-the-counter options don't work, you may need a prescription oral or topical antibiotic such as tetracycline or erythromycin. While they help prevent the bacteria that contributes to the acne, they don't do anything for the overproduction of oil that starts the whole acne process.

Bottom line: Try if your face doesn't clear with over-the-counter options

Retinoic acid. For more severe cases of acne, your doctor may prescribe a product containing a higher concentration of retinoic acid than you can get in the drugstore, such as Retin-A (tretinoin). These are available in creams or orally, but oral medications are used only for the most severe acne.

Bottom line: Next in line if antibiotics and milder remedies don't work

Estrogen. There's a reason some birth control pills are also approved for treating acne; the additional estrogen reduces the amount of available testosterone in your body, which in turn reduces sebum production.

Bottom line: Might consider low-dose-estrogen birth control pills—even if you don't need contraception—if your acne doesn't respond to other remedies

Spironolactone. This drug is used as a diuretic and blood pressure medication, but it also has some antiandrogenic effects that make it a good option for acne.

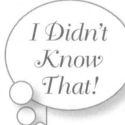

I Didn't Know That!

CALCIUM AND NAILS

Many women believe that extra calcium will translate into stronger nails. But a study published in the *New England Journal of Medicine* in 2000 found no truth to the claim. Researchers assessed changes in nail quality in 683 healthy postmenopausal women participating in a study on calcium supplementation to prevent osteoporosis. After taking about 800 milligrams of calcium or a placebo every day for a year, the women scored changes in the quality of their nails (including texture and brittleness). Most of the participants didn't notice any changes; of those who had, women in both groups reported that their nails had improved, meaning that calcium had no effect.

Bottom line: Spironolactone is generally used only for severe acne that hasn't improved with other options, particularly for women who don't want to—or can't—take oral tretinoin. It doesn't work for everyone, however. Ask your doctor to prescribe the lowest effective dose to reduce the risk of side effects, which may include menstrual irregularities, breast tenderness, low blood pressure when standing after sitting or lying down, headaches, fatigue, and dizziness. You shouldn't take it if you are pregnant, have kidney problems, or already experience abnormal menstrual bleeding.

HELP FOR YOUR NAILS

The same collagen loss that affects your face also leads to brittle nails. To handle the age-related brittleness of your nails, try these natural remedies. Give them time, however; it may take several weeks before you start to see significant results.

Moisturize like crazy. Slather vegetable oil on your hands before bed, then wrap them in plastic wrap or cover them with vinyl gloves. The hand coverings force the oil to penetrate your skin and keep the grease off your bedding, all the while preventing hands and nails from getting too dry.

Use acetone-free nail products. The acetone in many polish removers is incredibly drying. Speaking of drying, give your nails a break from nail polish, which is also drying.

Buy some biotin. Supplementing with this B vitamin (2.5 milligrams per day) can help strengthen nails. Other vitamins and supplements linked to healthier nails include vitamins A, C, D, E, B_{12}, and folic acid, and the minerals calcium, zinc, copper, iodine, manganese, and silica. Also, make sure that you're getting enough protein in your diet.

Wear rubber gloves. Overexposure to water from dishwashing and other chores can dry your hands and nails.

Stay warm. Temperature changes can make nails more prone to breakage, so wear your mittens when it's cold!

Supplement with gamma-linolenic acid (GLA). This fat helps strengthen skin, hair, *and* nails. Good sources are evening primrose and

When to Worry

Problems with your nails can be a sign of an underlying health condition. If you have any of the following or any other unusual nail condition, see your doctor.

Clubbing. If the tips of your fingers have gotten bigger, with the nail growing around the tip, you have clubbing. It can be a sign of a lung disease, inflammatory bowel disease, or liver disease, among others.

Yellow nails. Typically a sign of a respiratory condition. You may also find that your cuticles disappear and that the nail separates from the nail bed.

White or yellow spots. If you have white or yellow spots under the nail, you may have a fungal infection. If left untreated, the nail eventually thickens and crumbles. While antifungal medications are available to treat it, fungal infections tend to recur. So if you get one, see your doctor for a prescription treatment.

Pitting. It could be a sign of psoriasis or another skin condition.

Koilonychia (spoon nails). This condition means that the sides of your nails are turned toward the middle, creating a depression. It's often a sign of iron-deficiency anemia but may also indicate Raynaud's disease or lupus.

Terry's nails. Marked by a dark band at the top of the nail, this may signify liver failure, diabetes, congestive heart failure, or hyperthyroidism.

Beau's lines. White lines across the nail, an indicator of this nail disorder, may be a sign of Raynaud's disease or a severe systemic illness like uncontrolled diabetes.

Onycholysis. With this condition, the nail separates from the nail bed. It could indicate thyroid disease or psoriasis, or it could simply be a reaction to medication or products you're using on your nails.

Dark longitudinal streaks. These normally occur in dark-skinned people but could also be a sign of melanoma.

black currant oil, 500 milligrams of either twice daily. You can also up your omega-3 fatty acids, found in fatty fish like salmon and in fish oil supplements; flaxseed; and walnuts. And remember to give all supplements at least 3 months to show their effectiveness.

WHERE'D THE HAIR GO?

It's a hair-raising prospect: Nearly 40 percent of women lose noticeable amounts of hair after menopause—and even more notice that their once shiny, bouncy 'do isn't just turning gray, it's also looking dull, frazzled, brittle, and even lifeless during perimenopause and thereafter. But that's not all. Shifting hormones can virtually reprogram your body's hair patterns—slowing growth on your legs (and underarms and in your pubic area) while spurring the growth of unwanted strands on your face.

Researchers at England's Imperial College polled 941 postmenopausal women ages 45 to 94 about hair changes for a study published in the *British Journal of Dermatology* in 2011. The scientists discovered that midlife and menopause were hairy situations for plenty of women: Nineteen percent in their forties and early fifties reported that their hair was thinning all over their head—as did 37 percent of women over age 75. This is the type of thinning when your part suddenly seems wider . . . and you start to see more of your scalp than you'd like.

Another 9 percent of women were losing tresses along the hairline, where it meets the forehead—a trickier loss to camouflage. One in three said that their hair also felt drier. Meanwhile, 49 percent were contending with new hair on their chin, upper lip, or both.

Everyone loses 50 to 100 strands of hair per day, but it's wise to mention sudden or dramatic hair loss (like big piles in the drain after a shower or a hairbrush full of strands) to your doctor. These can be a sign of low iron, a side effect of medication (including for depression, arthritis, or high blood pressure, and even birth control pills). Hair loss may also be a symptom of lupus, an underactive thyroid, polycystic ovary syndrome (PCOS), or alopecia areata (an autoimmune disorder that causes hair to fall out), all of which require a medical diagnosis and treatment. Crash diets, skimping on protein for extended periods, scalp infections like ringworm, and severe stress can all trigger hair loss.

If you haven't yet reached menopause and your doctor diagnoses you with the female version of male-pattern baldness, you may be able to regrow hair by slathering your scalp with minoxidil (Rogaine), although studies find it usually doesn't work after menopause (more on that below). For most of us, however, plumping up and pampering the hair we have left is the best way to counter midlife hair blahs.

TLC FOR MIDLIFE HAIR

Love coloring, curling, straightening, flattening, shampooing, and blow-drying your crowning glory? Ease up. Too frequent washing, styling, and dyeing can cause harm. Chemical treatments and heat weaken the hair, causing it to break and fall out. Often it's a combination of treatments—keratin, coloring, and blow-drying, for instance—that does the most damage. Your best hair-protection strategy includes the following:

Go easy on your tresses. Avoid tools that overheat your hair. Set your hair dryer on cool and/or low settings, and minimize your use of flat irons, curling irons, and hot rollers. Don't dye your hair more than one or two shades beyond your normal color if possible: The more severe the color change, the more chemicals you require, which can make hair break. If you use hair gel or hair spray, comb it through before it dries; waiting until hair is hardened can cause more breakage.

Choose hair-care products designed for aging tresses. Shampoos and conditioners for mature hair promise volume, shine, and bounce without adding weight or skimping on the conditioning your hair needs. In a recent test of five sets of antiaging hair-care products, women between the ages of 40 and 60 reported that most made their hair look and feel soft, shiny, and manageable. Trading up to these age-appropriate products helps you avoid the pitfalls of using stuff that works on younger hair: Some volumizing shampoos skimp on conditioners, and some moisturizing products leave your locks limp, especially those with humectants, which grab moisture from the air. Rinse with warm or cool—not hot—water.

Dry and detangle gently. Don't rub or wring or twist your locks to dry them. Protect wet, breakage-prone hair by gently squeezing it the way your hairdresser does. Use a wide-toothed comb to remove tangles. Don't overcomb—too much combing or brushing can harm or lift the scales lining every shaft of hair, making it look dull and dry.

Pump up the volume. Make less hair look like more by asking your stylist to cut some short layers under the longer hair at the surface of your 'do. These support the rest of your hair, so it looks fuller. If you must use a hair dryer, try flipping your head over and drying hair from the inside— you'll spare your top hairs (which are exposed to more sun and styling

Goodbye, Unwanted Hair!

Tired of tweezing, waxing, or using other hair-removal products to get rid of excess hair on your chin or upper lip? Another option is laser hair removal, which uses a low-energy laser beam to disrupt the growth cycle of offending hair follicles.

Performed by plastic surgeons and dermatologists (licensed physician assistants or nurses may also do it, but make sure there's a physician on-site), this procedure works best for people with light skin and dark hair. Some lasers work well on darker skin, and medications can be applied to lighter hair to improve follicle destruction.

The procedure may take just a few minutes. You'll wear goggles and may have a numbing cream applied to the area first to minimize pain and stinging (be sure your doctor uses the lowest amount possible to avoid serious side effects). The result? Long-term improvement, but you may need several sessions to destroy most hair follicles and you may need additional visits for maintenance. Side effects can include blistering, discoloration after treatment, swelling, redness, and scarring.

products) and subtly puff up your look. Styling gels, foams, sprays, and mousses formulated for fine hair provide volume without unwanted weight.

Munch a tress-happy diet. While research doesn't show that any supplements or foods can reverse thinning hair, it makes sense to get plenty of the nutrients known to support the growth of healthy locks. These include B vitamins (such as B_6, biotin, and folate—found in foods like beans, peas, nuts, and eggs) and omega-3 fatty acids (found in salmon and other fatty fish, walnuts, canola oil, and fish oil and algal oil supplements), which contain fats your body uses to naturally moisturize hair and keep it shiny.

Ask your doctor about vitamin deficiencies. Dr. Ring says that she always checks for certain deficiencies in women with thinning hair, including protein, B vitamins, selenium, silica, magnesium, and vitamins A, C, and E. She also warns that too much vitamin A can actually trigger hair loss.

WHEN ALL ELSE FAILS . . . MEDICAL OPTIONS FOR HAIR LOSS

Women can have male-pattern baldness, too. While a woman won't go completely bald the way a guy would, this type of hair loss (known as androgenic alopecia) can be inherited from your mother's or father's family. But you're more likely to have it if both your parents also had hair loss. Telltale sign: thinning at the hairline at the top of your forehead. It can begin as early as your twenties. While the risk increases with age, it doesn't seem related to menopause.

A dermatologist diagnoses androgenic alopecia by examining your hair-loss pattern and taking a scalp biopsy. If the biopsy shows that the normal hair follicles have been replaced with miniature versions, you have it. The fix? Minoxidil is really the only good option for women. Finasteride isn't recommended due to side effects, and the drugs that are sometimes suggested if minoxidil doesn't work *may* slow hair loss in women but can cause cancer.

Minoxidil (Rogaine)

If you're not yet menopausal, you can slow hair loss by applying minoxidil (Rogaine) to your scalp twice a day. The drug works on both women and men, although women should use a lower-strength formula to prevent unnecessary side effects. (Don't use if you're pregnant, nursing, or trying to conceive.) It will take about 4 months to see noticeable results. Studies show, however, that Rogaine doesn't work after menopause.

In the end, though, unless you're willing to fork over the big bucks for major plastic surgery and hair replacement, the best thing you can do about your appearance is to remember that every wrinkle, every crease, and even every brown spot is a sign of the wonderful life you've led so far, a life that, hopefully, still holds enough laughter to deepen those creases at the corners of your eyes.

Part IV

Staying Healthy

Chapter 13

Protect Your Heart

Every minute of every day, heart disease kills another woman in America. In a single year, more than 400,000 women lose their lives to heart attacks, heart failure, and other cardiac troubles—more than the deaths from all cancers, accidents, breathing problems, and Alzheimer's disease in women combined. Thanks to the National Institutes of Health's splashy Red Dress campaign and other heart-health awareness efforts, more and more of us are clued in to the fact that heart health is a serious issue for women.

But there's still so much more we can do for ourselves—and for one another. What's standing in the way? These are big factors.

- **We downplay our own risk.** Your lifetime risk for developing heart disease is a scary 1 in 2. But just 31 percent of women know that heart disease is our leading cause of death.

◆ **We think of heart disease as a "man's problem."** Truth is, heart disease is a distinctly female concern, killing more women than men each year.

◆ **We overlook our stroke risk, too.** A stroke is like a heart attack in your brain. Most are caused by a clot blocking an artery that feeds brain cells. The same risks lead to both (high blood pressure, high cholesterol, and more), and the same preventive steps lower the risk for both. While 43 percent of all strokes happen to women, ours are more lethal: Sixty-one percent of stroke deaths are in women. And our risks are rising earlier in life than ever before—more than 100,000 women younger than age 65 have strokes each year, and 83,000 have heart attacks.

◆ **We ignore early warnings.** In a study at the University of California, Los Angeles, researchers found a troubling trend: The blood pressure of midlife women is rising twice as fast as that of men (by 8 to 10 points per decade, compared with 4 to 5 points for guys). Total cholesterol also rose faster in women than in men. All told, 36 percent of women in their forties and 54 percent in their fifties have high blood pressure; up to 30 percent have high cholesterol. The heart attack risk for midlife women has risen 10 percent in the past 20 years, while men's risk has dropped. And the risk for a midlife stroke is now twice as high among women as men.

◆ **Our doctors need education, too.** In one recent survey, New York-Presbyterian Hospital researchers found that fewer than one in five physicians knew that more women than men die each year from cardiovascular disease! Small wonder, then, that a woman's high blood pressure is less likely to be under control than a man's. Or that a woman's cholesterol levels are checked less often—and treated less aggressively. Or that women's heart attacks and strokes are often missed by doctors and emergency room staff because our symptoms don't look like a man's or because we seem too young for these serious problems.

A wake-up call? You bet. It's time to put the health of your cardio-vascular system—that's your heart plus your body's 60,000-mile-long network of arteries and veins—at the top of your to-do list. We know you're busy. Women responding to a recent American Heart Association survey reported that "family obligations and people to care for" got in the way of taking steps to prevent heart attacks and strokes. But can you really take care of everybody else if you don't pay attention to this risk?

We don't think so. Fact is, the fate of your heart and your brain really rests in your hands. Just 13 percent of cardiovascular health is determined by your genes, according to a recent Northwestern University study of 8,922 people (half of whom were women). That leaves 87 percent up to you.

"No woman is too young or too healthy to ignore her heart," says Susan Bennett, MD, director of the Women's Heart Program at George Washington University and a spokesperson for the American Heart Association's Go Red for Women campaign. "If you could peek into your heart right now, you would most likely see narrowing arteries and signs of atherosclerosis. Fighting heart disease isn't about getting a test once a year and then forgetting about it for the other 364 days. It's something women need to do every day."

MENOPAUSE AND YOUR RISK FOR HEART DISEASE, STROKE, AND HIGH BLOOD PRESSURE

Just 10 years ago, doctors still believed that the best protection for a midlife woman's heart and blood vessels was hormone replacement therapy (HRT) at menopause. Their logic? Estrogen pampers a woman's cardiovascular system before menopause—keeping "good" HDL higher and "bad" LDL lower, and helping arteries stay flexible to keep blood pressure healthier, too. So hormone therapy should keep a good thing going. It was such a dazzling "magic bullet" theory that, in the late 1960s, researchers gave estrogen tablets to men—8,341 of them to be precise, all heart attack survivors trying to avoid the next Big One. The experiment failed because the estrogen actually raised men's heart attack risk! But by 1992, doctors were writing nearly 32 million HRT prescriptions a year for women, and most believed it offered heart benefits along with hot-flash relief—even though experts at the National Institutes of Health warned that year that "we do not currently know whether estrogen will prevent cardiovascular disease."

Today we know that it decidedly doesn't. As we learned in Chapter 2, when taken orally, the estrogen in HRT makes your blood stickier and more likely to clot. It can triple heart disease risk and raises stroke risk by 9 to 31 percent. Researchers are still looking into whether hormone therapy may help a woman's heart health in the very early years of menopause, but so far the results are mixed. Positive trends are being seen in transdermal forms of hormones (those not taken by mouth, like a patch or gel), as well as in the use of bioidentical (rather than synthetic) forms of hormones (see Chapter 18 for more on these options).

Now when it comes to women's heart health, we're in the "beyond hormones" era. Heart experts know a lot more. For one, they now believe that declining estrogen may not be the whole reason that women's risk for cardiovascular disease triples between the ages of 45 and 55. This opens the door to new, effective lifestyle steps you can take to prevent problems. And new research in women (at last!) is revealing the best ways for women to use important medications that cut heart attack and stroke risk such as aspirin, cholesterol-lowering statins, and blood pressure drugs.

Here's what top women's heart-health experts now know about how midlife affects your cardiovascular health.

"Good" HDL shrinks. Your HDL—the "good" cholesterol that hauls the "bad" LDL to your liver for disposal—becomes smaller and less efficient at menopause. Since every 1-point rise in your HDL levels lowers heart disease risk by 3 percent, it makes sense to do all you can to pump up the size and the amount of HDL in your bloodstream with the most effective methods of all: aerobic exercise and smart eating.

"Bad" LDL gets worse. At menopause, your LDL also becomes smaller and denser—and better at burrowing into your artery walls to start growing nasty, gunky plaque. Keeping your LDL levels low—with a fiber-rich diet low in saturated fats, as well as exercise and a cholesterol-lowering statin if you need it—is important, too. A diet low in saturated fats and rich in good fats, like our 30-Day Slim-Down, Cool-Down Diet, can also make your LDL bigger and less lethal.

Insulin resistance and inflammation are on the rise. A drop in your metabolism (caused by a natural loss of muscle mass with age), plus a drop in estrogen, means more belly fat—which boosts the levels of inflammation and causes insulin resistance. Both encourage the growth of artery-clogging plaque and make plaque more likely to burst, leading to heart-damaging, brain-threatening blood clots. The fix? Produce, whole grains, exercise, and other Natural Menopause Solution healthy-living strategies cool off inflammation and help your body process blood sugar more efficiently.

Your arteries stiffen. Before menopause, estrogen helps keep blood vessels supple. Afterward, less flexibility means a higher risk for high blood pressure—a huge heart disease and stroke threat. Exercise combined with a low-salt diet rich in good fats (such as those from walnuts and pecans), potassium (think bananas and even coconut water), and plenty of fruits, vegetables, and whole grains has been proven to help.

You may become more "salt sensitive." Hormone drops at menopause can increase sodium's effect on your blood pressure even if you weren't salt sensitive before menopause, say researchers at the University of Miami. In a study of 40 women who'd had their ovaries removed during hysterectomies, 22 percent were salt sensitive before surgery, but that number rose to 52 percent 4 months after the procedures. It may not be the only reason high blood pressure risk increases during menopause, but it's a good reason to cut back on high-sodium fast food, many restaurant choices, and many processed foods.

That tummy pooch isn't just a fashion problem. Downshifting estrogen is a big reason more fat collects in your midsection at midlife. A waistline above 35 inches in women (and above 32 inches in women of

Asian descent) is a sign that there's fat *inside* your abdomen, wrapped around internal organs. Vicious visceral fat is a stronger stroke risk factor for women than men, tripling the risk for a brain attack at midlife. It also triples the risk for fatal heart disease, according to a Harvard Medical School study of 44,636 women. Deep belly fat quadruples your risk for high blood pressure and increases your LDL while it decreases your HDL levels by 30 to 100 percent. Our 30-day eating plan fights back with good fats like nuts and olive oil and with satisfying, fiber-rich whole grains, vegetables, and fruit—foods proven to target abdominal fat so you can lose it for good.

Higher anxiety = more harm. We're intrigued by recent research finding that levels of the stress hormone cortisol are higher in women around menopause—a discovery that may help explain why we often feel more stressed out at this time of life. Cortisol is a health problem because it tells your body to store more fat deep in your abdomen. But that's not all. High stress harms your heart—raising your blood pressure, boosting your LDL, and damaging artery walls so that plaque gains a toehold. Job strain alone can raise a woman's heart disease risk by 40 percent, researchers at Boston's Brigham and Women's Hospital reported recently. Extra cortisol also makes you extra hungry for high-fat, high-sugar foods. Easing stress with exercise and soothing yoga poses (like those you'll find in our 30-day workout plan) can help.

TESTS FOR HEART DISEASE AND STROKE RISK

Three standard checks—of your blood pressure, cholesterol and triglyceride, and blood sugar—can help you and your doctor determine your risks. But don't stop there. Pay attention to all of the factors listed above, then take the steps in our Natural Menopause Solution Prevention Plan to lower them.

Blood pressure. High blood pressure raises heart disease risk by 75 percent and causes half of all ischemic (clot-related) strokes. It stresses your heart, making it grow thicker and stiffer. Extra pressure also damages artery walls, speeding up the accumulation of plaque that can send a clot to your heart or brain. It can also mute your sensitivity to chest pain so that you don't notice warning signs of heart disease and could even suffer a "silent" heart attack.

How often should you be tested? Have your blood pressure checked at least every 2 years—and ideally at every doctor's visit.

Aim for: A reading below 120/80 mmHg—though there's evidence that a reading of 115/75 is even better. Between 120/80 and 139/89 is considered prehypertension and means you should do all you can with healthy lifestyle steps to lower your numbers. Higher than that is considered hypertension (high blood pressure). Your doctor may give you 6 months to lower it without drugs, then prescribe one or more medications if it's still elevated. (By the way, your blood pressure is considered low if the top number falls below 90 or the bottom number below 60. It's a problem if you're getting dizzy or faint. Low blood pressure can also be caused by infections or severe allergic reactions.)

For best results: Relax for a few minutes before your health-care practitioner wraps the blood pressure cuff around your arm (running from your car to the doctor's office can raise it temporarily). Sit with your feet on the floor, your back supported, and your test arm supported at heart level (on a surface or by the practitioner).

Cholesterol and triglycerides. High levels of "bad" LDL can double or even triple heart disease risk and raise stroke risk by 78 percent for women around menopause; low levels of "good" HDL can also double your heart disease risk and raise stroke risk by nearly 70 percent. High levels of triglyceride (another blood fat) also boost heart disease risk and can quadruple stroke risk in women, especially if your HDL levels are low.

How often should you be tested? Get a lipoprotein panel—a fasting blood test of your cholesterol and triglyceride levels—every 5 years if your levels are normal and more often (ask your doctor) if your levels are high and you're using lifestyle changes or drugs to improve them.

Aim for: LDL levels below 100 milligrams/deciliter (mg/dL)—lower if you have diabetes or are at high risk for cardiovascular problems because of a family history of early heart trouble or other factors, HDL levels above 60 mg/dL (higher is better), and triglyceride levels under 150 mg/dL.

For best results: Be sure to fast for 9 to 12 hours before taking the test. And ask your doctor to give you detailed test results: LDL, HDL, triglyceride. Just knowing your total cholesterol (the sum of your LDL, HDL, and another blood fat, called VLDL) won't tell you what you need to know about your "good" HDL and "bad" LDL.

Blood sugar. High blood sugar contributes to bigger deposits of heart-threatening plaque in artery walls and makes heart attacks and strokes more severe. Prediabetes boosts heart disease risk by 16 to 30 percent; type 2 diabetes raises heart attack and stroke risk two- to four-fold. Both also raise stroke risk significantly.

How often should you be tested? Get a fasting blood sugar test at age 45, sooner if you're overweight and have any other risk factors (see page 338 for more details).

Aim for: Fasting blood sugar below 100 mg/dL; 100 to 125 mg/dL is a sign of prediabetes, while 126 mg/dL and higher indicates diabetes.

For best results: Have your fasting check in the morning.

OTHER TELLTALE SIGNS

Plenty of other things can be warnings that you're at higher risk for heart disease or stroke. Pay attention to these.

Your weight. Extra weight means extra risk. A body mass index (BMI—a measure of your weight compared to your height) between 25 and 29.9 doubles heart disease risk and raises stroke risk by 11 percent; a BMI of 30 or higher triples heart disease risk and raises stroke risk by 41 percent. But weight isn't the whole story—even normal-weight women are at higher risk if they're carrying extra body fat around their midsection.

Your waist size. Heart attack risk doubles when your waistline expands beyond 34 inches and goes higher as your waistband stretches: One study found that for some women, a big waist tripled their risk. A tummy pooch, even if you're not overweight, signals the presence of visceral fat—active fat wrapped around internal organs that pumps hormones, deadly inflammatory chemicals, and fatty acids directly to your heart and liver and to every cell in your body, 24/7. This biologically busy blubber raises blood pressure, makes cells resistant to insulin (the hormone responsible for blood sugar absorption, a heart risk), and accelerates the growth of gunky plaque in artery walls.

Metabolic syndrome. Nearly half of all midlife women may have metabolic syndrome—a collection of warning signs that may seem like no big deal on their own but that added together could spell big trouble. Metabolic syndrome doubles heart disease and stroke risk. You have it if you have any three of five warning signs.

- A waist measurement of 40 inches or more for men, and 35 inches or more for women

- Triglyceride levels of 150 milligrams per deciliter (mg/dL) or above, or you're taking medication for elevated triglyceride levels

- HDL, or "good" cholesterol, below 40 mg/dL for men and below 50 mg/dL for women, or you're taking medication for low HDL levels

- Blood pressure of 130/85 or above, or you're taking medication for elevated blood pressure levels

- Fasting blood sugar levels of 100 mg/dL or above, or you're taking medication for elevated blood glucose levels

Smoking. Tobacco use quadruples a woman's risk for fatal heart disease. The more you smoke, the higher your stroke risk: One cigarette a day doubles it; two packs a day raises it ninefold. Chemicals in cigarette smoke damage arteries; make blood stickier and more likely to form clots; raise your blood pressure and cholesterol levels; and can make arteries in your heart spasm.

Your health history. Other health conditions—some of which affect women predominantly or exclusively—can also raise your heart disease and stroke risk significantly. Among them are

- Sleep apnea

- Migraines with an aura

- Blood-clotting disorders (having had several miscarriages or having deep vein thrombosis may be signs you have a clotting disorder)

- Preeclampsia during a pregnancy (high blood pressure and/or excess protein in your urine)

- Gestational (pregnancy) diabetes

- Polycystic ovary syndrome

- Lupus

- Rheumatoid arthritis

If you have any of these conditions, ask your doctor about the best ways to lower your heart attack risk. And make sure to do all you can with healthy lifestyle changes to further reduce your odds.

Your family's health history. Heart disease on your family tree can double the risk of heart disease and strokes. You share genes *and* a legacy of eating and exercise habits with your nearest and dearest. In a University of Texas Southwestern study of 2,404 people without known heart disease, a family history doubled a woman's odds for dangerous, undetected plaque lurking in the arteries of her heart. Having a parent with heart disease raises your risk by about 45 percent, but having a sibling with heart disease raises it even further. When researchers from the landmark Framingham Heart Study followed the health histories of 4,506 women and men, they found that those who had a brother or sister with heart disease had double the risk for developing it, too. Early heart disease in your family (before age 60 for women relatives) can increase your risk even if your cholesterol, blood pressure, blood sugar, weight, and waist size are normal. It's worth talking with your doctor about whether you're a good candidate for a more advanced heart-health check such as an exercise stress test or a coronary calcium scan, which can detect plaque in artery walls.

What's Your BMI?

Consult the chart below to find out your BMI. For women, a BMI of 18.5 and below is considered underweight; between 18.5 and 24.9 is normal weight; between 25.0 and 29.9 is overweight; and 30.0 and above is obese.

HEIGHT	WEIGHT (LBS)													
5'0"	97	102	107	112	118	123	128	133	138	143	148	153	158	163
5'1"	100	106	111	116	122	127	132	137	143	148	153	158	164	169
5'2"	104	109	115	120	126	131	136	142	147	153	158	164	169	175
5'3"	107	113	118	124	130	135	141	146	152	158	163	169	175	180
5'4"	110	116	122	128	134	140	145	151	157	163	169	174	180	186
5'5"	114	120	126	132	138	144	150	156	162	168	174	180	186	192
5'6"	118	124	130	136	142	148	155	161	167	173	179	186	192	198
5'7"	121	127	134	140	146	153	159	166	172	178	185	191	198	204
5'8"	125	131	138	144	151	158	164	171	177	184	190	197	203	210
5'9"	128	135	142	149	155	162	169	176	182	189	196	203	209	216
5'10"	132	139	146	153	160	167	174	181	188	195	202	209	216	222
5'11"	136	143	150	157	165	172	179	186	193	200	208	215	222	229
6'0"	140	147	154	162	169	177	184	191	199	206	213	221	228	235
6'1"	144	151	159	166	174	182	189	197	204	212	219	227	235	242
6'2"	148	155	163	171	179	186	194	202	210	218	225	233	241	249
BMI	19	20	21	22	23	24	25	26	27	28	29	30	31	32

THE NATURAL MENOPAUSE SOLUTION AND YOUR HEART

We love simple and elegant solutions, and here's a great one. The same healthy eating and exercise program that helps women lose weight, trim belly fat, and control menopausal symptoms—yes, we're talking about the 30-Day Slim-Down, Cool-Down Diet—can also lower your risk for the factors that lead to heart attacks and strokes.

Our test panelists are proof. Many saw their LDL and total cholesterol levels drop in just a few weeks on the plan. And blood pressure for many of them dropped to healthier levels, too.

Following the plan could help *you* lower your LDL, raise your HDL, and get a better grip on your blood pressure and blood sugar levels. But don't stop there. In this chapter you'll find additional steps aimed at keeping a woman's heart and blood vessels healthy. First, here's a recap of the plan's essentials and the heart-healthy benefits of this approach.

Plenty of fruits and vegetables. The Natural Menopause Solution eating plan loads your plate with produce—which is good news for your heart. Women who filled up on fruits and vegetables had levels of "bad" LDL that were 9.5 points lower than those who skimped, according to a Boston University study published in the *American Journal of Clinical Nutrition*. Every 1-point drop in your LDL levels lowers your heart attack risk by 2 percent.

How they help: Soluble fiber in produce blocks the reabsorption of LDL cholesterol found in digestive fluids back into your bloodstream. Fruits and veggies are also rich in antioxidants such as quercetin, which discourages the buildup of artery plaque.

Whole grains instead of refined grains. Choosing brown rice, whole grain bread, and other healthy grains is a key component of our eating plan—and a move that your blood vessels will cheer. In one study that followed 9,776 women and men for 19 years, it was found that those who got about 6 grams of soluble fiber a day (about the amount in a bowl of oatmeal, 1/2 cup of barley, and a pear) had a 15 percent lower risk for heart disease than those who got less than 1 gram a day. And in a Harvard School of Public Health study, women who ate the most whole grains had a 40 percent lower risk of stroke than those who ate the least.

How they help: Whole grains also cool inflammation; just two servings a day reduced deaths from inflammation-related diseases by 30 percent over 17 years, the Iowa Women's Health Study found. They also combat insulin resistance and spikes in insulin that encourage the growth of artery plaque. And whole grains like oatmeal and barley are packed with a special soluble fiber called beta-glucan. Simply starting the day with oatmeal could lower your LDL by 7 points.

More good fats, fewer bad fats. Good-for-you monounsaturated fats (think nuts, avocados, and olive and canola oil) and omega-3s (found in fatty fish like salmon, as well as walnuts and canola oil) are among the luscious luxuries of the 30-Day Slim-Down, Cool-Down Diet. And your heart will love them, too. In one study, researchers found that eating just 14 walnut halves a day helped women lower their LDL levels by 10 percent and boost their HDL levels by 18 percent. According to another study, having fish one to three times a month cut women's risk for heart disease by 21 percent.

Quick Tip
RESTAURANT CONFIDENTIAL

To keep your weight in check and your heart healthy, skip these fatty foods.

Butter, creamy salad dressings, and cheesy toppings. Keeping your daily intake of saturated fat to less than 7 percent of your daily calories—that's about 1 tablespoon of butter or a slice of Cheddar cheese plus ½ cup of ice cream, if you eat 1,800 calories a day—can lower your LDL by 9 to 11 percent.

Fried fish. Enjoying broiled or baked fish one to four times a week could cut your stroke risk by 27 percent. But having fried fish (like fish sticks, a fast-food fish sandwich, or the fried-fish special at the local diner) could raise your stroke risk by a whopping 44 percent.

Trans fats. Still found in some baked goods, french fries, and other fried items on restaurant menus, trans fats can boost your heart attack risk by as much as 50 percent. More and more establishments are banning this Frankenfat, but it's often impossible to tell from the menu whether an eatery has made the switch. Since these foods are also high in empty calories, just saying no is a good idea.

How they help: Monounsaturated fats can help lower LDL, raise HDL, and calm blood pressure. Omega-3s, meanwhile, help prevent blood clots, inflammation, and irregular heart rhythms.

Less sodium. The fresh, unprocessed foods of the 30-Day Slim-Down, Cool-Down Diet are naturally low in blood pressure–raising sodium. Cutting back is a powerful move. In a Duke University study of people with high blood pressure, 71 percent of those who ate less sodium (but made no other menu changes) brought their blood pressure under control.

How it helps: Extra sodium prompts your body to pump more water into your bloodstream in an attempt to dilute it. The outcome? Your blood volume increases, and the force of blood moving through your arteries increases, too. Too much sodium, research suggests, can also stiffen arteries, further raising blood pressure. Cutting back on it stops all of these bad effects.

Plenty of calcium. This bone-building, hot flash–calming mineral is one of our Flash-Fighting Four. It's also a heart-healthy superstar. In the Women's Health Study—a national look at the health of more than 28,000 women—researchers found that women who got about 1,100 milligrams of calcium a day from food were 11 percent less likely to develop high blood pressure, compared with women who got less than 560 milligrams a day.

How it helps: Calcium may help regulate blood pressure by keeping your arteries flexible, keeping the body's sodium and potassium levels in a healthy balance, encouraging weight loss, and perhaps even discouraging insulin resistance.

Exercise every day. Daily walks plus regular strength training help you blast fat on the Natural Menopause Solution exercise plan. Your heart loves this duo, too. Regular exercise reduced heart disease risk by 40 percent in one study of more than 27,000 midlife and older women, say researchers from Brigham and Women's Hospital in Boston. And it can cut stroke risk by 25 to 50 percent.

How it helps: Exercise encourages more fat particles in your bloodstream to mature into HDL, *and* it makes HDL bigger. That protects your

LOOK BEYOND THE SALT SHAKER

About 80 percent of the sodium in a woman's diet doesn't come from the salt shaker—it's hidden in processed foods and in restaurant and fast foods. Big sources include canned beans and soups; microwaveable entrées and side dishes; bottled salad dressings; canned vegetables; snack foods; as well as cold cuts, hot dogs, and other processed meats. Eating fresh, unprocessed foods (and choosing low-sodium and no-salt-added items) can make a big difference.

arteries from a buildup of gunky plaque. Regular exercise also reduces inflammation, discourages blood clotting, and lowers blood pressure.

Feeling good. The Natural Menopause Solution can help you feel more confident, serene, peaceful, and happy. More and more research shows that feeling good isn't just a nice extra—it's positively powerful heart protection. Depression, which boosts bodywide inflammation and makes blood more likely to clot, quadruples a woman's risk for heart disease and raises the risk for a fatal heart attack fourfold. It also increases stroke risk by 20 to 30 percent. Stress harms blood vessels by raising blood pressure and damaging artery walls. The good news? There's plenty of evidence that stress- and depression-lifters like love and friendship pamper your arteries.

How it helps: Learning to let anxiety and stress roll off your back, in whatever way works best for you, could cut your stroke risk by an extra 24 percent, say researchers from the UK's University of Cambridge. Relaxation exercises have the power to lower levels of "bad" LDL cholesterol, studies suggest. And learning a stress-reducing set of moves, such as tai chi or yoga (part of the 30-day exercise plan) could reduce LDL cholesterol by as much as 26 percent over time.

OTHER IMPORTANT STRATEGIES

These additional strategies offer further protection against heart attacks and strokes.

Stop smoking—even if you're "just" a social smoker. Smoking raises your risk for heart disease and stroke by raising blood pressure, tightening arteries, and making blood stickier and more likely to clot. It also damages fragile artery walls, opening the door for plaque buildup. Cigarette smoking doubles, triples, or even quadruples your risk for developing heart disease, and once you have the disease, smoking doubles your risk for sudden cardiac death. Studies also show that smoking just one to four cigarettes a day can triple a woman's risk.

How it helps: By quitting, you allow your cardiovascular system to work normally again. Heart disease and stroke risks start dropping almost immediately and fall by 30 percent within a year. Your risks drop to normal within 10 to 14 years.

What you should know: Nicotine replacement products (like gum and patches), the anticraving drugs bupropion (Wellbutrin) and varenicline (Chantix), counseling, and phone support can all help you quit successfully. While you're at it, steer clear of secondhand smoke, too. It can boost your risk by 25 to 30 percent.

Take fish oil or algal oil capsules. Packed with heart-healthy omega-3 fatty acids, fish oil or algal oil capsules can fill gaps if you don't always manage to eat fish two or more times a week. Getting plenty of omega-3s could reduce your risk for fatal heart disease by up to 30 percent, say researchers at Louisiana's Ochsner Medical Center who reviewed dozens of good-fat studies. It may also reduce stroke risk, by decreasing atherosclerosis and regulating off-beat heart rhythms that can send blood clots to your brain.

How it helps: Omega-3s keep cell membranes healthy. This improves artery flexibility and maintains optimal electrical activity in the heart muscle so that your heartbeat stays normal, too. Omega-3s also protect

(continued on page 330)

Happier and Healthier…
THE NATURAL MENOPAUSE SOLUTION WAY

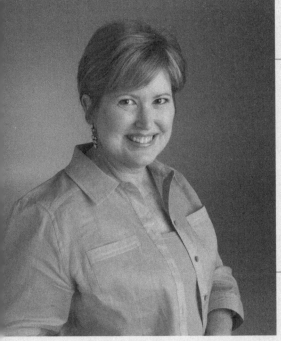

MARIE FRITZ

Age: 56

Pounds lost: 4½

Inches lost: 5

Major changes: Total cholesterol dropped 30 points. Lost 1½ inches in the waist. No more heartburn!

"It's Time to Make My Well-Being a Priority"

"I started 'menopausing' 11 years ago," Marie says. "I've gotten some mean hot flashes, and I have night sweats—especially if I've been stressed out during the day. But my worst symptoms have been heartburn and insomnia. I've asked a number of women, who've told me they've gotten heartburn more often since menopause, too. I sleep on four pillows and even raised the head of my bed up on 2-by-4-inch boards to help ease the heartburn, but it would still get so bad that my neck and the base of my skull ached."

Marie was pleasantly surprised that she's had "no heartburn whatsoever" since starting the 30-Day Slim-Down, Cool-Down Diet. She also lost 1½ inches from her waist—enough to notice that she could move into the soothing poses of the plan's yoga routine with new ease. "To me, losing belly fat was the most important thing," she says. "I get compliments about the way I look. My clothes fit better.

"Belly fat, stiff hips, and a bad back from an injury several years ago meant I had a hard time even bending over to tie my shoes. As I kept doing the walking and yoga routines, I became more flexible; I could move better. I really think at this point in life, if you don't keep moving, you can become very stiff. I love the way being flexible again feels!"

Marie's cholesterol had always stayed within a healthy range, but at a doctor's appointment a few months before starting the program, she got unwelcome news. "My doctor said, 'Uh-oh, you're inching toward the danger zone. We have to watch this,'" she recalls. "Heart disease runs in my family. When I saw the numbers, I thought, 'I don't want to be a statistic.'" In just 30 days on the plan, Marie inched back down toward the safe zone, with a 30-point drop in total cholesterol and a 13-point reduction in the heart-threatening LDL. "I know heart health is something I have to be serious about as I get older. I don't like to take any type of medication, so getting this improvement with diet and exercise alone was really great."

A family trip to Arizona during her first week on the plan put Marie and the 30-Day Slim-Down, Cool-Down Diet to the test. Both passed with flying colors. She brought flaxseed with her and bought ingredients to make the Slimming, Cooling Smoothie in the well-equipped kitchen of the Frank Lloyd Wright–designed home she and her family had rented. "I altered the recipe till it tasted best for me. I found that almond milk was good in it, and so was adding half a banana. All of the menopausal women in our group loved it! I would have a cup before going out for walks and felt really filled up."

Huffing and puffing through 1 mile when she started the program, Marie has built up endurance—and a new love for walking. She now takes 4-mile interval walks at a local park. She's set her sights on hiking during a vacation in North Carolina and hopes to start trekking sections of the Appalachian Trail with her husband. She's already bought her hiking shoes. "Being on the plan helped me switch my priorities," she notes. "I realized I've only got this body I'm in now. If I don't take care of it, nobody else will. It's time to make my well-being a priority."

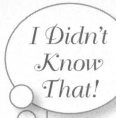

GOOD FATS AND GOOD CHOLESTEROL

Good fats have the power to get your cholesterol levels into a healthier balance. In one study of 322 people, researchers from Israel, Germany, and the United States found that a diet rich in good fats lowered "bad" LDL levels by 5.6 points, raised "good" HDL levels by a respectable 6.4 points, and reduced heart-threatening triglycerides by 22 points—tricks that a low-fat diet *didn't* do.

plaque in artery walls from breaking open, which can cause heart-threatening, brain-threatening blood clots to form.

What you should know: Most women should aim for 1,000 milligrams of omega-3s per day. Some experts recommend getting at least 600 milligrams as DHA, the form of omega-3s that your body uses most easily. Research shows that most fish oil capsule makers refine the oils to remove toxins. But if you're concerned or you're a strict vegetarian, try algal oil DHA capsules instead. They're made from the same algae that fish use as the raw material for "producing" omega-3s.

LDL on the high side? Try foods fortified with sterols and stanols. These natural compounds, added to cholesterol-lowering margarines and even some brands of cow's milk and rice milk, can reduce your LDL levels even more than a healthy diet alone can. In one study, people with normal cholesterol levels who used margarines fortified with sterols and stanols saw their bad cholesterol decrease by 7 to 11 percent after 3 months.

How they work: Sterols and stanols are called phytosterols and come from the membranes in plant cells. Chemically similar to the cholesterol your body makes, they get absorbed into your digestive system instead of heart-threatening cholesterol—thereby lowering LDL levels in your bloodstream.

What you should know: Aim for up to 2 grams of sterols and stanols a day, about the amount in 2½ tablespoons of fortified margarine or two 8-ounce glasses of fortified orange juice. Eat an extra serving of red, yellow, or orange fruit or vegetables a day if you do. These compounds can reduce the absorption of heart-friendly carotenoids from the foods you eat.

Ask your doctor about low-dose aspirin. Taking one 81-milligram aspirin a day could help protect you from a stroke. Thought it was a heart helper? Doctors thought so, too. But then a study at the University of Buffalo in New York of 51,000 women and 44,000 men revealed that its benefits are gender-dependent. For men, it helped prevent heart attacks; for women, it cut stroke risk by 17 percent.

How it helps: Aspirin makes platelets in your blood less sticky, so they won't form clumps and clots.

What you should know: Aspirin can also increase your risk for ulcers and serious gastrointestinal bleeding, so it's important to clear this strategy with your MD first. Taking aspirin seems to reduce stroke risk best in women over age 65, but it may help you if you're younger and at higher than normal risk due to high blood pressure, out-of-rhythm heartbeats called atrial fibrillation, or a family history of strokes.

Taking a Statin? Add Fiber

If you're taking a statin to reduce your LDL cholesterol, pairing it with a fiber supplement could give you bigger benefits. A study of 68 people with moderately high LDL levels (161–186 mg/dL) at Robert Wood Johnson Medical School in New Brunswick, New Jersey, found that those who took simvastatin alone cut their LDL by 29 percent. Adding a teaspoon of ground psyllium (Metamucil) in water three times a day pushed their levels down by 35 percent.

ASK ABOUT MEDICATIONS

If your cholesterol or blood pressure doesn't come down to a healthy level after 3 to 6 months of serious healthy lifestyle changes—like following the Natural Menopause Solution—it's time to talk to your doctor about taking a prescription medication. Cholesterol-lowering statins and blood pressure–lowering drugs can all help—but only if you take them. While doctors are increasingly aware of women's cardiovascular risks, many still overlook midlife threats. Know your numbers, and don't brush off signs of trouble.

Chapter 14

Sidestep Diabetes

*I*t's a hidden female health crisis, a life-threatening diagnosis that sends out whispered warnings years in advance. Yet too often, midlife women and our doctors miss telltale signs of diabetes risk that are hiding in plain sight.

Type 2 diabetes is a high blood sugar problem that affects 12.6 million American women. Dealing with diabetes is a daily concern, a balancing act that juggles food, exercise, blood sugar tests, and sometimes medications. Coping can be stressful and time consuming, but it's more than just a hassle. Diabetes raises your risk for heart attacks and strokes; boosts your odds for brittle-bone fractures and fatal cancers; and leads to vision loss, kidney failure, and a shocking number of amputations each year.

Millions of midlife women are at risk for diabetes—and the number grows along with rising weight and expanding waistlines. You've no doubt heard about the diabetes epidemic that's sweeping the nation. But you may not have heard about these shadow epidemics. First comes insulin resistance, which develops years before your blood sugar creeps upward. Sixty-eight million Americans are insulin resistant, up from 47 million just a few years ago. Next (if you do nothing) comes prediabetes, when blood sugar begins to rise past normal. Five years ago, 57 million Americans had prediabetes; today that number is 79 million.

No woman wants to hear that she's on the road to diabetes—and perhaps that's one reason so few of us hear from our doctors that we have one of these conditions. But if you have prediabetes, your odds for developing full-blown type 2 diabetes in the next 5 to 10 years are as high as 50 percent. We think you'd rather know about this when there's still time to reverse it.

The rest of the story is that you can prevent or delay diabetes, and the best way to do it is with the same strategies that help you lose weight and stay comfortable and serene as menopause approaches. It's another reason we're so excited about the Natural Menopause Solution.

"Reducing your risk can be as simple as losing just 7 percent of your body weight—something you can do with a healthy diet and a half hour of exercise every day," says Virginia Peragallo-Dittko, RN, CDE, director of the Diabetes Education Center at Winthrop-University Hospital in Mineola, New York, home to one of the nation's first diabetes prevention programs for people with prediabetes. "That's very freeing—you can avoid a big health problem with small changes. You don't have to get back to your high school weight or exercise for hours every day. Small changes get you there."

MENOPAUSE, MIDLIFE, AND DIABETES RISK

Hundreds of midlife women slashed their diabetes risk in a landmark, government-funded study called the Diabetes Prevention Program. For 3 years, women and men with prediabetes either followed a healthy eating and exercise plan, took a blood sugar–lowering drug, or did nothing. Ultimately, the diet and exercise group cut their risk for developing full-blown diabetes by 58 percent—far better than the other groups. Ten years later, this group was still far ahead.

That's great news for midlife women, because midlife is when insulin resistance rises sharply. In one study of 12,861 people published in the journal *Archives of Internal Medicine*, just 5 percent of women in their twenties and 11 percent in their thirties were insulin resistant. But the numbers soared to 33 percent of women in their forties, 49 percent in their fifties, and 63 percent age 60 and older. If you're overweight and/or have a wide waistline, your risk for insulin resistance is 5 to 15 times higher than it is for a woman at a healthy weight and waist size. (Insulin resistance is also a big component of metabolic syndrome, which can threaten your heart, too.)

What's the connection between midlife, menopause, and this silent problem? Researchers think that shifting hormones may interfere with your body's ability to obey insulin's signals. But the biggest cause is belly fat. The more deep abdominal fat you have—and women have more at midlife thanks in part to falling estrogen levels—the more insulin resistant you are, report researchers from Laval University in Quebec. And the higher your risk for diabetes. In fact, belly fat is a bigger risk factor for diabetes than simply carrying excess weight.

Before menopause, estrogen encourages your body to store more fat on your butt and hips. But as estrogen plummets, fat moves front and center (and you find yourself shopping for forgiving elastic-waist pants!). It turns out other hormones shove fat toward your belly, too. New research suggests that levels of the stress hormone cortisol, which also directs your body to store more fat in your abdomen, rise at menopause, according to an Italian study published in the March 2011 issue of the journal *Menopause*.

This fat is nasty stuff. It collects deep in your abdomen, twining itself around your internal organs and hooking itself up to the major blood vessel, the portal vein, that serves your liver. This active fat pumps fatty acids, hormones, and proteins into your bloodstream 24/7 that interfere with your liver's important role in healthy blood sugar control and that encourage insulin resistance throughout your body.

You may never want to wear a bikini again, but striving for a flatter tummy (a goal you can reach on the Natural Menopause Solution) is a worthy target for any midlife woman who wants to lose weight all over and stay healthier.

TESTS FOR DIABETES

Your past affects your risk for insulin resistance, prediabetes, and full-blown diabetes, too. If you're among the 2 to 10 percent of women who had gestational (pregnancy) diabetes, your odds for eventually developing diabetes are at least 50 percent, yet doctors often fail to test blood sugar frequently in this group of women. Polycystic ovary syndrome—a fertility problem that involves insulin resistance, higher than usual testosterone levels, and sometimes ovarian cysts—also raises risk.

Here's how to tell where you and your blood sugar stand.

A fasting blood sugar test. One of two tests that doctors use to diagnose diabetes and prediabetes, a fasting blood sugar test reveals how much sugar remains in your blood when you haven't eaten in 8 to 12 hours.

How often should you be tested? Get a fasting blood sugar test at age 45, sooner if you're overweight and have any of these risk factors: You don't exercise; you have high blood pressure or cholesterol; you've had gestational (pregnancy) diabetes or have a family history of diabetes; you gave birth to a baby weighing 9 pounds or more; you have polycystic ovary syndrome; or you are of African American, Latino, Asian American, Native American, or Pacific Islander descent.

Aim for: Fasting blood sugar below 100 milligrams/deciliter (mg/dL). A reading of 100 to 125 mg/dL is a sign of prediabetes; 126 mg/dL and higher indicates diabetes. (Your doctor will probably test twice to confirm a diagnosis.)

For best results: Have your fasting check in the morning; studies show that a.m. results are more accurate than later checks because they pick up overnight blood sugar highs related to insulin resistance in your liver (an early indication of diabetes risk).

An A1C test. Long used by people with diabetes (and even by some people with prediabetes) to track long-range blood sugar, the A1C is now considered a good screening test. The bonus: No fasting required. In 2010, the American Diabetes Association endorsed this easier screening test. It's not perfect, but if you can't manage a fasting test, it's a good alternative.

Aim for: An A1C of 5.6 or lower. You may have prediabetes if your A1C is 5.7 to 6.4 percent. You may have diabetes if your A1C level is 6.5 percent or higher.

For best results: If you have iron deficiency anemia, a B_{12} deficiency, or chronic liver or kidney disease, an A1C won't give reliable results for diagnosing diabetes. If you have any of these conditions, talk with your doctor about whether they may be affecting your A1C results and whether you should do extra daily blood sugar checks to see if your numbers are trending higher or lower than your A1C shows.

Oral glucose tolerance test. If you ever had a diabetes check during pregnancy, you've had an oral glucose tolerance test (OGTT). It can be a more sensitive way to detect prediabetes and diabetes and to assess whether prediabetes is progressing toward diabetes. For these reasons, the American Diabetes Association says that it can be used in place of a fasting blood sugar check.

For an OGTT, you must fast for 8 to 12 hours; then at the doctor's office or the lab, you'll drink a very sweet beverage containing 75 milligrams of glucose. Your blood will be drawn after 1 hour and again after 2 hours. Blood sugar levels of both blood samples (and of a sample taken at the start of the test) will be checked to see how your body handles blood sugar immediately after a test meal.

Ask your doctor about checking your insulin levels along with your blood sugar levels. This can detect even earlier signs of insulin resistance—when your body is processing blood sugar quickly by raising your insulin levels.

Aim for: Levels below 140 mg/dL. If your results are between 140 and 200 mg/dL, you may have prediabetes (also called impaired glucose tolerance). Levels above 200 mg/dL are in the diabetic range; doctors usually test twice to confirm a diagnosis of diabetes.

For best results: Fast as directed by your doctor.

OTHER TELLTALE SYMPTOMS

Many of the telltale signs of rising diabetes risk are the same as warning signs for heart disease. The reason? These conditions travel together in your body because they're caused by many of the same factors: overweight, inactivity, and excess abdominal fat. If you have any of these, talk with your doctor about whether you should have your blood sugar levels checked.

Metabolic syndrome. As we discussed in Chapter 13, nearly half of all midlife women may have metabolic syndrome. See page 320 to find out if you're one of them.

Your waist size. Simpler than figuring out all of the other risks of metabolic syndrome, researchers say that a woman with a waist measuring more than 35 inches is five times more likely to have insulin resistance than a woman with a slimmer midsection. That's because a wide waist is a sign of deep abdominal fat, which encourages insulin resistance by pumping fatty acids, hormones, and inflammation-boosting compounds into your bloodstream.

THE NATURAL MENOPAUSE SOLUTION AND DIABETES PREVENTION

One reason the Natural Menopause Solution is so adept at melting away stubborn excess pounds is its stellar ability to reverse insulin resistance. We talked earlier in this book about how that can help with weight loss for women around menopause. But insulin resistance, as you now know, is also the prime problem behind type 2 diabetes. Here's how the elements of our plan discourage this devastating blood sugar problem, too.

SLASH DIABETES RISK BY GIVING UP "LIQUID CANDY"

Sugary sodas, fruit punch, sweetened iced tea, and even an overload of fruit juice can all push your risk for prediabetes and diabetes sky-high. Just one 12-ounce can of soda a day increased the risk for metabolic syndrome—the insulin resistance underlying prediabetes and diabetes—by 44 percent, according to a recent, headline-grabbing study at Boston University School of Medicine.

Better sleep. Surprised that a great night's sleep—something you can achieve with the research-proven remedies in our plan—is also a diabetes stopper? In a study at Boston's Brigham and Women's Hospital of more than 70,000 female nurses, those who got fewer than 5 hours of sleep a night were 57 percent more likely to develop type 2 diabetes than were those who got 7 to 8 hours.

How it helps: Getting your fill of deep sleep helps your body regulate blood sugar better, say University of Chicago researchers. Regularly missing out on slow-wave stages of sleep has the same effect on your body's insulin sensitivity as gaining 20 to 30 pounds would, they report in a 2007 study published in the *Proceedings of the National Academy of Sciences.*

A rainbow of fresh produce. At every meal the fruits and vegetables you'll find in our plan also take aim at diabetes and at the health warning signs that precede it. In a recent study of 486 women published in the *American Journal of Clinical Nutrition*, those who ate the most fruit were 34 percent less likely to have metabolic syndrome than women who had little fruit, and those who had the most vegetables cut the risk by 30 percent compared with women who ate the least amount of veggies. Meanwhile, adding just one serving of leafy greens a day reduces your risk for metabolic syndrome by 9 percent; boosting your fruit intake by 3 servings a day lowers your risk by 18 percent, say Tulane University researchers who looked at the diets and blood sugar levels of 71,346 women for a 2008 study in the journal *Diabetes Care*.

How it helps: Produce is packed with fiber, which helps slow the rise in blood sugar after you eat, so your body can process it in a healthier way. It also supplies nutrients like magnesium that are essential for healthy blood sugar absorption. And there's new evidence, reported by Italian researchers at a recent conference of the Endocrine Society, that cell-protecting antioxidants in produce also help your body become more sensitive to insulin.

Hearty whole grains. By making the switch from refined grains to whole grains on the 30-Day Slim-Down, Cool-Down Diet, you'll reap big blood sugar benefits. Simply replacing white rice with brown rice—and getting two or more servings per week—could cut diabetes risk 11 percent, say Boston researchers who tracked 157,463 women for a study presented

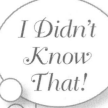

I Didn't Know That!

SURPRISING SYMPTOMS OF DIABETES AND INSULIN RESISTANCE

Blood sugar problems are usually dangerously symptom-free but not always. Watch out for these stealth symptoms.

Patches of thickened, velvety, or darker skin on the neck, underarms, or groin. Called acanthosis nigricans, this skin discoloration is a sign of insulin resistance.

Unusual fatigue, excessive thirst and urination, blurred vision, unexpected weight loss. These can be signs of high blood sugar—call your doctor right away.

at an American Heart Association scientific conference in 2010. In a German study, researchers who followed 25,067 women and men for 7 years recently found that those who got the most fiber from whole grains were 27 percent less likely to develop diabetes than those who got the least, according to a report in the journal *Archives of Internal Medicine*.

How it helps: Fiber helps control blood sugar levels after a meal. Whole grains also contain small but important amounts of good fats, protein, and nutrients like magnesium that can help your body process blood sugar more effectively. People who eat a lot of fiber may also have less abdominal fat!

More calcium-rich, low-fat dairy products. Dairy products can help whittle your waistline on our plan, but that's not all. Low-fat or fat-free dairy defends against diabetes, too. Two servings a day cut the risk for insulin resistance by a whopping 62 percent, reports a British study published in the *Journal of Epidemiology and Community Health*. At least a dozen other studies confirm dairy's protective effects, say researchers from Quebec's Laval University.

How it works: The calcium, vitamin D, magnesium, and other minerals in dairy—and featured among our Flash-Fighting Four—help your body "listen" to insulin's signals.

A focus on good fats. Nuts, olive oil, and more—the good fats you'll find in our eating plan—also have diabetes-fighting power. Women who ate about an ounce of nuts or a serving of peanut butter five times a week were 21 percent less likely to develop diabetes than nut avoiders were, according to a Harvard School of Public Health study published in the *Journal of the American Medical Association*. And Spanish researchers have found that people who consume olive oil also have lower risk.

How it helps: Monounsaturated fats keep the walls of cells healthy so that they can obey insulin's signals and quickly bring blood sugar inside, say Italian researchers who reviewed the good news about these good fats for the journal *Clinical Nutrition*.

Less saturated fat. Your waistline, your heart—and your blood sugar—will love the low levels of saturated fat and trans fats in our plan. In the landmark Diabetes Prevention Program, people lowered their

It Worked for Me!

**Mimi Kolb, 49, lost 5½ pounds and 5½ inches—
and her blood sugar and cholesterol levels improved.**

At 49, Mimi is in perimenopause—and coping with hot flashes and night sweats that seem to come and go. "In the past I've had days and days of frequent hot flashes and night sweats," she says. "I've also had times that were flash free. After the first week on the Natural Menopause Solution, I haven't had any hot flashes or night sweats—it could be because of the ingredients in the diet, the exercise plan, the weight I lost, or all three."

Mimi loves her flatter belly and is thrilled about having less back fat. "The yoga-with-weights routine helped tone my upper body, including my back," she notes. As a result she's been able to go "shopping" in her own closet, rediscovering clothes that had been too snug but now fit again. "My clothes look better, and I'm wearing things that I hadn't been able to wear comfortably for a while. I love that!"

Almond butter—an ingredient in the Slimming, Cooling Smoothie that's on the 30-Day Slim-Down, Cool-Down Diet menu every day—was an unfamiliar food for Mimi that she quickly grew to love. "I didn't want to put it into the smoothie; I just wasn't too sure about it," she recalls. "So I ate a little with a spoon or fork every day. It was a good thing to have right before

risk for diabetes dramatically, in part by slashing saturated fat to 7 percent of total calories.

How it helps: Saturated fat interferes with your body's ability to process blood sugar. In a Swedish study of 76 women and 86 men published in the journal *Diabetologia*, people who ate saturated fats instead of monounsaturated fats saw their insulin sensitivity fall by 24 percent.

No processed meats. Steering clear of processed meats (hot dogs, lunch meat, commercial sausage, etc.) is a cornerstone of our plan and,

I exercised. And then I made my smoothies without it. Sometimes I varied the fruit in the smoothie, too—like with peaches instead of the pineapple."

Regular butter may have been one of the toughest ingredients for her to give up. "I used to go through a stick of butter a week," she says. "But I quickly got used to the good fats in this eating plan. And I appreciated that every meal was spelled out for me—there was no guesswork. If you like to cook, it's a great plan; the recipes are delicious. They seemed a little complicated at first, but they really are easy to prepare. I really enjoyed the shrimp with coconut rice and the turkey sausage. The homemade turkey sausage met with my husband's approval, and a friend of mine and her son said they really liked the cranberry breakfast cookies." Mimi discovered that the eating plan is also very portable—she stayed on track during a beach vacation on the Outer Banks of North Carolina and on a weekend in New York City. "I cooked with some health-conscious friends, and I found that if I looked, I could find foods that work with the plan on the restaurant menu, too."

After just 4 weeks on the plan, she not only lost weight and inches, but her blood sugar and cholesterol levels nudged downward, too. "My doctor and I are watching my cholesterol, which is just a little bit high," Mimi says. "My doctor said it's a hereditary thing and that medicine would help to fix it, but I'd rather not take medication. Seeing that diet and exercise could make a difference so quickly will motivate me to keep going. There's also some diabetes in my family, so seeing lower numbers for my fasting blood sugar was also a good sign. I wasn't at risk yet, but I don't ever want to be."

it turns out, helps you sidestep diabetes. In one Harvard School of Public Health study, people who munched on hot dogs, bologna, and bacon five or more times a week increased their risk for diabetes by 19 percent.

How it helps: Skipping this stuff keeps an overload of nitrite preservatives out of your body. That's a good thing, because nitrites may switch off or even destroy insulin-producing cells in your pancreas, according to researchers.

Walking and weights. Every time you hit the pavement for a Natural Menopause Solution walk, rejoice—with every step you're also battling diabetes. In a Harvard School of Public Health study of 40,000 women, those who walked briskly for 30 minutes a day and limited sitting time in the evenings (they watched TV for 10 or fewer hours a week) were 43 percent less likely to develop diabetes than women who walked less and sat more.

How it works: Exercise packs a four-way punch against diabetes: It helps you lose weight, shrinks abdominal fat, makes your muscles sip more blood sugar around the clock, and makes muscle fibers more sensitive to insulin.

ANOTHER IMPORTANT STRATEGY

Supercharge your diabetes-prevention efforts with this additional strategy.

Take mini breaks. Could getting up from your office chair for a drink of water or walking around the living room during TV commercials lower your risk for diabetes? You bet. Getting up for as little as a minute a few times a day (more is better) could help keep your blood sugar 18 percent lower, trim an inch from your waistline, and help you stay slimmer, report Australian researchers who compared the health and break times of 168 women and men in a 2008 study in the journal *Diabetes Care.*

Why it helps: Sitting for hours at a time shuts off a key enzyme in your muscles called lipoprotein lipase, which helps control your blood sugar and promotes fat-burning, say researchers at the University of Missouri–Columbia. This shutdown happens after an hour or two of sitting, even in people who exercise regularly. Mini breaks rev it up again.

What you should know: Just a minute or two of movement every hour is all it takes, the Australian researchers say. At work, try standing when you're talking on the phone, taking a 1-minute stroll down the hallway, or even marching in place a few times an hour. At home, use TV commercial breaks to do quick chores, exercise, or walk around. Better yet, do something else entirely: In one study, people who cut their TV time in half (from 5 to $2\frac{1}{2}$ hours a day) burned an extra 800 calories a week doing everyday stuff like playing board games, knitting, playing the piano, and having fun with the family.

Chapter 15

Prevent Cancer

When it comes to stopping the second-biggest killer of midlife women, we bet you know the drill by heart—put annual mammograms and pelvic exams on your don't-miss list, do breast self-exams, slather on sunscreen, and sign up for a colonoscopy once you've celebrated your 50th birthday. Smart steps like these are a big reason that cancer deaths among women have fallen a whopping 14 percent since 1990, according to the American Cancer Society.

As more women get on board, more lives are being saved. But thanks to conflicting headlines about cancer prevention that so often lead the nightly TV news, a sneaky new cancer risk—confusion—may be silently *boosting* your odds of getting one of the cancers that affect women most often. (In order, these are breast cancer, lung cancer, colorectal cancer, and gynecologic cancers—of the cervix, ovaries, uterus, and vagina.)

These days, one in three women say they're confused about how often to have mammograms. Half of all women in their forties and nearly 40 percent over age 50 avoid this essential breast check (leading to 20,000 unnecessary deaths per decade). One in nine skip Pap tests for cervical cancer. Many more are uncertain about whether they need annual pelvic checks. Plenty of us don't get needed skin cancer exams. And we postpone colon cancer screenings even though they can outright prevent the third-leading cancer in women from ever taking hold in your body.

One in three of us don't know that cancer risk rises with age (a 70-year-old woman's risk is 13 times higher than it was when she was 39). At the same time, we're not taking lifestyle steps that bolster protection: More than half of us don't know that extra pounds; too little exercise; and too much alcohol, red meat, and processed meats raise cancer risk, according to a recent national survey conducted by the nonprofit American Institute for Cancer Research. And even though you've probably heard that fruits, vegetables, and whole grains may reduce colon cancer risk, fewer than one in three of us get enough of these goodies daily. Confusion about cancer prevention may explain why one in two women think nothing can be done to head off this killer, the same survey found.

"We can't control our age, but we can control our cancer risk," notes AICR dietitian Alice Bender, RD, MS. "That's what more and more research is showing, and that's what people of all ages need to understand. Evidence from the lab and the clinic suggests that these Americans can significantly lower their risk. 'It's never too late' is good news for Americans worried about their cancer risk. We should take that to heart and feel empowered by it."

In other words, the last thing you should do is throw up your hands in frustration and scream, "Forget it!" Don't wait until questions about the perfect way to prevent cancer stop swirling. And don't give in to feeling powerless. Because you're not. While researchers hammer out the fine print, your best bet is to forge ahead with steps proven to discourage the development and growth of cancer and to maximize early detection (which leads to better treatment and survival). This is especially true for some of the most common and most feared cancers women face at midlife and beyond.

In this chapter we've gathered the latest evidence and the best expert advice—cutting through conflicting research and advice about tests, early-warning symptoms, lifestyle-based prevention strategies, and drugs and supplements that may lower risk. Your next move? Make these steps a part of your life, confident that you're doing all you can to stop cancer in its tracks.

MIDLIFE, MENOPAUSE, AND CANCER RISK

Menopause itself doesn't increase your risk for cancer. But many of the risk factors for common cancers *are* related to menopause. You've probably heard that women who take hormone replacement therapy (estrogen plus progestin) for more than 4 years face a higher risk for breast cancer. And if you have dense breasts, which make detecting problems on a mammogram more difficult, HRT could quadruple your breast cancer risk, report researchers at the University of California, San Francisco, who reviewed 1.3 million mammograms for a 2011 study.

Here are a few other factors that increase your odds of getting cancer.

Your age. Most cancers take years or even decades to develop and to grow to a detectable size. That's why your risk for cancers of the breast, colon, and ovaries, for example, increases with the number of candles on your birthday cake—and why many screening tests for cancer are recommended for women starting in their forties and fifties.

For instance, 70 percent of breast cancer cases are diagnosed in women over age 50, and half in women age 65 or older. (Of course, you should stay alert to symptoms no matter what your age and talk to your doctor about earlier screening if you have a family history of certain cancers or other risk factors we'll talk about later in this chapter.)

Your waist size and weight. As you've learned from earlier chapters (and probably from your own experience!), a woman's weight and waist size tend to creep upward at midlife thanks in part to menopause-related hormone shifts, age-related loss of calorie-burning muscle mass, rising levels of stress due to a busy life, and habits that leave us sitting (and eating) more and moving less. For example, a big weight gain before menopause (35 to 50 pounds or more from your twenties through your fifties) could double your risk for breast cancer, according to a National Cancer Institute study that's tracking 72,000 midlife women. Being overweight or obese at midlife doubled the risk for cancers of the uterus (endometrium) and the esophagus, according to the United Kingdom's landmark Million Woman Study. Extra weight also raised odds for leukemia, multiple myeloma, and non-Hodgkin's lymphoma, as well as cancers of the kidneys and the pancreas. And it can double the lung cancer risk in nonsmokers and former smokers.

The cancer-weight link seems to be deep abdominal fat—and, indeed, a wide waistline has been shown to increase risk. In a Harvard School of Public Health study of 47,382 women, postmenopausal women with waists measuring 36 inches or more were 83 percent more likely to develop breast cancer, as compared with those with smaller midsections. Excess abdominal fat alters body chemistry in ways that keep more cancer-fueling estradiol (a form of estrogen) in circulation, the researchers say. It also boosts levels of insulin, which encourages the growth of cancer cells, say researchers from the University of North Carolina at Chapel Hill in a study of weight and cancer risk published in the *American Journal of Epidemiology*.

Your activity level. Staying active—with daily walks, strength training, and plenty of everyday activity like gardening, playing with your kids or grandchildren, dancing, walking your dog, playing tennis, or following your bliss in other ways that involve movement—could reduce your breast cancer risk by 29 percent, according to American Cancer Society researchers in a study of more than 72,000 women that was published in the journal *Cancer Causes and Control*. In other research, American and Italian scientists estimate that boosting activity levels could prevent 14 percent of colon cancers and 22 percent of uterine cancers. Yet 60 percent of us aren't getting enough activity, and one in four isn't getting any at all, according to the Centers for Disease Control and Prevention. Yes, inactivity levels rise at midlife and beyond—in part because we're busy juggling family, work, and community commitments and in part because loss of precious muscle mass begins to take a subtle toll by making everyday activity and exercise just a little bit more of an effort (a great reason to try the Natural Menopause Solution yoga-with-weights routine to rebuild and hold on to muscle)!

These aren't the only factors that raise cancer odds, of course. Other important, non-menopause-related risks include:

Your family history. Cancer in first-degree relatives could double your risk for melanoma and quadruple your odds for colon cancer. If you're a carrier of the breast cancer genes BRCA1 or BRCA2, your odds for breast and ovarian cancer may be two to seven times higher than average. Talk to your doctor about genetic testing for these if you have two first-degree relatives (mom, sister, daughter) diagnosed with breast cancer before age 50; or three first- or second-degree (grandmothers, aunts) diagnosed at any age with breast cancer or other breast or ovarian cancer patterns in your family or if you're of Ashkenazi Jewish descent and have even one first-degree relative with breast or ovarian cancer.

Smoking. Heard that smoking doesn't affect a woman's breast cancer risk? Turns out that's wrong. In 2011, West Virginia University researchers who checked the health histories of 76,628 women found that in women who were at a normal weight or somewhat overweight, smoking increased the breast cancer risk by 16 to 62 percent (the more you smoke and the more years you smoke, the higher your risk). Cigarettes also increase the risk for cancers of the lungs, esophagus, larynx (voice box), mouth, throat, kidneys, bladder, pancreas, stomach, and cervix, as well as for acute myeloid leukemia.

Alcohol. While one drink a day can lower a woman's risk for heart disease, even one glass of wine, one beer, or one cocktail a day may be responsible for 13 percent of all cancers of the breasts, liver, and digestive system in women, say researchers from Britain's University of Oxford, who traced the diets and the cancer histories of volunteers in the landmark Million Women Study. But according to the American Cancer Society, one drink raises most women's risk just slightly, while three to five drinks daily boost it by 50 percent.

A diet low in produce and whole grains and high in red meat, processed meats, saturated fat, and salt. Your diet can help protect you from—or raise your risk for—cancers of the breasts, colon, esophagus, stomach, and more. Smart choices lower your risk in many different ways, says an expert panel put together by the American Institute for Cancer Research to look at links between diet and cancer. For example, eating plenty of fiber-rich fruit, vegetables, and whole grains will probably lower your risk for cancers of the colon and esophagus. Avoiding big portions of animal fats (like butter, cheese, and fatty meats) can help reduce breast cancer risk. And foods packed with DNA-protecting antioxidants seem to lower the risk for cancers of the mouth, esophagus, lungs, stomach, and pancreas. Excess sodium boosts stomach cancer risk, too. Yet just 13 percent of women eat even the minimum amount of fruit (about 1½ cups) daily, and only 19 percent munch the minimum amount of veggies (about 2 cups) recommended by the US government for good health, according to the latest national survey of America's eating habits.

CANCER TESTS

Here's what you need to know about the best ways to quickly spot—and protect yourself from—the cancers most common to midlife women.

Mammogram. Despite all the pink-ribbon attention breast cancer gets (and we're all for raising awareness as well as funding more research!), a woman's lifetime risk of getting breast cancer now stands at one in seven. Your best defense? Catch this all-too-common cancer early, and your chances for survival are 100 percent. Ask about a digital mammogram—which, like a conventional mammogram, uses x-ray images but on a computer, so they can be checked more closely—if you are under age 50, haven't reached menopause, or have dense breasts. Extra glandular tissue makes dense breasts more cancer prone and makes detection more difficult.

How often should you be tested? The American Cancer Society recommends annual mammograms for women beginning at age 40, while the

US Preventive Services Task Force's new guidelines say that women at average risk should have a mammogram every 2 years between the ages of 50 and 74. Talk to your doctor about what's best for you, taking into account your breast cancer risk, such as having a family history of breast and/or ovarian cancer. For example, if a parent or a sibling had breast cancer, you should start getting mammograms at an age that's 10 years younger than the age of the youngest family member when she was diagnosed (but not before you're 25 in most cases and not later than 40). Ask about magnetic resonance imaging (MRI) checks, which are more expensive than mammograms and invasive (a dye is injected into your body) but have the best track record for detecting tiny, early cancers and precancers. If you've had breast cancer or a precancer, your doctor will tell you how often to have a mammogram.

If your mammogram reveals anything unusual, an ultrasound (which uses sound waves to detect problems) may be the next step. Meanwhile, don't rely on thermography (which uses temperature differences to spot potential issues) to screen for breast cancer. Experts say it's not as effective as a mammogram, but it may help doctors get more information once a lump or tumor has been discovered.

For best results: When you make your appointment, find out if the mammogram center has a record of your previous mammograms; if not, call the centers where you've had the test done in the past and ask to have the results sent in time for your upcoming exam. Comparing mammograms helps the radiologist interpret the results. Skip deodorant, talcum powder, and lotion under your arms and on your breasts on the day of your mammogram—they can look like calcium spots (a type of precancer) on the x-rays. Afterward, call your doctor's office or the test center for the results; while most mammograms find no problems at all, don't assume that silence means that everything's normal. Too busy to make an appointment? Sign up for automatic phone/e-mail/snail mail reminders at your doctor's office—a little nudging increased the percentage of women who made it to their annual breast checks by up to 25 percent, according to a Kaiser Permanente study.

Clinical breast exam. Also called a CBE, this is a doctor's check of your breasts, and it usually happens during your annual gynecologic checkup. While a mammogram is your first-line screening check for breast cancer, an annual CBE is worth getting, just to cover all your bases.

How often should you be tested? You should have a CBE yearly, starting at age 25. If you're at a high risk for breast cancer, some experts recommend having a CBE every 3 to 6 months, beginning at an age that's 10 years younger than your youngest close relative was when she was diagnosed with breast cancer. If you've had breast cancer or a precancer, follow your doctor's recommendation for when to get a CBE.

For best results: Ask your doctor to show you how to perform a breast self-exam during or right after your CBE.

Breast self-exam. Once considered a cornerstone of breast cancer detection, breast self-exams (BSEs) may not add much extra protection if you're getting regular mammograms and CBEs. But we've all heard stories of women who found their own breast cancers, so it makes sense to get in the habit of doing self-exams so that you can spot or feel any changes quickly and take action.

How often should you do one? A monthly BSE is a great idea if you feel motivated to do one; something less formal—checking your breasts every once in a while when you take a shower or get dressed—is okay, too. Most changes aren't cancer, but be sure to contact your doctor if you notice new swelling; a lump, skin irritation, or dimpling; nipple pain or a nipple that's turned inward; redness or scaliness of the nipple or breast skin; or a discharge other than breast milk, according to the American Cancer Society.

For best results: Regular checks are optional but give you one big advantage: You'll know the difference between normal, no-worries bumpiness and something new.

Pap test. Since its introduction in the 1940s, this important cancer check has reduced deaths from cervical cancer by more than 70 percent in the United States; but 10,000 women still develop cervical cancer each year, and 3,600 die. Cervical cancer is caused by 15 different strains of the human papillomavirus; it can take decades for an infection to grow and disrupt cells in ways that lead to cancer. That's why the average age for a cervical cancer diagnosis is 50—which means women around menopause still need this critical exam.

For the test, a tiny sample of cells is taken from the surface of your cervix (the lower end of your uterus) and examined for signs of abnormal cells that are precancerous or cancerous. It can also spot infections and inflammation that might need treatment.

How often should you be tested? Guidelines from the American College of Obstetricians and Gynecologists recommend that women begin Pap test screening at age 21, be screened every 2 years through age 30, and then be screened every 3 years as long as their last three test results have been normal. You may need more frequent checks if you have a history of precancer or cervical cancer, are HIV-positive, or were exposed to the drug DES before you were born.

For best results: Ask your doctor if you also need an HPV test, which checks the same cell sample used for the Pap test for the presence of most of the high-risk HPV strains that raise cancer risk. While most HPV infections are temporary (your body fights them off), a persistent infection with a cancer-causing HPV strain increases your risk for cell changes that can lead to cancer. An HPV test fills in important gaps: Pap tests miss 40 percent of precancers, while an HPV check can spot trouble years earlier. If the results of both tests are normal, your risk for cancer is so low that some experts say it's okay to wait 3 years before being tested again. (An HPV vaccine, which protects against most high-risk strains, is recommended for women younger than age 26, but so far it hasn't been approved for older women.)

Colon check. Colonoscopy and a handful of other colon exams can spot precancers before they burrow into the lining of your intestines—meaning that this test can actually *prevent* cancer, saving up to 11,700 American lives a year. Yet because just half of us get this important test, tens of thousands of women develop this cancer—and die needlessly—every year.

How often should you be tested? It depends on your colon cancer risk and on which test you choose. Speak with your physician to decide which test is best for your health condition and history. Here are the details.

- **Colonoscopy.** The gold standard colon check, it allows your doctor to view the entire colon with an endoscope, a flexible tube with a light and a camera attached. You'll need to do a 1-day bowel cleanse the day before the procedure so that nothing blocks the view, but the bonus is that your doctor can remove any precancerous polyps she finds (with other colon exams, the patient has to come back for a colonoscopy to remove the polyps). Most people need rechecks every 10 years if the results are normal.

- **Virtual colonoscopy.** No invasive endoscope needed; a virtual colonoscopy uses a computed tomography scanner to take 3-D images of your colon from the outside. If all's well, you'll need a repeat in 5 years. Downside: You'll still need the colon cleanse and a regular colonoscopy if your doctor finds a polyp.

- **Sigmoidoscopy.** This procedure checks just the lower portion of the large intestine. You'll still need bowel prep, but because this test is less extensive, you'll need a repeat in 3 to 5 years if your results are normal. Combining sigmoidoscopy with an annual fecal occult blood test (FOBT) is even better; more cancers and precancers are found this way than by either test alone.

- **Fecal occult blood test (FOBT).** This is a "wipe and toss" test that you'd take in the privacy of your own bathroom. It finds hidden blood in your stool, which can be a warning sign for polyps. You have to avoid some foods beforehand that can give false-positive readings, and the test has to be repeated annually. A newer type called a fecal immunochemical test (FIT or iFOBT) is more accurate and doesn't limit your food intake.

- **Double-contrast barium enema (DCBE).** For this procedure, your colon is filled with air and liquefied barium, then scanned via an x-ray machine. But it misses half of all precancers that a colonoscopy will find, so it has fallen out of favor.

Some people need earlier testing. For example, if you're African American, you're at higher risk for colorectal cancers and should start testing at age 45. Get a colonoscopy every 5 years starting at 40, or younger if you've had colon cancer in the past or have a first-degree relative who did. You may also need earlier testing if a parent or a sibling had a precancerous polyp (check with your doctor), or if you have a chronic inflammatory bowel disease, such as ulcerative colitis or Crohn's disease.

For best results: For colonoscopy and sigmoidoscopy, don't skimp on bowel prep. The liquid diet and laxatives aren't fun, but the last thing you want to hear is that your doc couldn't see everything—or that you'll need a second look after a better cleanse. In one recent study, researchers at Columbia University Medical Center in New York reviewed 3,047 colonoscopies and found a high rate of missed cancers and precancers in people who hadn't prepped properly.

Skin check. Even though you know your own skin well, your doctor's the expert when it comes to skin cancer. In one study of 126 people with melanoma, published in the *Archives of Dermatology* in 2009, doctors spotted more early-stage cancers than patients had and found them even sooner, when these potentially fatal cancers were smaller, had invaded less of the skin, and were easiest to treat.

How often should you be checked? Have an annual full-body skin exam if you are over age 30, have ever had a serious sunburn, have a weird-looking mole, have a family history of melanoma, or have a personal history of any skin cancer.

For best results: Embarrassed about baring all? Get over it. Feeling shy is a top reason that people skip skin checks, but not getting checked could be deadly. It's also wise to check your own skin in a full-length mirror once a month (use a handheld mirror or enlist your partner to check hard-to-see areas like your back, your head, and the back of your legs). Learn to recognize your moles, blemishes, freckles, scars, and other marks so you can notice any changes in the future. And take trouble spots to your doctor right away. These include skin growths that increase in size and look pearly, translucent, tan, brown, black, or multicolored; any mole, birthmark, beauty mark, or brown spot that has changed color, size, thickness, or texture; a mole or other mark that has an irregular border and is bigger than ¼ inch (the head of a pencil eraser); a sore or spot that itches, hurts, bleeds, scabs over, and doesn't heal within 3 weeks.

Annual pelvic exam. There's no screening test for ovarian cancer, the fifth most common cancer among women and the most deadly reproductive-system cancer. Every year about 22,000 women are diagnosed with the disease, and 15,500 die. If you are at high risk—because genetic testing shows that you have a mutation that boosts your odds for ovarian cancer such as a BRCA1 or BRCA2 mutation—talk to your doctor about getting regular checks of your ovaries with a transvaginal ultrasound, plus a blood test for CA-125, a protein that's elevated in women with ovarian cancer. Otherwise, experts say, your best catch-it-early strategy is an annual pelvic exam as well as awareness of ovarian cancer's whispered, easy-to-miss symptoms.

During a pelvic exam, your doctor checks your vagina, cervix, uterus, fallopian tubes, ovaries, and rectum. She does this by inserting one or two gloved and lubricated fingers in your vagina and using her other hand on your abdomen to feel the position, size, and shape of your ovaries and uterus. She'll also examine your vagina and cervix.

How often should you be checked? Schedule a pelvic exam every year with your gynecologist, family doctor, or internist.

For best results: Keep in mind that many women who are diagnosed with ovarian cancer report vague, hard-to-place symptoms beforehand. Often these telltale signs are misdiagnosed by family doctors and by digestive specialists and urologists as irritable bowel syndrome or a urinary tract infection—losing valuable time. Experts recommend consulting your gynecologist if you're experiencing symptoms such as a swollen or bloated abdomen; increased girth around your middle; persistent pain or pressure in your abdomen or pelvis; an inability to eat or feeling full quickly; changes in urination like a sudden urgent need to go to the bathroom or frequent urination; new problems with constipation or diarrhea; and unexplained vaginal bleeding.

Lung cancer screening. In the summer of 2011, news of an important breakthrough in lung cancer screening made headlines around the world: Catching this often-aggressive form of cancer early, with a computerized tomography scan, slashed death rates by 20 percent. That's great news, because lung cancer is the leading cause of cancer deaths among American women. The earlier this cancer can be caught, the better your chances for survival—your chances are about 50 percent if it's found before it spreads, 2 percent if it's found later.

The study, which tracked 53,000 midlife women who had been pack-a-day smokers for at least 30 years, found that helical CT scans discovered tumors that conventional x-rays had missed. The women had annual checks—something that's not yet covered by many insurance companies but that some hospitals are beginning to offer at a lower price to people at risk for lung cancer.

Does that include you? People at high risk for lung cancer include women over age 60 who currently smoke or are former smokers, those who've already had lung tumors, and those with chronic obstructive pulmonary disease (COPD)—a progressive breathing problem most often caused by smoking. If that's you, talk to your doctor about the pros and cons of lung cancer screenings with a helical or spiral CT scan or, if this isn't available in your area or isn't affordable, via sputum (sputum cytology) or a chest x-ray.

One problem with all of these tests: false-positive results—signs of trouble that turn out to be nothing when checked with a biopsy. In the new National Lung Screening Trial, one in five scans produced false-positive results. This can result in unnecessary fears and even be dangerous, because a lung biopsy is an invasive procedure that can cause a collapsed lung or infection.

How often should you be checked? That's a question to ask your doctor. Since the news that lung screenings are helpful is so recent, it's not yet clear how often they should be repeated.

For best results: Contact your doctor if you have the potential warning signs of lung cancer. These include coughing that won't go away or gets worse over time; chest pain; wheezing, hoarseness, or shortness of breath; weight loss and appetite loss; coughing up blood; an unexplained fever; and repeat bouts of pneumonia or bronchitis. Eight out of 10 cases of lung cancer are smoking related; the best way to lower your risk is to quit.

THE NATURAL MENOPAUSE SOLUTION AND CANCER PREVENTION

The healthy components and results of the Natural Menopause Solution are also important, research-proven strategies for lowering your risk for most types of cancer. Here's how the plan helps.

A healthier body weight. You'll drop extra pounds on the 30-Day Slim-Down, Cool-Down Diet. This can lower cancer risk, too. Added weight may increase your risk, thanks to the connection between abdominal fat and insulin resistance. When researchers at Harvard School of Public Health checked the health and weight of 80,000 female nurses, they found that those who had gained 55 pounds or more after age 18 had a 45 percent increase in breast cancer risk after menopause, as compared with women whose weight stayed at healthy levels through their twenties, thirties, and forties. In another study, women who had gained more than 60 pounds after age 18 tripled their risk for invasive breast cancer, compared with women who'd put on 20 pounds or less. Extra pounds also lower your odds for survival. In a recent study of 3,995 women with breast cancer, researchers at California's City of Hope National Medical Center found that overweight women were 69 percent more likely to die than women at a healthy weight.

How it helps: Higher insulin levels (as your body tries to force blood sugar into resistant cells) can spur the growth of cancer cells. And more body fat means higher levels of estrogen, which spur estrogen-sensitive breast cancer.

Movement every day. The daily walks, regular strength training, and yoga on our 30-day exercise plan will keep you in motion and reduce the risk for several types of cancer. Four hours a week of aerobic exercise (walking, taking a class at the gym, riding an exercise bike) could lower breast cancer risk by a respectable 15 to 20 percent. At the same time, you'll reduce your risk for colon cancer by 25 percent and lower your odds for lung cancer and endometrial cancer.

How it helps: Getting physical may reduce your risk by helping to control your weight and belly fat levels. It may also slow tumor development by reducing levels of estrogen, insulin, and a compound called insulin-like growth factor I (IGF-I). Exercise also boosts immunity—a strong immune system battles cancer at its earliest stages.

Plenty of produce. Our plan, with its emphasis on fresh fruits and vegetables, offers protection against many cancers, including those of the mouth, pharynx, larynx, esophagus, stomach, lungs, pancreas, and prostate. (Surprisingly, fruits and veggies may not lower your breast cancer risk directly—though by helping control your weight and belly fat, they can have an impact.)

How it helps: The vitamins and minerals in produce bolster your immune system, but that's just the beginning. Biologically active phytochemicals—beneficial compounds in fruits and vegetables—protect the DNA in your cells from the damage that kick-starts cancer. Sulforaphane, found in broccoli, cabbage, and cauliflower, whisks cancer-promoting substances out of the body. Carotenoids, found in yellow, orange, and red fruits and vegetables, also shield DNA and may even help smokers lower their lung cancer risk (though beta-carotene supplements have the opposite effect). And indole-3-carbinol—found in cruciferous veggies like kale, mustard greens, and radishes—discourages tumor growth and may even reverse early precancerous changes in cervical cells.

Whole grains every day. From whole wheat bread and quinoa to barley and oatmeal, whole grains show up in nearly every Natural Menopause Solution meal. And they're building a track record as colon cancer fighters (despite earlier reports to the contrary). The World Cancer Research Fund concluded in 2011 that the evidence that fiber protects against colon cancer is "convincing." In a National Cancer Institute study of the diets of more than 34,000 people, those who downed the most fiber were 27 percent less likely to have precancerous colon growths than those who consumed the least. Fiber from whole grains (as well as fruit) was the most protective.

How it helps: Fiber speeds the passage of food through your digestive system, preventing cancer by getting potentially harmful substances out of the way quickly. It also helps control your weight.

A cutback in saturated fat. You'll enjoy good fats instead of gobs of cheese, full-fat milk, butter, ice cream, and fatty red meats on the 30-Day Slim-Down, Cool-Down Diet. That's good news, because the saturated fat in those foods is emerging as a cancer bad guy. In the largest study ever to look at the link between dietary fat and breast cancer, researchers from the National Cancer Institute found that women whose diets included the most fat were at a 15 percent higher risk than those who ate the least. And in a Harvard School of Public

I Didn't Know That!

THE DOWNSIDE OF THAT GLASS OF WINE

A glass of wine, a cold beer, or a cocktail a day may lower heart disease risk, but it could increase a woman's risk for breast and colon cancer. One drink a day doubled women's risk for hormone-sensitive breast cancers in the landmark Women's Health Initiative study, say researchers at the Fred Hutchinson Cancer Research Center in Seattle. And in the UK's Million Women Study, just one drink a day was responsible for 13 percent of cancers of the breasts, liver, rectum, mouth, throat, and esophagus. Other studies suggest that it may also boost colon cancer risk.

Alcohol may increase cancer risk by damaging DNA. Researchers suspect that it also acts as a solvent, dissolving other harmful chemicals (like the toxins in tobacco smoke) and carrying them into cells. In addition, alcohol can raise estrogen levels and, as a result, increase breast cancer risk.

What to do? If you enjoy alcohol or want to drink to help lower your heart disease risk, stick with a glass a day at most. If you're concerned about cancer, skipping alcohol may be a wiser move.

Health study of 88,751 women, those who consumed the most saturated fat raised their colon cancer risk by 89 percent compared with those who got the least.

How it helps: Researchers aren't sure why eating animal fats may raise cancer risk; in fact, the real culprits could be the hormones found in fatty meats and full-fat milk products.

Environmental Toxins and Your Cancer Risk

From cancer-causing formaldehyde in hair-care products to cell-damaging compounds in the crunchy char on grilled meat to carcinogens in the air we breathe, dozens of compounds in the air, water, food, and personal-care products may increase your long-term risk for cancer. In 2010, the President's Cancer Panel raised new alarms, saying that scientists and lawmakers had downplayed the environmental threat. While some experts believe that about 5 percent of cancers are triggered by toxins, the panel said the real number is probably far higher.

The panel suggested taking these steps to help reduce your—and your family's—exposure.

- **Take off your shoes when you come indoors.** You'll avoid tracking in cleaning products, lawn-care chemicals, and other toxins.

- **Install water filters on the faucets in your home.** While the EPA regulates nearly 100 chemicals that could end up in drinking water, thousands more aren't, according to a 2009 *New York Times* investigation. Hundreds of these chemicals may be associated with an increased risk of cancer.

- **Use water bottles made of stainless steel** or of plastics that are free of bisphenol A (BPA) and phthalates, hormone-disrupting chemicals that can leach from the container into the water.

Fewer processed meats. You won't miss processed meats, such as hot dogs, deli meats, and sausage, on our eating plan, which is filled with more healthful protein sources. Processed and red meat are also emerging as cancer risks. Eating beef, pork, or lamb daily can raise your risk for colon cancer 2½ times higher than it is for a woman who eats these red meats less than once a month, say researchers who tracked the diets

- **Choose organic foods whenever possible**, and wash all produce before eating to remove any pesticide residue. When you can, choose meats, poultry, eggs, and milk products from farm animals that were raised without antibiotics and growth hormones. Can't buy all organic? One great strategy is to focus your organic budget on pesticide-free versions of the "dirty dozen"—fruits and vegetables that the watchdog Environmental Working Group has found have the highest levels of pesticides. In 2011, these were peaches, apples, sweet bell peppers, celery, nectarines, strawberries, cherries, pears, imported grapes, spinach, lettuce, and potatoes. (Find up-to-date lists at www.ewg.org.) These nonorganic foods, the group says, are consistently clean (low to no detectable pesticide residues): onions, avocados, sweet corn, pineapples, mangoes, asparagus, sweet peas, kiwifruit, bananas, cabbage, broccoli, and papaya.

- **Buy soaps, shampoos, cosmetics, and household cleaning products carefully.** Check the National Institutes of Health's Household Products Database (www.householdproducts.nlm.nih.gov/index.htm) and the Environmental Working Group's Skin Deep Cosmetics Database at www.ewg.org/skindeep/ to help you find less toxic alternatives.

- **Reduce your radiation exposure.** Use a hands-free headset with cell phones, and discuss imaging tests with your doctor to be sure that they're medically necessary. Also, check radon levels in your home; this colorless, odorless gas that seeps in from some types of rocks can increase lung cancer risk.

and health histories of 88,751 midlife women. In a British study of more than 35,000 women, those who ate the most processed meat saw their breast cancer risk rise 64 percent higher than it was for those who skipped it, while eating red meat several times a week raised the risk by about 20 percent.

How it helps: Red meats may raise cancer risk because they contain more saturated fat. Processed meats may increase the odds due to high levels of sodium or preservatives.

OTHER IMPORTANT STRATEGIES

Adopting these additional strategies can help you keep your risk for cancer as low as possible.

Kick the habit. Want to reduce your odds for at least eight types of cancer with one healthy move? Quit smoking today. Smoking cigarettes increases your risks for cancers of the breasts, lungs, esophagus, cervix, throat, kidneys, bladder, and pancreas, according to the National Cancer Institute. The risk may be higher for some people, depending on genetics. In an Emory University review of 50 studies, researchers found that smokers who'd inherited a gene that slowed down the way their bodies neutralized the toxins in cigarette smoke had a risk for breast cancer that was 2.4 times higher than for those whose bodies neutralized the toxins quickly.

How it helps: Quitting stops your exposure to more than 7,000 noxious chemicals in tobacco smoke, including 68 known carcinogens such as arsenic, benzene, and vinyl chloride.

What you should know: Steer clear of secondhand smoke, too. In one review, researchers from the California Air Resources Board found that exposure to secondhand smoke raised breast cancer risk by up to 90 percent. Thirdhand smoke—exposure to nicotine and other tobacco-smoke residue on indoor surfaces and even on a family member's or a friend's clothing—may also raise risk. Since this residue clings to furniture, drapes, carpets, and walls (it doesn't leave if you air out a room after a smoker's been puffing away), your best protection is to keep your home (your car, too!) smoke free.

Consider chemoprevention. If you're at high risk for breast cancer or have been diagnosed with breast cancer recently and finished treatment, your doctor has probably mentioned medications that could reduce your odds for a recurrence or for a new cancer.

In one landmark study, women at high risk who took tamoxifen cut their odds for developing breast cancer over the next 7 years by 42 percent. And when researchers funded by the National Institutes of Health followed thousands of women who'd been treated for estrogen receptor–positive breast cancer, just 10 percent of those who took Herceptin (trastuzumab) plus tamoxifen saw the cancer spread after 4 years, compared with 26 percent who received tamoxifen alone. After just 2 years, Herceptin cut the risk of cancer deaths by 33 percent.

How it works: These drugs lower the cancer risk by blocking the effects of estrogen on breast tissue.

What you should know: Chemoprevention does have side effects. Tamoxifen raises the risk for endometrial cancer and blood clots; and Herceptin increases your risk for congestive heart failure. If you're not yet menopausal, taking these drugs could send your body into premature menopause.

Chapter 16

Build Strong Bones

*I*magine being tiny enough to walk around inside your own bones. You might think you were visiting the most beautiful, intricate—and busy—cave on earth. You'd scramble through tunnels with lacelike, crystalline walls, stroll through soaring archways, and watch construction crews constantly tear apart sections of bone and then rebuild them (kind of like an endless highway improvement project).

If your fantastic voyage coincided with the hormonal shifts of menopause, you'd also spot trouble brewing. Now, wrecking crews are working faster and faster while the bone-building brigade slows down. As a result, your skeleton's strong, flexible architecture grows weaker as your bones' internal supports grow thinner and more sparse. From the outside, you'd never feel a thing. But your risk for a life-altering fracture is rising fast. Small wonder that half of all women over age 50 will have a bone fracture in their lifetime.

It's a sobering prospect. Bone fractures later in life can lead to chronic pain, loss of mobility, and even early death. The solution, however, isn't simply promising to take more calcium after menopause. New research shows that smarter timing = stronger bones. Taking bone health seriously *during* perimenopause may be more crucial than experts ever realized for maintaining strong bones in the years to come. And a string of recent studies is revealing the best way to do just that—with an optimal combination of food, supplements, and physical activity.

If you're not taking steps to baby your bones now, if you haven't updated your bone-health strategy in a few years, or if recent headlines questioning the value of calcium have led you to toss this important supplement in the trash (or leave it on the kitchen shelf), keep reading. What you learn could save your life.

BEYOND ESTROGEN: NEWS ABOUT HORMONES AND HEALTHY BONES

Conventional wisdom says it's smart to get extra serious about bone density *at* menopause. That's when bone density drops like crazy. Women build bone into their thirties, then start losing it in their forties. But when estrogen levels fall sharply at menopause, bone loss doubles or triples for the next 5 to 6 years, especially in the most fracture-prone sections of your spine. The fallout: You could lose 15 percent of your bone mass in the first 5 years of menopause alone. After that, losses occur at a slower rate; by age 80, you could lose 40 percent of your peak bone mass. By age 59, 4 percent of women have osteoporosis—seriously weakened bones that are at risk for fracture—and seven times that number have troubling signs of dangerous bone thinning, called osteopenia, according to a 2010 study published in the *Journal of Bone and Mineral Research*, by researchers from the Centers for Disease Control and Prevention. By age 80, 52 percent of women will have osteoporosis. After your 50th birthday, bone loss means that your risk for a fracture doubles every 7 to 8 years—unless you do something about it.

The risk is highest for Caucasian and Asian women and lowest for African American and Latino women, but nobody's skeleton is made of steel. A bone fracture is a life-altering event that brings disability and often a loss of precious independence. It can also kill you: Breaking your hip increases your risk of dying within 4 years sixfold, and breaking one or more of the vertebrae in your spine boosts the risk of dying eightfold, according to the North American Menopause Society.

But in the past few years, researchers have turned their attention to the bone weakening that begins years before a woman's last period. It turns out that bone loss accelerates a few years before menopause, even before your estrogen levels drop. That means that something else is at work on midlife bones; and so far, scientists think the prime suspect may be inhibin, another hormone produced by your ovaries. Normally, inhibin helps bones by balancing the work of osteoclasts (bone cells that dissolve bone) and osteoblasts (bone cells that rebuild bone). When levels fall, the bone dissolvers take center stage.

That's powerful motivation to bolster your bone health today. But the truth is that, wherever you are in your menopause journey, it's the right time to do all you can to baby your bones. There's even evidence that avoiding osteoporosis could help you live 5 years longer, say Australian researchers. Yet many women find out they have brittle bones only after a bad break that leads to a hospital stay—and often the inability to remain independent in their own home. "This is a hidden disease in that the diagnosis 'osteoporosis' is rarely recorded as the main reason for a hospitalization. Most people are unaware they even have the disease until they suffer a fracture," notes researcher Wendy Max, PhD, codirector of the Institute for Health & Aging at the School of Nursing at the University of California, San Francisco. "With the aging of the baby boomers, we have to educate women about the risks of osteoporosis at early ages to prevent illness and disability at later ages."

THE CALCIUM QUESTION

In May 2011, newspapers around the world ran headlines like these: "More Calcium Doesn't Mean Stronger Bones," "US Recommendations for Calcium May Be Too High," and "Extra Calcium May Not Do Older Women Much Good." If you didn't read any further, you might think those big white calcium tablets—or that glass of milk you sip each morning—isn't doing much for you. But don't assume that means calcium is a dud. The study, from Sweden's Uppsala University, found that getting more than about 1,140 milligrams of calcium a day didn't provide extra protection against fractures. The best amount for fracture prevention? About 750 to 1,140 milligrams of calcium per day—the amount you'd get from a healthy diet containing two to three servings of dairy. Adding vitamin D boosted protection.

The truth is, most of us need more, not less, calcium than we're getting. When University of Connecticut researchers looked at the calcium intakes of 9,475 people, they found that women shortchanged themselves at every stage of life, according to a study published in the February 2011 issue of the *Journal of the American Dietetic Association.* Women in their thirties got about 730 milligrams of calcium a day, dropping to 671 milligrams for women in their forties, and to about 640 milligrams for those in their fifties and sixties. Considering that national guidelines call for 1,000 milligrams a day before age 50 and 1,200 milligrams a day after that, we're all missing the mark!

Pairing calcium with vitamin D is even better for bones. Your body can't absorb calcium without the help of vitamin D. This is more important than ever at midlife because as estrogen levels fall, so does the effectiveness of an enzyme that activates vitamin D. While the Institute of Medicine recently increased daily D recommendations to 600 IU, the National Osteoporosis Foundation says that taking 1,000 IUs of D a day is even better (and it's safe). Daily calcium (with vitamin D) could reduce your bone-fracture risk by an impressive 25 percent, researchers from Australia's University of Western Sydney reported in a study in the journal *Lancet.* Other research shows that getting calcium plus D can improve bone mineral density in your spine, thighbones (femurs), and arms.

In fact, calcium plus D may mean you won't need a bone-building prescription drug. When nutritionists at the University of Illinois at Urbana–Champaign reviewed studies looking at the success of calcium plus vitamin D for increasing bone density and preventing fractures, they found convincing evidence. The combination is so effective, says Karen Chapman-Novakofski, PhD, a professor of nutrition, that many people should consider starting there before trying bone-building bisphosphonate drugs. (Of course, this is a decision to make with your doctor.) And calcium and vitamin D are two of our Flash-Fighting Four, which is great news for your bones.

"I suspect that many doctors reach for their prescription pads because they believe it's unlikely that people will change their diets," she notes. But for many people, "prescription bone-building medicines should be a last resort. Bisphosphonates, for instance, disrupt normal bone remodeling by shutting down the osteoclasts, the cells that break down old bone to make new bone. When that happens, new bone is built on top of old bone. Yes, your bone density is higher, but the bone's not always structurally sound."

HOW ARE YOUR BONES?

Simply having 40 or more candles on your birthday cake is a potent risk factor for osteoporosis. If you have one or more of the following extra risk factors, your doctor may recommend that you get an early bone mineral density test to check the state of your skeleton. You may be at higher risk for brittle bones if you:

- Had a low trauma bone fracture as an adult, such as from a minor fall

- Are a cigarette smoker

- Have a low body weight

- Are weak and frail (for example, you can't get out of a chair by yourself)

- Have used drugs like the corticosteroid prednisone, the blood thinner heparin long term, or antiseizure drugs

- Have a digestive-system condition that interferes with the absorption of nutrients, such as Crohn's or celiac disease

- Have rheumatoid arthritis, hyperparathyroidism, kidney disease, severe liver disease, or alcoholism; even regularly having more than two drinks a day raises risk

- Don't get much calcium (from food or supplements) on a daily basis

- Don't do much weight-bearing exercise such as walking, dancing, or lifting weights

- Are or have engaged in intense exercise (such as marathon running), which reduces estrogen levels

- Have had an eating disorder, which can also reduce estrogen levels or interfere with calcium absorption

- Have spent long periods of time on bed rest, which accelerates bone loss

Experts recommend that all women get a bone density scan at age 65, though you should be screened earlier if you have any risk factors and your doctor agrees that your bones may be in peril. The gold standard bone check is called a DEXA (short for dual-emission x-ray absorptiometry) scan, which uses x-rays to measure bone density. Other bone tests, like a screening test of your heel or wrist using ultrasound (you can often find these checks for free or at low cost at health fairs), aren't as accurate but can help you and your doctor assess your bone health and your need for a DEXA. (Don't worry; the test is quick and painless, and the radiation exposure is tiny—one-tenth as much as from a chest x-ray.)

Don't get us wrong. A DEXA scan of your spine or hip isn't perfect. It can't assess all-round bone strength, 70 percent of which comes from bone density and 30 percent of which comes from the architecture of your bones—something a DEXA scan can't see. But it can help your doctor determine whether your bones are healthy or in danger. The results of a DEXA scan are usually given as a T-score, which compares your bone density to that of healthy young women. A T-score of -1 or greater is normal; -2.5 or lower is osteoporosis; and between -2.5 and -1 is considered osteopenia.

If your DEXA shows that you have low bone density, your health-care provider will also do a FRAX test. This online calculator (you can check it out yourself at www.shef.ac.uk/FRAX/) predicts your fracture risk over the next 10 years, based on bone density plus key signs of bone health that a scan simply can't see—such as your age, weight, smoking and drinking habits, family and personal history of fractures, and whether or not you use oral corticosteroids (such as for asthma or other breathing problems) or have rheumatoid arthritis. (If you have slightly low bone mass, having one or more of these risks could double or triple your fracture odds.) If your bone density score is -1 or lower, or if your FRAX score shows that your risk for a hip fracture over the next 10 years is 3 percent or higher, your doctor may suggest bone-building drugs.

If you have osteoporosis or osteopenia, it's important to work with your doctor to do all you can to safeguard your bones. Talk with her before starting an exercise program—heavy weight lifting or a too-vigorous aerobic routine could trigger a fracture. But if you have osteopenia or if your bone density is within the normal range, the Natural Menopause Solution bone-health strategy could help you hold on to more bone as you age—and even help you build new bone. Our 30-day workout routine includes upper- and lower-body exercises that are important for strengthening the bones in your arms, legs, hips, and more.

HOW THE NATURAL MENOPAUSE SOLUTION HELPS YOUR BONES

Did you know that the Natural Menopause Solution can also keep your bones strong? These components can help.

Interval walks. Weight-bearing exercise, such as brisk walking, reduced risk for a bone fracture by 41 percent in one study at Brigham and Women's Hospital in Boston. Picking up the pace of your walks just a little (as you will on the 30-Day Slim-Down, Cool-Down Diet's interval walks) could make your bones stronger, say researchers at the University of Michigan–Ann Arbor. In a study published in the journal *Bone*, postmenopausal women who increased their walking pace slightly (they walked about 2.8 miles at a pace of 16½ minutes per mile) built more bone than women who stuck with a slower pace. The study authors say the extra force stimulated better bone growth.

How it helps: With every footstep, the impact of weight-bearing exercise stimulates your bones to produce more osteoblasts—the cells that build bone. Walking is especially good at bolstering bone density in your hips and spine—two of the most common places where brittle bones shatter.

Strength training. Lean, sexy muscle isn't the only perk you'll get from our plan's yoga-with-weights routine. Strength training also keeps your bones strong. In an Italian study published in the *Journal of Aging and Health*, women who strength-trained three times a week for 6 months lost significantly less bone than women who didn't work out. A University of Arizona study of 140 postmenopausal women even found gains in bone density with strength training—especially in their hips, where the bones support more weight than anywhere else in the body.

How it helps: When you do strength-training exercises, you work your muscles as well as the tendons that connect muscles and bones. As tendons tug on bone, they stimulate bone growth.

Calcium and vitamin D. Two of our Flash-Fighting Four are also bone-friendly essentials. Getting your calcium from a mix of foods and supplements is a proven winner—women who did this had stronger bones than those who relied on supplements or on food alone, according to a Washington University School of Medicine study that was published in the *American Journal of Clinical Nutrition*. But calcium alone won't cut it. According to Harvard Medical School experts, vitamin D may "be the most important variable in preventing osteoporosis." In a Harvard School of Public Health study of 77,337 postmenopausal women, published in the *American Journal of Clinical Nutrition*, those who got just 500 IU of vitamin D a day were 37 percent less likely to have broken a hip than women who got 140 IU. In the Swedish study mentioned earlier in this chapter,

Can Yoga Build Bone?

Maybe. Yoga experts say poses that strengthen areas most likely to fracture—your hips, spine, and wrists—could help you maintain bone density. In a pilot study conducted by physical therapists in New York City, people who performed a 10-minute yoga routine daily saw significant improvement in bone density at the hips and spine. Poses that can help these areas—and that you'll find in our Natural Menopause Solution yoga routine—include Chair Pose, Hero Pose, and Warrior Pose.

women who got calcium plus D had lower fracture risk than those who got the same amount of calcium alone.

How they help: Calcium is an important building block for the scaffolding that keeps your skeleton strong. You need D on board in order for calcium from food and supplements to be absorbed into your bloodstream. In your bones, you need D for healthy bone "remodeling"—it activates osteoclasts, which dissolve bone, and helps bone-building osteoblasts mature.

Nutrient-rich produce and whole grains. Add yet another talent to the many that fruits, vegetables, and whole grains boast. These healthy foods lower your fracture risk, too. In a McGill University study of 3,539 postmenopausal women, researchers found that fracture risk fell by 14 percent for those who ate 40 percent more of these healthy foods and 28 percent for those who ate 80 percent more, compared with those who ate the least. And in a Tufts University study of 1,164 women and men, researchers found that more produce meant higher bone density.

How they help: Grains, leafy greens, and other produce deliver nutrients that help calcium and D work even better—including magnesium, potassium, and vitamin K. Vitamin K, found in green leafy vegetables like lettuce, is crucial for bone mineralization—the process that adds calcium phosphate crystals to make bones strong and hard. Potassium (found in produce like bananas, tomatoes, oranges, apples, broccoli, and cantaloupe) protects your bones by helping your body hold on to more calcium. And magnesium (one of our Flash-Fighting Four, found in whole grains, bananas, spinach, beans, and lentils) plays a role in keeping bones strong yet flexible.

SKIP THESE BONE ROBBERS

Following the 30-Day Slim-Down, Cool-Down Diet is the best foundation for building and strengthening your bones. But be careful not to sabotage your efforts. Take steps to rid your life of the following common, bone-harming stuff:

Cola—regular or diet. In a 2006 Tufts University study of 1,413 women, those who drank diet or regular cola three or more times a week for 5 years had bone density that was 3.7 to 5.4 percent lower than those who sipped colas once a month or less. This may be due to phosphoric acid, an ingredient unique to colas. As your body breaks it down, the acidity of your blood rises. Your body uses calcium and/or magnesium to neutralize it—pulling calcium from your bones if necessary.

Control it: The occasional cola is okay. One a day or several each week might be a problem, however.

Too much salt. In one study of 4,000 older women and men from Hong Kong, those with the saltiest diets had the lowest bone density. Researchers estimate that getting an extra teaspoon of salt per day leads to an extra loss of 1 percent of bone density per year. More sodium in your bloodstream leads to more calcium lost in your urine. In one University of California, San Francisco, study, women lost 33 percent more calcium and 23 percent more of a bone protein called NTX (a sign of bone loss) in their urine on a high-salt diet than on a low-salt diet.

Control it: Just 22 percent of the sodium in our diets comes from our salt shakers. The rest is found in processed and packaged foods like soups, condiments, breads, and snack foods. And many restaurant and fast-food choices are also high in sodium. Read nutrition information when grocery shopping, and choose low-sodium options (like fruit salad, fresh green salad, and menu items without sauces) to get a handle on salt.

Excess protein. In one Purdue University study of 54 postmenopausal women, those who followed a diet high in animal protein lost 1.4 percent of their bone density, while those who ate plant-based proteins like beans and tofu lost little or none. Munching lots of meat may encourage faster and more extensive bone turnover. A high-meat diet may also make your blood more acidic, which prompts your body to go looking for calcium to buffer it.

Control it: Eating protein from a variety of sources is a good idea, researchers say. And while it's okay to bump up your protein a little to boost satisfaction and hold on to muscle mass, avoid eating animal protein–heavy foods on a daily basis.

Smoking. Compared with nonsmokers, women smokers lose bone faster and reach menopause an average of 2 years sooner than nonsmokers, which means they go into the early menopausal years of rapid bone loss earlier in life, too. As a result, by age 60 your fracture risk is 17 percent higher, and by age 80 it's 71 percent higher than a nonsmoker's. We're not entirely sure why that is, but there's evidence that smokers don't absorb as much calcium from food and may have lower estrogen levels before menopause, which could lead to lower bone density.

Control it: Quit!

Too many alcoholic beverages. Alcohol increases your odds for falls and thus for fracture risk. More than one drink a day or more than seven per week boosts your risk for a hip fracture by 70 percent or more and your risk of any bone fracture by 35 percent. Two or more drinks within 6 hours raises your risk for a bone-threatening fall by 20 percent.

Control it: Stick with one drink or less per day.

BONE-BUILDING DRUGS

If the best drug-free strategies for protecting your skeleton (outlined above) aren't enough, your doctor may recommend bone-building medications. These drugs include the following:

Bisphosphonates. The most widely prescribed bone-building medication for women (and men) with or at risk for osteoporosis, these drugs include alendronate (Fosamax), ibandronate (Boniva), risedronate (Actonel), and zoledronic acid (Reclast). Studies show that bisphosphonates can reduce your risk for fracturing one or more vertebrae in your spine by 40 percent to 70 percent and can cut your chances for breaking a bone in your hips, arms, wrists, or elsewhere due to osteoporosis by 40 to 50 percent. Taking one for 2 to 6 years can increase the density of your bones by 1 to 4 percent. Bone density can improve by 5 to 10 percent if you take these drugs for 7 to 10 years. That may sound small, but consider this: Do nothing and you'll lose 1 to 2 percent of bone density every year.

How they work: Bisphosphonates slow down the natural pace of bone loss in your body by interfering with the work of bone-dissolving osteoclast cells in your skeleton. They also shorten the lives of these cells. But they don't interfere with natural bone rebuilding, so your body can "catch up" and gain bone density.

What you should know: For best absorption, take most bisphosphonates first thing in the morning, with a glass of water, then wait $\frac{1}{2}$ to 1 hour before eating or drinking anything or taking other drugs or supplements. Some delayed-release types taken once a week or once or twice per month should be taken right after breakfast (follow your doctor's directions). Common side effects include nausea, constipation or diarrhea, dry mouth, and burping.

Bisphosphonates can also be given as an injection once a year or once every 2 years—zoledronic acid (Reclast)—or four times a year—ibandronate (Boniva). You may have flulike symptoms, a fever, a headache, and muscle pain for a few days after an infusion.

You've probably heard warnings on the news about thighbone fractures and jawbone problems with bisphosphonates. These are rare side effects that happen in less than 1 percent of patients, so don't let fears make you quit these drugs on your own. Talk with your doctor right away, however, if you feel unusual bone, joint, or muscle pain or have any troubling side effects.

Experts recommend that women (and men) with osteoporosis continue taking bisphosphonates indefinitely and that people at risk for osteopenia review their treatment with their doctor regularly. Since bisphosphonates linger in bone for 5 to 10 years after you quit taking them, you may be able to stop or take a "drug holiday" after about 5 years of use without endangering your bones.

Raloxifene (Evista) is a type of drug called a selective estrogen receptor modulator (SERM), or an estrogen antagonist. Marketed as a way to get the bone-friendly benefits of estrogen without hormone replacement therapy's health risks, it can protect you from some types of fractures. In one 2-year study of 601 women with low bone density, raloxifene increased spine and hipbone density by more than 1 percent; in another, 3 years of use increased bone density by more than 2 percent and reduced the risk for spine fractures by 55 percent. However, the National Osteoporosis Foundation says that so far there's no evidence it helps prevent fractures of the hips or other bones.

How it works: SERMs work like bisphosphonates, helping increase bone density by slowing down bone loss. In addition, SERMs can reduce your risk for invasive breast cancer by about 65 percent—and for that reason this drug is sometimes prescribed for women at high risk for breast cancer.

What you should know: For bone benefits, take raloxifene every day. You shouldn't take it if you're at risk for a stroke—because you have heart disease, atrial fibrillation (out-of-rhythm heartbeats), have had a mini stroke (called a transient ischemic attack, or TIA), or have already had a stroke. Stop taking it right away, and call your doctor if you have any symptoms that might mean you have a blood clot, such as leg pain, a warm feeling in your lower leg, swelling in your hands or anywhere in your legs or feet, chest pain, shortness of breath, or sudden vision changes.

Raloxifene may also cause hot flashes, sweating, and sleep problems.

Calcitonin (Fortical and Miacalcin) is the synthetic version of a hormone made naturally by your thyroid gland that helps control the way your body uses calcium and builds bone. It isn't as effective as bisphosphonates for preventing fractures but may be a good option if you have osteoporosis, can't or choose not to use bisphosphonates or raloxifene, and are 5 years or more into menopause. Studies show that this drug can increase bone density at the spine by 3 percent. In one study of 1,255 women, those who used calcitonin nasal spray for 5 years saw the risk for spinal fractures fall by 33 percent. But it didn't seem to protect against fractures in other places. It has not been proven to protect or build bone in early-postmenopausal women.

What you should know: Calcitonin is available as a nasal spray (Miacalcin Nasal Spray, Fortical Nasal Spray) and as an injection (marketed as Miacalcin Injection). Side effects for calcitonin injections include nausea, local inflammation at the injection spot, and flushing of the face or hands. A runny nose, a sinus infection, and irritated nasal passages may occur with the nasal sprays.

Teriparatide (Forteo), a parathyroid hormone, is unique: It's the first FDA-approved osteoporosis drug that builds bone rather than simply

Should You Try Ipriflavone?

Touted in health food stores and online as the latest bone builder for women, supplements containing ipriflavone—a synthetic version of a plant estrogen found in soy—claim to slow bone loss and even to stack up new bone. How good is it? In one 2-year study of 198 postmenopausal women, those who took it with daily calcium supplements saw bone density increase by 1 percent; those who didn't had a nearly 1 percent decline. The difference seems tiny, but experts at Boston's Beth Israel Deaconess Medical Center say it could "add up to a lot of bone over time."

Most, but not all, ipriflavone studies have found a small benefit; a few did not. One reason: This compound seems to work best when taken with 1,000 milligrams of daily calcium. But it can cause side effects such as stomach pain, diarrhea, and dizziness.

The biggest caution: If you're considering taking ipriflavone, talk to your doctor about monitoring your white blood cell count. There's some evidence that ipriflavone can decrease this important part of your immune system if taken for longer than 6 months. If you have a weakened immune system, this supplement may not be right for you.

It Worked for Me!

**Deborah Schrader, 49, lost 1 pound and 7¾ inches—
and improved strength and flexibility.**

"When you're approaching your 50th birthday, losing a couple of pounds is a victory," says Deb. "It used to be that if I just focused on cutting calories, weight loss was easy. Now it's more difficult. This program gave me the jump-start I needed to lose inches!"

Two months before her 50th birthday, Deb's final weigh-in for the test panel showed that she'd shed less than a pound—but lost $1\frac{1}{2}$ inches from her waist and $1\frac{1}{2}$ inches from her hips. "I've gone down almost a full size," she says happily. "Part of the credit goes to the yoga-with-weights routine. I know that a woman's muscle mass declines with age, which slows down your metabolism unless you do something about it. You have to fight it, and now I am."

The deep-down *ahhhh* of yoga also helped her sleep by helping to relieve stress and improving her flexibility so she had less neck and shoulder pain. "Back in the old days, I could sleep through the night. Now I'm getting back to that. And my hot flashes have been minimal."

Building strength and improving flexibility were important to Deb for another reason: keeping her bones fracture free. "My mother had two falls that led to broken hips. I know that things can snowball with extra pounds and reduced muscle strength as you get older. And my own workouts in the past focused more on my abdominal muscles and core, kind of neglecting my legs. Now I'm stronger all over."

slowing bone loss. It may be a good choice for you if you've had a brittle-bone fracture, have very low bone density, or are still losing bone or having fractures despite taking other types of osteoporosis drugs. In one study of postmenopausal women who'd had a spinal fracture, teriparatide increased bone density by 8.6 percent in the spine and 3.5 percent in the hips and cut the risk for spine fractures by 65 percent and hip fractures by 53 percent.

How it works: This drug stimulates bone-building osteoblast cells, so they work harder. The result: a stronger support system inside your bones.

What you should know: To take teriparatide, you must give yourself a daily injection with a special injection pen that's loaded with the right dose of medicine. You may get muscle cramps and feel nauseated or dizzy. You can take this drug for up to 2 years.

Hormone replacement therapy (HRT). One of hormone replacement therapy's real talents is its ability to bolster women's bones after menopause. Studies show that 5 years of HRT use increases the bone density in your spine by 4.5 percent and in your hips by 3.7 percent. In the landmark Women's Health Initiative study, HRT also protected women against fractures of the spine, hips, and other spots.

How it works: By boosting estrogen levels in your body, HRT helps tip the balance of bone building and bone breakdown in a positive direction so that bone density increases.

What you should know: The protection comes with a high price. Since HRT can raise your risk for breast cancer, stroke, heart disease, and dangerous blood clots in your lungs and legs, the North American Menopause Society says that, for most women, HRT is not a great option when used solely for bone health. And taking lower-dose formulas for as short a period of time as possible for menopausal symptoms, such as hot flashes, night sweats, and sleep problems, may not offer the bone protection found in studies that used older, higher-dose formulas.

The bottom line? If you've been using HRT and you and your doctor think you're a good candidate for continuing, it may help your bones— but get a bone density scan to be certain. If you're taking a low dose for menopausal symptoms, don't assume that your bones are safe. Talk about your risk with your doctor. And if you've decided to quit HRT, ask your doctor how to continue protecting your bones. Bone density drops rapidly and fracture risk rises when you stop taking these hormones.

Part V

Putting It All Together

Chapter 17

The Natural Menopause Solution Journal

W e think you'll notice—and be thankful for—the changes you experience on the Natural Menopause Solution, whether it's the jeans that are no longer quite so snug, the first full night of blessed sleep you've had in months, or simply a sense of calm energy. But some improvements happen more gradually, so it can be motivating to write down your symptoms to track your progress over time. Plus, logging what you eat and when you exercise can keep you accountable and help you pinpoint what may trigger food cravings or hot flashes and which remedies are really working.

First, we've given you a spot to assess your current weight, health measures, and menopausal symptoms. Then, we've provided daily logs to record your meals, workouts, and symptoms. Photocopy these as many times as you need.

BEFORE YOU GET STARTED

Before you begin the Natural Menopause Solution, record your current measurements below. Seeing the changes in these numbers will help keep you motivated—and if you aren't making as much progress as you'd like, this info can cue you to modify the program to maximize your results. Take your measurements again after you've completed the 30-Day Slim-Down, Cool-Down Diet or anytime you'd like to check in.

Accurately measuring your own limbs and torso can be a challenge, so we recommend that you get a friend to help. To get the most accurate results while measuring, make sure to stand up straight, shoulders back, arms relaxed, and follow these guidelines for measuring each part of your body.

- **Chest:** Measure at the fullest point of your bust.

- **Waist:** Measure at the narrowest part of your torso (usually about 2 inches above your belly button).

- **Hips:** Measure at the fullest part, and make sure the tape measure is parallel to the floor all the way around your hips.

- **Arms and thighs:** Measure at the fullest part of each, when the limb is relaxed, with arms hanging down and feet shoulder-width apart.

TODAY'S DATE/ TIME:		**CHEST:**	
HEIGHT:		**WAIST:**	
WEIGHT:		**HIPS:**	
BODY MASS INDEX (BMI)*:		**LEFT THIGH:**	
		RIGHT THIGH:	
		LEFT BICEPS:	
		RIGHT BICEPS:	

*See chart on page 322 to find your BMI.

For the following measurements, you will need to see your doctor. Since it's a good idea to check in with him or her before you start any diet or fitness program anyway, now's a good time for a checkup! You may also want to make an appointment for a few weeks down the road so the two of you can review your success.

BLOOD PRESSURE:	
FASTING BLOOD GLUCOSE AND/OR A1C LEVEL:	
HDL CHOLESTEROL:	
LDL CHOLESTEROL:	
TOTAL CHOLESTEROL:	
TRIGLYCERIDES:	

Finally, fill out the following questionnaire to gauge the frequency and severity of common menopausal symptoms you may be experiencing. This quick quiz will help you see all the ways midlife hormonal shifts are affecting you. Retake it after 30 days to see which symptoms have improved. You can also use your results to pinpoint symptoms that need more help, such as the solutions in Part III.

1. I have hot flashes and/or night sweats
    ☐ Rarely or never
    ☐ Once a month
    ☐ Several times per month
    ☐ Once a week
    ☐ Several days a week
    ☐ At least once a day
    ☐ Several times a day

2. The intensity of my hot flashes and/or night sweats is usually

☐ Mild

☐ Moderate

☐ Intense

3. My hot flashes and/or night sweats bother me

☐ Not at all

☐ A little

☐ Moderately

☐ A lot

4. I get a good, refreshing night's sleep

☐ Rarely or never

☐ Once a month

☐ Several times per month

☐ Once a week

☐ Several nights a week

☐ Every night

5. I wake up (not due to night sweats) and have trouble falling back to sleep

☐ Rarely or never

☐ Once a month

☐ Several times per month

☐ Once a week

☐ Several nights a week

☐ Every night

6. I wake up (not due to night sweats) and can't fall back to sleep
   - ☐ Rarely or never
   - ☐ Once a month
   - ☐ Several times per month
   - ☐ Once a week
   - ☐ Several nights a week
   - ☐ Every night

7. The quality of my sleep interferes with my daily life because it affects my mood, focus, and mental and physical energy
   - ☐ A little
   - ☐ Somewhat
   - ☐ A lot

8. I have food cravings that aren't related to hunger
   - ☐ Rarely or never
   - ☐ Once a month
   - ☐ Several times per month
   - ☐ Once a week
   - ☐ Several days a week
   - ☐ Every day

9. My food cravings are
   - ☐ Mild
   - ☐ Moderate
   - ☐ Intense

10. In the past month, my mood has generally been
    - ☐ Almost always unhappy
    - ☐ More often unhappy than happy
    - ☐ More often happy than unhappy
    - ☐ Almost always happy

11. In the past month, I have been

☐ Almost always stressed

☐ More often stressed than calm and relaxed

☐ More often calm and relaxed than stressed

☐ Almost always calm and relaxed

12. In the past month, I have been

☐ Almost always fatigued

☐ More often fatigued than energetic

☐ More often energetic than fatigued

☐ Almost always energetic

13. In the past month, I would

☐ Almost always forget things (words, names, where I put the car keys, etc.)

☐ Forget things more often than in the past

☐ Sometimes forget things

☐ Rarely or never forget things

14. My interest in sex during the past month has been

☐ Lower than usual

☐ About the same as ever

☐ Strong

15. Other menopausal symptoms that I've noticed in the past month:

_____

_____

_____

_____

My Natural Menopause Solution Food Log

DATE:

MEAL TYPE/ TIME	FOOD EATEN (INDICATE FOODS AND QUANTITIES)
BREAKFAST (GOAL: 350 calories)	
LUNCH (GOAL: 450 calories)	
DINNER (GOAL: 450 calories)	
SNACK OR DESSERT (GOAL: 250 calories)	

MY DAILY DOSE: The Flash-Fighting Four

☐ Lean Protein   ☐ Calcium   ☐ Vitamin D   ☐ Magnesium

THOUGHTS/OBSERVATIONS/CHALLENGES:_____

_____

_____

_____

_____

My Natural Menopause Solution *Workout Log*

DATE:

TYPE OF WALK	# MINUTES	YOGA ROUTINE	WEIGHT USED	MUSCLE MOVES OR MODIFICATIONS

THOUGHTS/OBSERVATIONS/CHALLENGES:_____

_____

_____

_____

_____

_____

_____

My Natural Menopause Solution *Symptoms Log*

DATE:

1. How many hot flashes and/or night sweats have I had in the past 24 hours? ____

2. How severe were they?

   ☐ Mild

   ☐ Moderate

   ☐ Intense

3. How much did my hot flashes and/or night sweats bother me in the past 24 hours?

   ☐ Not at all

   ☐ A little

   ☐ Moderately

   ☐ A lot

4. I had a good night's sleep last night. ☐ Yes ☐ No

5. I woke up (not due to night sweats) and had trouble falling back to sleep. ☐ Yes ☐ No

6. I woke up (not due to night sweats) and couldn't fall back to sleep at all. ☐ Yes ☐ No

7. How was my mood in the past 24 hours?

   ☐ Mostly unhappy

   ☐ On an even keel

   ☐ Mostly happy

8. How was my stress level in the past 24 hours?

☐ Low

☐ Normal

☐ High

9. How was my energy in the past 24 hours?

☐ Low

☐ Normal

☐ High

10. Have I had trouble remembering things in the past 24 hours?

☐ Lots of trouble

☐ Some trouble

☐ No trouble

THOUGHTS/OBSERVATIONS/CHALLENGES:_____

_____

_____

_____

_____

_____

Chapter 18

If You Need More Help

Y ou remember reading about HRT back in Chapter 2. Interestingly enough, in the 10 years since those negative study results began trickling out, the pendulum has swung slightly in the other direction. And while we aren't using hormones in the same way we did before the Women's Health Initiative (WHI), women *are* still requesting them and doctors *are* still prescribing them.

That's because later analyses of the WHI revealed that most of the negative outcomes occurred only in older women, not in younger post-menopausal women (ages 50 to 59). Hormone therapy even seemed to provide some cardiovascular protection in younger women, particularly estrogen-only therapy, possibly because these women were less likely to have any heart problems to begin with.

We also recognized that hormone therapy should be individualized for each woman, something the WHI never did. For instance, a 115-pound woman experiencing severe hot flashes may need a different dose and preparation than a 175-pound woman whose major problems are low libido and insomnia. "In my mind, I think that we have finally come to a point of reason or moderation, and a focus on greater individuality when it comes to hormone therapy," says Melinda Ring, MD, the medical advisor for *The Natural Menopause Solution*. "We are in a much better place than we were a decade ago."

What does this mean for you? If you find that the natural relief in this book doesn't alleviate all your menopause-related difficulties, you may want to talk to your doctor about hormones. Today, rather than recommending hormone therapy for pretty much any woman, major medical organizations like the North American Menopause Society and the Endocrine Society agree that hormone therapy for women in their fifties, and for fewer than 10 years after menopause, can provide significant benefits if women can't find relief in other ways. However, those who are more than 10 years past menopause should not start on hormone therapy, given what we know about the risks.

"There is a tipping point where the risks start to outweigh the benefits," Dr. Ring says. "The [risks] are not insignificant things. I think there are a lot of benefits [to supplemental hormone therapy], and as long as we stay in the safe age range for women, their overall quality of life, as well as important long-term factors such as cardiac and diabetes risks, will be improved by using it just around the time of menopause."

BIOIDENTICAL VERSUS SYNTHETIC HORMONES

Although we don't know exactly why the WHI showed the cardiovascular risks it did, researchers have their theories. One is that the synthetic estrogen and progestin used in Prempro and Premarin played a role. For instance, there is some evidence that the conjugated equine estrogen used in the WHI and many other studies of hormone therapy binds to cellular receptors that promote breast cell division, while the

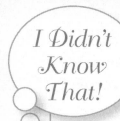

THE *GOOD* NEWS ABOUT THE WHI

If you find that you need to take hormone therapy, you don't have to completely freak out about it. In fact, what often gets lost in the rhetoric about the risks of this therapy are some of its benefits. In fact, the Women's Health Initiative (WHI) found the following:

Breast cancer. A study published in a 2011 issue of the *Journal of the American Medical Association* reported that women in the estrogen-only arm who took the hormone for an average of 7 years reduced their risk of breast cancer by 21 percent. In addition, a study published in the *New England Journal of Medicine* showed that the risk of breast cancer associated with combination hormone therapy dropped significantly once the women stopped taking the hormones and returned to premenopausal risk levels within 5 years.

Colon cancer. Women taking Prempro reduced their risk of colon cancer by 37 percent. That means that in 10,000 women, 6 fewer women would develop the disease.

Heart disease. Women in the estrogen-only arm of the study had lower coronary artery calcium, a marker of heart disease risk, than women who didn't take the drugs. They also had no increased risk of heart disease compared with women not taking estrogen therapy.

Osteoporosis. Women taking Prempro reduced their risk of hip fractures 33 percent. So out of 10,000 women taking the drug, 10 would have a hip fracture compared with 15 in 10,000 women who were not taking the drug. On the estrogen-only side (Premarin), 6 fewer women would have a hip fracture each year.

This is not an insignificant benefit, says Dr. Ring, given recent concerns about the most common antiosteoporosis drugs—bisphosphonates, like Fosamax (alendronate) and Actonel (risedronate)—that may cause strange fractures when taken for long periods of time. If women can put off using those drugs for 5 or 10 years because they are taking estrogen therapy, they may reduce their risk of the fractures.

bioidentical hormone estradiol, which links to cell receptors that prevent breast cells from dividing, may actually prevent breast cancer development.

That's why more women—and doctors—are turning to bioidenticals, hormones that are, quite literally, identical to the hormones your body makes. They are usually derived from yeast, bacteria, or animal cells in which the DNA for the hormone has been inserted. Basically, the cells are turned into little hormone factories.

Ever since actress Suzanne Somers published a book promising that compounded estrogen and progesterone would restore a woman's youth with fewer health risks than the FDA approved forms of the hormones, bioidentical hormones have been the hot thing. The reality is that the term *bioidentical* refers to the three types of estrogen produced in your body (E1 estrone, E2 estradiol, and E3 estriol) as well as one type of progestin called progesterone. Estradiol is the estrogen found in abundance when a woman is in her reproductive years and that plummets during perimenopause. While combinations of all three types of estrogens can be ordered through compounding pharmacies, estradiol is also available in medications from drug companies. Similarly, bioidentical progesterone is available either through a compounding pharmacy or through pharmaceutical companies in the drug Prometrium.

The difference is that the compounding pharmacy formulation is individualized in terms of dose and strength; it may also be mixed with other ingredients like testosterone. But because the product the pharmacist puts in your hand is not FDA approved or assessed for purity, safety, and effectiveness, it may be *less* effective and safe than those sold by drug manufacturers. That's why you should discuss your options with a doctor who is well versed in menopausal hormone therapy. Together you can decide what's right for you: a custom compounded estrogen formulation or a commercially available form. If you do use a compounded formula, make sure that it's from an experienced compounding pharmacy with strict quality control measures in place.

Overall, the evidence for bioidenticals has been increasing in recent years. For instance, four studies of women who'd switched from the synthetic progestin medroxyprogesterone acetate (MPA) to natural progesterone found that both their symptoms and their quality of life improved more when they switched, while the number of side effects dropped.

In another study, of 176 women, that compared symptom improvement in women whose therapy included MPA or progesterone, those taking progesterone had worse sleep, sexual functioning, and aches and pains than the MPA group. They also had a much higher improvement in anxiety, depression, menstrual bleeding, and cognitive difficulties (memory, information processing, etc). Overall, 65 percent of the women said the progesterone combination was better than the MPA combo.

Then there's the issue of how the hormones are supplied to your body. Systemic estrogen is metabolized through the liver, which is also where blood clotting agents are produced; perhaps the estrogen heightened their effect, making blood more likely to clot and lead to heart disease, stroke, or blood clots to the lung.

So when Dr. Ring prescribes estrogen therapy for her patients, she typically recommends an estrogen formulation that isn't cleared by the liver. That means a vaginal ring, an intravaginal tablet, or a suppository; a cream or lotion; or a patch. She also recommends that women use estradiol. There are several pharmaceutical branded products made with estradiol, but she sometimes prescribes a version produced in a compounding pharmacy. These pharmacies make customized drugs, such as mixing a testosterone gel with an estrogen cream for women who need testosterone for sexual desire problems (more on testosterone and sexual desire on page 277).

For women who need progesterone with their estrogen to protect their uterus (and help with the many other functions of progesterone in the body), Dr. Ring also prescribes bioidentical prescriptions, either the FDA-approved micronized (meaning finely ground) oral Prometrium tablets, or, if you need a dose that isn't available, a formulation prepared through a compounding pharmacy. If the woman has had a hysterectomy, she might instead use a progesterone cream or drops placed under the tongue. Several very low dose progesterone creams are available over the counter for perimenopausal women who aren't taking estrogen, though they're not strong enough to protect the uterus when used with estrogen.

Since the WHI, drug manufacturers have also introduced products with much lower doses of estrogen and progesterone, and doctors began prescribing the medication for shorter periods, just long enough to help women get through the worst of their menopausal symptoms.

TESTING HORMONE LEVELS

Wouldn't life be wonderful if you could just spit onto a glass slide and voilà! your doctor could magically tell you whether or not you are close to menopause and/or you might need supplemental hormones? No more needles!

Yeah, well. It would also be wonderful if kitchen faucets poured out dark chocolate, but that isn't going to happen. Although you can buy kits that use your saliva to test your hormone levels—something many Web sites, books, and even health professionals claim provides an accurate measurement of your blood hormone levels—the reality is that there is scant scientific evidence for their use.

In order for a test to be accepted by medical professionals, it has to be accurate. And we still don't have a saliva test that is accurate. The American College of Obstetricians and Gynecologists (ACOG), the FDA, the North American Menopause Society (NAMS), the Institute for Clinical Systems Improvement, and the American Association of Clinical Endocrinologists (AACE) all warn that the tests are not valid. Why? Hormone levels are about as steady as your emotions in midlife. Everything from diet to time of day to the type of hormone under investigation can affect the result. In fact, here's what the FDA had to say on the topic in 2010: "There is no scientific basis for using saliva testing to adjust hormone levels. Instead, practitioners should adjust hormone therapy dosages based on a patient's symptoms."

In reality, there *are* ways to get an accurate reading on your hormonal status at midlife, says Dr. Ring. But they involve those aforementioned needles to collect blood for analysis. "I only use salivary testing when I need to map hormone levels over a month," primarily in younger women who are having fertility problems or irregular periods, she says.

For menopausal women, she does what most physicians do—orders blood tests during the week after ovulation, known as the luteal phase, if a woman is still menstruating. Dr. Ring checks estradiol and progesterone levels and levels of follicle-stimulating hormone (FSH)—the hormone that triggers the growth of egg-containing follicles on the ovaries, and testosterone. She also measures both free testosterone—which is the amount available for your body to use—and total testosterone; some of the hormone is bound up with other proteins and not available for use, kind of like the money in your 401(k).

She also checks the ratio of estrogen metabolites (known as the 2/16 hydroxyestrone ratio). A low ratio is associated with an increased risk of estrogen-dependent diseases, such as breast cancer, although low rates don't mean a woman has or will get breast cancer. That ratio can also be increased through many of the lifestyle recommendations you find throughout *The Natural Menopause Solution* such as exercise and a healthy diet, including increased consumption of healthy fats like those found in flaxseed oil, nuts, olive oil, and salmon and of cruciferous vegetables such as broccoli, cauliflower, Brussels sprouts, and kale (which all contain the phytochemical indole-3 carbinol).

Dr. Ring also checks levels of DHEA-sulfate and pregnenolone, hormones important in the production of *other* hormones, like estrogen and testosterone, and cortisol, the so-called stress hormone, if she suspects that stress is playing a role in a woman's symptoms. Other blood tests that your doctor should order when evaluating your menopausal status include thyroid, liver, and kidney function tests, and glucose tests to rule out other medical conditions that may have similar symptoms.

THE BOTTOM LINE

So what should you do about hormone therapy for *you*? That's an answer you'll come to as you work your way through *The Natural Menopause*

Solution. We have literally hundreds of natural remedies throughout the book for everything from hot flashes to insomnia and vaginal dryness. We strongly recommend that you try some of them first.

If, however, they don't work for you and your symptoms are still disconcerting, then it's time to talk to your doctor about other options, whether that means hormone therapy or another medical option. If you are considering hormones, ask your doctor these questions.

1. Is there anything in my medical history that precludes my taking hormone therapy?
2. Which type of hormone therapy do you recommend? Why?
3. Is that the lowest effective dosage?
4. What side effects can I expect?
5. How long should I take it?
6. How long until it starts working?

The bottom line on hormone therapy for menopausal symptoms is that there's no such thing as one size fits all. If you do turn to hormone therapy, that's okay; we want you to feel good and be happy, and sometimes a little estrogen or progesterone is what you need. Just remember: Keep it short, avoid oral forms of estrogen, and make it bioidentical.

Index

Underscored page references indicate boxed text. **Boldface** references indicate illustrations.

A

A1C tests, 337
Abdominal fat. *See* Belly fat
Acanthosis nigricans, 340
Acetone, 303
Acne, 299–303
Actonel, 377
Acupuncture/acupressure, 203–4, 229, 288
Aerobic exercise, 148, 158
Age
  cancer risk and, 348
  of menopause, average, 10–11
Air conditioning, 190
Alarm clock placement, 225–26
Alcoholic beverages
  eating plan recommendations, 63
  health risks, 350, 361, 376
  incontinence and, 284
  sleep problems and, 224
Alendronate, 377
Algal oil, 330
Alprazolam, 222, 252
Alternative medicine, 30–31

Ambien, 234
Amitriptyline, 233
Anaerobic exercise, 148
Androgenic alopecia, 308
Annual pelvic exams, 347, 357
Antibiotics, 287, 301–2
Anticonvulsants, 223
Antidepressants, 209, 211–12, 233, 246–47, 253
Antihistamines, 233
Antioxidants, 296
Anxiety, 247–53, 266, 317, 326
Aphrodisiacs, 274
Apigenin, 233
Appetite signals, 215, 218. *See also* Cravings
Applied relaxation, 249–50
ArginMax for Women, 277
Arm Raise, 176, **176**
Artery flexibility, 316
Aspirin, heart health benefits, 331
Ativan, 234, 252
Auricular acupressure, 229
Avocados, good fats in, 52
Azelaic acid, 299

B

P

Paced breathing, 190–91

Packaged foods. *See* Processed foods

Pain

chronic, sleep problems and, 223–24

medications for, 222, <u>224</u>

during ovulation, 6

during sex, <u>264–65</u>

Pancakes

Lemon-Ricotta Pancakes, 94

Panic attacks, 248

Pap tests, 347, 353–54

Paroxetine, 209, 211, 253

Passionflower, 251

Pasta

Beef 'n' Broccoli Pasta Salad, 101

Pasta with Garlicky White Clam
Sauce, 127

Pasta with Gorgonzola-Walnut Sauce,
113

Paxil, 209, 211, 253

Pelvic exams, annual, 347, 357

Pelvic muscles, 266, 285

Peptide YY, 157

Percutaneous nerve stimulation, 290

Perimenopause, <u>10–12</u>, 213–16, 248, 367,
397

Periodic limb movements of sleep
(PLMS), 222

Personality, insomnia therapy and,
<u>230</u>

Pessaries, 288

Pesticides, in foods, <u>54</u>, <u>363</u>

Phosphatidylserine, 258

Phosphoric acid, 375

Physical appearance

hair care, 305–9

libido and, 273

nail care, 303–5

skin care, 294–303

sleep and, 216

Phytoestrogens, 45, 57, 60, 197, <u>198</u>,
199

Phytosterols, 330

Pillows, 190

Pitting, of nails, <u>304</u>

Pizza

Pita Pizzas, 107

Plastic surgery, 297–99

Plastic water bottles, <u>362</u>

PLMS, 222

PMS, <u>12</u>, <u>240</u>, 248

Polycystic ovary syndrome, 320–21, 336

Portion sizes, 62

Positive thinking, as hot flash remedy,
191–92

Postmenopause, 6, <u>11</u>, <u>263</u>

Potassium, 374–75

Poultry. *See also* Meat

buying recommendations, <u>363</u>

as lean protein, 44–46

recipes

Chicken Adobo, 118

Chicken Salad Pita, 104

Chicken Stew with Almond
Couscous, 120–21

Gingered Turkey Meat Loaf, 116

Homemade Turkey Sausage, 91

Pita Pizzas, 107

Roasted Turkey Breast with
Vegetables, 114

Spiced Chicken with Lentils, 119

Turkey Cutlets with Cranberry Wild
Rice, 115

UTI risk and, <u>287</u>

Pramipexole, 222

Prediabetes, 319, 334, 336–38, <u>339</u>

Preeclampsia, 320–21

Pregnancy, 17, <u>263</u>, 321, 336

Premarin, 18, 19–21, 269–70, 395, <u>396</u>

Premenopause, <u>11</u>, 185, 213–16, 217

Prempro, 19–21, 395

Preservatives, 49, 343

Pristiq, 209

Probiotic suppositories, <u>287</u>

Processed foods

health effects, 295–96

meats, 48–49, 63, 342–44, 363–64

sodium in, 63, <u>326</u>, 375

Wressell, Amy, 37, <u>83</u>
Wrinkles, 296, 297–99, <u>298</u>

X

Xanax, 222, 252
Xyrem, 223–24

Y

Yellow nails, <u>304</u>
Yoga
  benefits of, 151–53, 276–77, <u>374</u>
  equipment for, 164
  routine, with weights
    overview, 9, 170–71
    pose descriptions, 171–81, **171–81**
  as therapy for
    anxiety, 250
    hot flashes, 193
    insomnia, 226–27

Yogurt
  recipes
    Creamy Maple Sauce, 144
    Creamy Orange Dressing, 102
    Mixed-Fruit Cup, 87
    Nutty Berry Fool, 141
    Slimming, Cooling Smoothie, 85
    Strawberry-Almond Smoothie, 86
  substitutions for, 62
  UTIs and, <u>287</u>

Z

Zaleplon, 234
Zestra, 268
Zinc, 300
Zoledronic acid, 377
Zoloft, 211–12, 246, 253
Zolpidem, 234

About the Authors

Prevention® is the #1 healthy lifestyle brand and the largest health magazine in the United States, with a total readership of nearly 11 million.

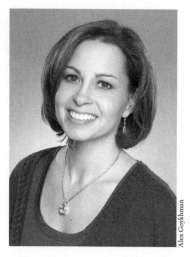

Alex Goykhman

Melinda Ring, MD, serves as the medical director of Northwestern Integrative Medicine. She is board-certified in internal and integrative medicine, the innovative practice of combining conventional Western medicine with safe, evidence-based complementary and alternative medicine (CAM) therapies to improve the health of her patients.

Dr. Ring received her bachelor's degree from the University of Michigan and earned her medical degree and residency from the University of Chicago. Following residency, she completed the Fellowship in Integrative Medicine at the University of Arizona. She was mentored by a distinguished faculty including Andrew Weil, MD.

She is a clinical assistant professor in the Department of Medicine at the Northwestern Feinberg School of Medicine. Her expertise is reflected in her contribution to textbooks, lectures, and research articles in the field of women's health and integrative medicine. Dr. Ring strives for a balanced life of work, family, and play with her husband, two energetic sons, and their funny canine companions.